Common Procedures— Common Problems

Editor

MARK D. MILLER

CLINICS IN SPORTS MEDICINE

www.sportsmed.theclinics.com

Consulting Editor
MARK D. MILLER

April 2018 • Volume 37 • Number 2

ELSEVIER

1600 John F. Kennedy Boulevard • Suite 1800 • Philadelphia, Pennsylvania, 19103-2899

http://www.theclinics.com

CLINICS IN SPORTS MEDICINE Volume 37, Number 2
April 2018 ISSN 0278-5919, ISBN-13: 978-0-323-58326-8

Editor: Lauren Boyle
Developmental Editor: Donald Mumford

Clinics in Sports Medicine (ISSN 0278-5919) is published quarterly by Elsevier Inc., 360 Park Avenue South, New York, NY 10010-1710. Months of issue are January, April, July, and October. Business and Editorial Offices: 1600 John F. Kennedy Blvd., Ste. 1800, Philadelphia, PA 19103-2899. Customer Service Office: 3251 Riverport Lane, Maryland Heights, MO 63043. Periodicals postage paid at New York, NY and additional mailing offices. Subscription prices are $357.00 per year (US individuals), $664.00 per year (US institutions), $100.00 per year (US students), $405.00 per year (Canadian individuals), $820.00 per year (Canadian institutions), $235.00 (Canadian students), $475.00 per year (foreign individuals), $820.00 per year (foreign institutions), and $235.00 per year (foreign students). Foreign air speed delivery is included in all *Clinics* subscription prices. All prices are subject to change without notice. **POSTMASTER:** Send address changes to *Clinics in Sports Medicine*, Elsevier Health Sciences Division, Subscription Customer Service, 3251 Riverport Lane, Maryland Heights, MO 63043. Customer Service (orders, claims, online, change of address): Elsevier Health Sciences Division, Subscription Customer Service, 3251 Riverport Lane, Maryland Heights, MO 63043. **Tel: 1-800-654-2452 (U.S. and Canada); 314-447-8871 (outside U.S. and Canada). Fax: 314-447-8029. E-mail: journalscustomerservice-usa@elsevier.com (for print support); journalsonlinesupport-usa@elsevier.com (for online support).**

Reprints. For copies of 100 or more of articles in this publication, please contact the Commercial Reprints Department, Elsevier Inc., 360 Park Avenue South, New York, NY 10010-1710. Tel.: 212-633-3874; Fax: 212-633-3820; E-mail: reprints@elsevier.com.

Clinics in Sports Medicine is covered in *MEDLINE/PubMed (Index Medicus) Current Contents/Clinical Medicine, Excerpta Medica,* and *ISI/Biomed.*

Contributors

CONSULTING EDITOR

MARK D. MILLER, MD
S. Ward Casscells Professor, Head, Department of Orthopaedic Surgery, Division of Sports Medicine, University of Virginia, Charlottesville, Virginia, USA; Team Physician, James Madison University, Director, Miller Review Course, Harrisonburg, Virginia, USA

EDITOR

MARK D. MILLER, MD
S. Ward Casscells Professor, Head, Department of Orthopaedic Surgery, Division of Sports Medicine, University of Virginia, Charlottesville, Virginia, USA; Team Physician, James Madison University, Director, Miller Review Course, Harrisonburg, Virginia, USA

AUTHORS

ANNUNZIATO AMENDOLA, MD
Chief, Division of Sports Medicine, Professor of Orthopedic Surgery, Duke University Medical Center, Duke Sports Science Institute, Durham, North Carolina

CHRISTOPHER A. ARRIGO, MS, PT, ATC
Owner, Clinical Director, Advanced Rehabilitation, Tampa, Florida; Special Consultant for Throwing Injuries, Lafayette Medical Director, MedStar Sports Medicine, Washington, DC

JUSTIN H. BARTLEY, MD
Sports Medicine and Shoulder Surgery Fellow, Department of Orthopedic Surgery–Sports Medicine, University of Colorado Boulder, CU Sports Medicine and Performance Center, Boulder, Colorado

LORENA BEJARANO-PINEDA, MD
Research Fellow, Division of Foot and Ankle Surgery, Department of Orthopedic Surgery, Duke University Medical Center, Durham, North Carolina

MATTHEW H. BLAKE, MD
Department of Orthopaedic Surgery and Sports Medicine, Avera McKennan Hospital & University Health Center, Sioux Falls, South Dakota

STEPHEN F. BROCKMEIER, MD
Associate Professor, Department of Orthopaedic Surgery, University of Virginia, Charlottesville, Virginia

AARON CASP, MD
Resident, Department of Orthopaedic Surgery, University of Virginia, University of Virginia Health System, Charlottesville, Virginia

JAMES E. CHRISTENSEN, MD
Sports Medicine Fellow, Department of Orthopaedic Surgery, University of Virginia, Charlottesville, Virginia

JESSICA DiVENERE, BS
Research Assistant, Department of Orthopedic Surgery, University of Connecticut, Farmington, Connecticut

FRANK WINSTON GWATHMEY, MD
Assistant Professor, Department of Orthopaedic Surgery, University of Virginia, University of Virginia Health System, Charlottesville, Virginia

JOEL B. HULEATT, MD
Orthopedics and Sports Medicine, University of Connecticut School of Medicine, Farmington, Connecticut

DARREN L. JOHNSON, MD
Professor and Chairman, Department of Orthopaedic Surgery, Director of Sports Medicine, University of Kentucky College of Medicine, Lexington, Kentucky

JEREMIAH D. JOHNSON, MD
Resident, Department of Orthopedic Surgery, University of Connecticut, Farmington, Connecticut

SANJEEV KAKAR, MD, MBA
Department of Orthopedic Surgery, Mayo Clinic, Rochester, Minnesota

WILLIAM N. LEVINE, MD
Frank E. Stinchfield Professor and Chairman, Department of Orthopedic Surgery, NewYork-Presbyterian/Columbia Orthopedics, New York, New York

STEPHANIE LOGTERMAN, MD
Resident, Department of Orthopedic Surgery, University of Colorado Denver, Denver, Colorado; Department of Orthopedic Surgery, University of Colorado, Anschutz Medical Campus, Aurora, Colorado

HARRISON S. MAHON, MD
Department of Orthopaedic Surgery, University of Virginia, Charlottesville, Virginia

NIV MAROM, MD
Hospital for Special Surgery, New York, New York

ROBERT G. MARX, MD
Hospital for Special Surgery, New York, New York

AUGUSTUS D. MAZZOCCA, MD, MS
Professor and Chairman, Department of Orthopedic Surgery, University of Connecticut, Farmington, Connecticut

ERIC C. McCARTY, MD
Chief of Sports Medicine and Shoulder Surgery, Department of Orthopedic Surgery–Sports Medicine, University of Colorado Boulder, CU Sports Medicine and Performance Center, Boulder, Colorado

MATTHEW D. MILEWSKI, MD
Division of Sports Medicine, Boston Children's Hospital, Boston, Massachusetts

MARK D. MILLER, MD
S. Ward Casscells Professor, Head, Department of Orthopaedic Surgery, Division of Sports Medicine, University of Virginia, Charlottesville, Virginia, USA; Team Physician, James Madison University, Director, Miller Review Course, Harrisonburg, Virginia, USA

CARL W. NISSEN, MD
Elite Sports Medicine, Connecticut Children's Medical Center, Farmington, Connecticut

NICHOLAS PULOS, MD
Department of Orthopedic Surgery, Mayo Clinic, Rochester, Minnesota

NAOMI ROSELAAR, BS
Hospital for Special Surgery, New York, New York

JOSEPH J. RUZBARSKY, MD
Hospital for Special Surgery, New York, New York

FELIX H. SAVOIE, MD
Ray Haddad Professor and Chairman, Department of Orthopaedics, Tulane University, New Orleans, Louisiana

BRIAN SHIU, MD
Fellow, Department of Orthopedic Surgery, NewYork-Presbyterian/Columbia Orthopedics, New York, New York

JULIAN J. SONNENFELD, MD
Resident, Department of Orthopedic Surgery, NYP/Columbia University Orthopedics, New York, New York

ARMANDO F. VIDAL, MD
Associate Professor, Department of Orthopedic Surgery – Sports Medicine, University of Colorado Boulder, Boulder, Colorado; CU Sports Medicine Center, Denver, Colorado

KRISTINA LINNEA WELTON, MD
Sports Medicine and Shoulder Surgery Fellow, Department of Orthopedic Surgery – Sports Medicine, University of Colorado Boulder, CU Sports Medicine and Performance Center, Boulder, Colorado

KEVIN E. WILK, PT, DPT, FAPTA
Associate Clinical Director, Champion Sports Medicine, A Select Medical Facility, Director, Rehabilitation Research, American Sports Medicine Institute, Birmingham, Alabama

JAMES D. WYLIE, MD, MHS
Department of Orthopedic Surgery, Fellow, Boston Children's Hospital, Boston, Massachusetts

Contributors

MARK D. MILLER, MD
S. Ward Casscells Professor, Head, Department of Orthopaedic Surgery, Division of Sports Medicine, University of Virginia, Charlottesville, Virginia, USA; Team Physician, James Madison University, Director, Miller Review Course, Harrisonburg, Virginia, USA

CARL W. NISSEN, MD
Elite Sports Medicine, Connecticut Children's Medical Center, Farmington, Connecticut

NICHOLAS PULOS, MD
Department of Orthopedic Surgery, Mayo Clinic, Rochester, Minnesota

NAOMI ROSELAAR, BS
Hospital for Special Surgery, New York, New York

JOSEPH J. RUZBARSKY, MD
Hospital for Special Surgery, New York, New York

FELIX H. SAVOIE, MD
Ray J. Haddad Professor and Chairman, Department of Orthopaedics, Tulane University, New Orleans, Louisiana

BRIAN SHIU, MD
Fellow, Department of Orthopedic Surgery, NewYork-Presbyterian/Columbia Orthopedics, New York, New York

JULIAN J. SONNENFELD, MD
Resident, Department of Orthopedic Surgery, NYP/Columbia University Orthopedics, New York, New York

ARMANDO F. VIDAL, MD
Associate Professor, Department of Orthopaedic Surgery – Sports Medicine, University of Colorado Boulder, Boulder, Colorado; CU Sports Medicine Center, Denver, Colorado

KRISTINA LUTZ WELTON, MD
Sports Medicine and Shoulder Surgery Fellow, Department of Orthopaedic Surgery – Sports Medicine, University of Colorado, Boulder; CU Sports Medicine and Performance Center, Boulder, Colorado

KEVIN E. WILK, PT, DPT, FAPTA
Associate Clinical Director, Champion Sports Medicine, A Select Medical Facility; Director, Rehabilitation Research, American Sports Medicine Institute, Birmingham, Alabama

JAMES D. WYLIE, MD, MHS
Department of Orthopedic Surgery, Fellow, Boston Children's Hospital, Boston, Massachusetts

Contents

The elbow is one of the more difficult joints in which to obtain good results. Common issues include placement of correct portals, neuropraxia, ankylosis, heterotopic bone formation, and simple failure of the procedure. Common solutions include portal placement safeguards, nerve protection, early motion and cryocompression, oral or injectable steroids, radiation therapy, secure stabilization, and postoperative protection and rehabilitation based on available evidence and imaging.

Injuries to the hands and wrist are common in athletes. Injuries include acute fractures, dislocations, and ligamentous and tendon injuries, as well as more chronic injuries, such as sprains and strains. Complications in the treatment of sports injuries of the hand and wrist may be divided into 2 categories: incorrect or delayed diagnosis and iatrogenic injury related to treatment. This article highlights common sports injuries of the hand and wrist and their complications and includes tips for successful management.

The use of hip arthroscopy continues to expand. Understanding potential pitfalls and complications associated with hip arthroscopy is paramount to optimizing clinical outcomes and minimizing unfavorable results. Potential pitfalls and complications are associated with preoperative factors, such as patient selection, intraoperative factors such as iatrogenic damage, traction-related complications, inadequate correction of deformity, and nerve injury, or postoperative factors, such as poor rehabilitation. This article outlines common factors that contribute to less-than-favorable outcomes.

 Video content accompanies this article at http://www.sportsmed. theclinics.com.

Anterior cruciate ligament (ACL) reconstruction is one of the most commonly performed procedures in the United States. Although complications are rare in ACL surgery, failure to appreciate them can lead to significant patient morbidity in the short and long terms. More common complications in ACL reconstruction include tunnel malposition, infection, tunnel osteolysis, fixation failure, fracture, arthrofibrosis, graft site morbidity, and deep vein thrombosis or pulmonary embolism. Tunnel malposition is the most common technical error in ACL reconstruction leading to failure. Proper planning during the index surgery can help prevent these complications, especially when related to tunnel malposition.

The multiple ligament injured knee presents a challenge with regard to management and treatment. Immediate management of the acute injury requires special attention and thorough examination because knee dislocations have been associated with significant complications. Treatment options range from closed reduction and immobilization to surgical repair and/or reconstruction of the injured ligaments. This article focuses on complications that may result from surgical treatments of the multiple ligament injured knee and ways of prevention. These complications include vascular and neurologic complications, venous thromboembolic events, arthrofibrosis, compartment syndrome, wound problems, heterotopic ossification, fractures and avascular necrosis, tunnels positioning complications, and malalignment.

The rates of arthroscopic meniscus repair continue to increase with excellent reported outcomes. Complications, sometimes catastrophic, following meniscus repair may occur. The rate of postoperative complications may be reduced by adequate diagnosis, appropriate patient selection, meniscus repair selection, surgical techniques, and postoperative management. When complications occur, the provider must identify and take steps to rectify as well as prevent further complications from occurring. This article details the common diagnostic, technical, and postoperative pitfalls that may result in poor patient outcomes.

Focal cartilage defects in the knee are commonly found on MRI and arthroscopically. When these lesions are symptomatic and fail nonoperative management, several surgical strategies are available. Common surgical techniques include reparative (ie, microfracture) and restorative procedures (ie, autologous chondrocyte implantation, particulated juvenile allograft cartilage, osteochondral autograft transfer, and osteochondral allograft). These surgical procedures have shared and novel complications associated with their use. This article provides a detailed, case-based discussion of common complications encountered in surgical procedures for focal cartilage defects of the knee, highlighting causes, clinical recognition, and how to address and avoid these complications.

Participation in sports activity has increased significantly during the last several decades. This phenomenon has exposed orthopedic sports medicine surgeons to new challenges regarding the diagnosis and management of common sport-related injuries. Arthroscopy is becoming more commonly used in many of the surgical procedures for these injuries and carries the risk of complications. Wound and nerve complications make up the bulk of complications in most procedures. This article describes these complications associated with the common surgical procedures related to foot and ankle sport-related injuries and how to address and prevent them.

Joel B. Huleatt, Carl W. Nissen, and Matthew D. Milewski

The treatment of sports injuries in the skeletally immature has a unique set of complications. Growth deformity may occur after anterior cruciate ligament reconstruction; therefore, skeletal age is used to help guide the choice between physeal sparing and transphyseal techniques. Arthrofibrosis after tibial spine fracture fixation can be reduced by initiating immediate range of motion and should be treated early and cautiously to avoid iatrogenic fracture. Nonunions of medial epicondyle elbow fractures are more common with nonoperative treatment but seldom lead to clinical problems outside of certain athletes. Risks of OCD fixation are specific to the material of screw used.

Kevin E. Wilk and Christopher A. Arrigo

There are numerous complications that can occur after a musculoskeletal injury or surgery in the sporting population. Prevention of the most frequent complications is the key in any successful rehabilitation program, but occasionally problems do occur. A thorough well-designed postoperative or postinjury rehabilitation program may prevent these problems. However, if complications do arise, a team approach among the parties involved in the process to develop an evidenced-based treatment program designed for the underlying complication can successfully treat these issues. The authors discuss the complications seen in sports injuries to the knee, shoulder, elbow, and foot/ankle joints of the body.

CLINICS IN SPORTS MEDICINE

RELATED INTEREST

Orthopedic Clinics, October 2016 (Volume 47, Issue 4)
Sports-Related Injuries

THE CLINICS ARE AVAILABLE ONLINE!
Access your subscription at:
www.theclinics.com

CLINICS IN SPORTS MEDICINE

Preface

Common Procedures—Common Problems: It's Complicated

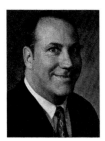

Mark D. Miller, MD
Editor

Several years ago, I put together an Instructional Course Lecture (ICL) entitled "Common Sports Medicine Procedures: Hero and Goat." The idea was that the faculty would present their best and worst cases for each commonly performed sports medicine procedure. The course was a success, but the ICL organizers wanted more on complications. I struggled with this at first because no one wants to broadcast their failures. Nevertheless, I ultimately recognized that if others could learn from my mistakes, then they wouldn't have to learn the same lesson the hard way. Will Rogers is credited with the following observation: "There are three kinds of men. The ones that learn by readin'. The few who learn by observation. The rest of them have to pee on the electric fence for themselves." It is our hope that this issue of *Clinics in Sports Medicine* will help you avoid the latter!

This issue is a top to bottom approach to sports medicine complications, with an emphasis on the shoulder and the knee, which represents the majority of our practices. Please recognize that although the authors are not responsible for all of the complications presented, it is a humbling experience to "air your dirty laundry" and in some cases, the authors have included their own complications. Shoulder instability, rotator cuff repair, and coracoclavicular reconstruction are covered in the first three articles. This is followed by elbow and wrist/hand complications. Hip arthroscopy, a relative newcomer to the sports medicine world, has its own unique complications, many associated with a tight space and a steep learning curve, and merits its own article. Four articles on knee procedures follow: anterior cruciate ligament reconstruction, multiple ligament knee injuries, meniscal treatment, and articular cartilage repair/reconstruction. The issue concludes with articles on foot and ankle surgery, pediatric sports medicine procedures, and complications related to rehabilitation.

As Consulting Editor for *Clinics in Sports Medicine*, I usually ask experts in each area to serve as the Guest Editor for each issue. Although I certainly don't want to be

Clin Sports Med 37 (2018) xiii–xiv
https://doi.org/10.1016/j.csm.2018.01.001
0278-5919/18/© 2018 Published by Elsevier Inc.

considered the expert in surgical complications (especially among my patients), in the spirit of Will Rogers, I volunteered to put this treatise together myself. So…start readin' and watch out for those electric fences!

Mark D. Miller, MD
Division of Sports Medicine
University of Virginia
James Madison University
UVA Department of Orthopaedic Surgery
400 Ray C. Hunt Drive, Suite 330
Charlottesville, VA 22903, USA

E-mail address:
mdm3p@virginia.edu

Shoulder Instability
Common Problems and Solutions

William N. Levine, MD*, Julian J. Sonnenfeld, MD, Brian Shiu, MD

KEYWORDS

- Shoulder • Surgery • Instability • Complications • Common

KEY POINTS

- Complications can be divided into 3 phases—preoperative, intraoperative, and postoperative.
- The recognition of preoperative significant bone loss is critical to avoid arthroscopic failures.
- Meticulous intraoperative technique is important to avoid complications.
- Postoperative rehabilitation is integral to ensuring success.

INTRODUCTION

The shoulder joint has a minimally constrained design that provides for function and mobility at the expense of stability. Surgeons have devoted themselves to restoring stability of the unstable shoulder while maintaining a pain-free, maximal range of motion. Both open and arthroscopic techniques for operative shoulder stabilization have evolved with their inevitable complications. With time, glenohumeral instability has become the subject of much analysis and unresolved controversy. This factor has led to the development of more than 150 different procedures aimed at tackling this issue, each with varying degrees of success.

There has been a significant amount of basic science and clinical research assisting our understanding of the causes and effects of shoulder instability. Advanced imaging techniques and arthroscopic techniques have also been instrumental in furthering our understanding. Despite improvement in outcomes following primary stabilization surgery, a 3% to 25% instability recurrence rate represents the most challenging postoperative complication.[1–3]

The complications arising from shoulder instability can be organized along the treatment continuum into 3 categories: preoperative, intraoperative, or postoperative. Although most complications occur in the postoperative period, they may be related to errors or decisions made during the preoperative or intraoperative periods. An

Department of Orthopedic Surgery, NYP/Columbia University Orthopedics, 622 West 168th Street, PH-1130, New York, NY 10032, USA
* Corresponding author.
E-mail address: wnl1@cumc.columbia.edu

Clin Sports Med 37 (2018) 161–177
https://doi.org/10.1016/j.csm.2017.12.001
0278-5919/18/© 2017 Elsevier Inc. All rights reserved.
sportsmed.theclinics.com

accurate assessment of the unstable shoulder preoperatively and identifying key radiographic features are essential for a successful treatment plan. The use of appropriate intraoperative techniques and strategies, including soft tissue mobilization, fixation methods, and management of capsular and/or bony defects, will determine the likelihood of success. Postoperative rehabilitation is equally important in regaining motion in the shoulder while avoiding potential complications. We present common surgical failures that arise during each of these 3 phases, why they may occur, and the means to avoid these complications to improve patient's outcomes.

PREOPERATIVE PHASE

The prevention of complications in the preoperative setting begins with appropriate diagnosis and establishment of clear surgical indications. The first step toward establishing an accurate diagnosis of shoulder instability involves taking a thorough history and performing a systematic physical examination. This is supplemented with additional imaging studies such as plain radiographs, computed tomography (CT) scans, MRI, or arthrography.

Failure to Appreciate Bone Loss

Bone loss of the glenoid and humeral head has been shown to be an important predictor of clinical failure after arthroscopic shoulder soft tissue stabilization surgery.[4–6] Several aspects of the patient history are critical, because some key clues from the shoulder instability history may signal the presence of glenoid bone loss. What degree of trauma, if any, was involved? Glenoid bone loss is suspected in the patient who sustains a high-energy injury, especially if the shoulder becomes dislocated with the arm in abduction and extension at the time of injury.[7] High-energy trauma tends to create more extensive injury to surrounding tissues, such as the rotator cuff or articular cartilage. How and by what method was the shoulder reduced? Bone loss, either glenoid or humeral sided, should always be suspected in the patient who sustains a shoulder dislocation that is not amenable to spontaneous reduction in the field or requiring a sedated reduction in the emergency department. What is the frequency of recurrence? Patients with glenoid bone loss often note that it has become progressively easier to subluxate the glenohumeral joint and often have a long history of either shoulder instability symptoms or coping with this injury.[7,8]

Additionally, an athletic history is important because the patient may not experience clear dislocation or subluxation, and only complain of pain or weakness when they bring their arm to maximum external rotation in abduction.[9] If the patient is a throwing athlete, the actual phase of throwing associated with the instability can help in identifying the direction of instability, along with whether or not there is bone loss.[8] Although these questions seem standard for any initial patient interview for a shoulder injury, the answers to these questions may rule out a patient for surgery or otherwise assist the surgeon in avoiding intraoperative and postoperative complications.

A thorough physical examination to compare the affected shoulder with the unaffected shoulder will serve as the internal control for the normal evaluation. With the patient in the supine position, and the scapula stabilized against the examination table, patients will typically experience apprehension to dislocation at varying degrees of shoulder abduction and external rotation. A positive apprehension test at small degrees of abduction and external rotation may indicate glenoid bone loss, because the humeral head in this scenario is easier to subluxate over the glenoid rim.[7,10]

Patients may experience improvement with the Jobe relocation maneuver.[11] A subtle indication of glenoid bone loss on examination is significant anterior translation or clunk during anterior load-and-shift testing as compared with the contralateral shoulder.[10] The instability examination should be completed with Gagey hyperabduction testing, where an increase in abduction on the affected side can be indicative of injury to the inferior glenohumeral ligament complex. Assessment for a sulcus sign and a posterior jerk test are also important in distinguishing between inferior instability and posterior instability, respectively.[12–14]

Imaging of the patient with bone loss in shoulder instability begins with standard radiography. Preoperative radiographs include the anteroposterior, scapular-Y, and axillary views. The plain radiographs allow for assessment of the normal glenoid rim and humeral head. Specifically, the axillary view assesses glenohumeral joint congruency and humeral head impression fractures. The most useful view for the detection of bony Bankart lesions is the West Point view.[15] Humeral head bone loss is best assessed with the Stryker notch view to identify Hill-Sachs lesions with high sensitivity.[16,17]

CT is the preferred modality to determine the extent of bone loss in the humeral head and/or glenoid, especially with advanced software that allows for 3-dimensional reconstructions. Plain radiographs often will underestimate the extent of the osseous involvement.[18] Multiplanar reformatting and 3-dimensional reconstructions are considered the gold standard for glenoid imaging because of the available humeral subtraction technique.[19] This technique allows for an accurate en face view of the glenoid surface, providing an opportunity to assess the location and size of bone loss on both the glenoid and humeral sides (**Fig. 1**).

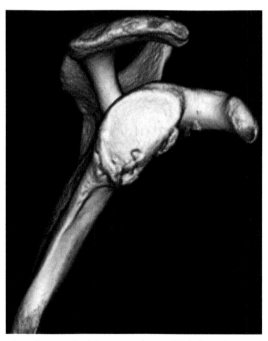

Fig. 1. Three-dimensional computed tomography sagittal view demonstrating high-quality en face assessment of glenoid. (*Courtesy of* Columbia University Center for Shoulder, Elbow, and Sports Medicine, New York, NY; with permission.)

In a study of 100 consecutive shoulders with unilateral recurrent anterior disloca-tions, Sugaya and colleagues[20] evaluated the morphology of the glenoid rim with 3-dimensional CT imaging. Bony deficiency of the glenoid was found in 90% of the shoulders. In addition, 20% to 25% of patients with anterior instability and glenoid bone loss that undergo repair will have diminished results and higher chance of recur-rent instability.[21] Therefore, it is imperative to precisely determine the amount of gle-noid bone loss in the unstable shoulder to determine the optimal treatment plan.

Glenoid bone loss can be quantified on 3-dimensional CT imaging by modeling the inferior two-thirds of the glenoid surface as a true circle, with the center of this circle at the "bare spot."[20,22,23] The amount of glenoid bone loss can be calculated using one of a variety of methods[20,24–27] (**Fig. 2**). Losses of less than 15% of the width of the glenoid (<3 to 4 mm from the anterior rim) are often insignificant in most patients, and can be managed with standard soft tissue instability repair. Defects of 15% to 30% (between 4 and 9 mm of bone remaining anterior to the bare spot) are relevant in the majority of patients. Finally, losses of greater than 30% (<4 mm of bone left anterior to the bare spot) are critically significant and require bony augmentation procedures.[28]

Although MRI provides useful information about soft tissue anatomy, including the glenoid labrum, chondral surfaces, glenohumeral capsuloligamentous structures, and the rotator cuff, it can also demonstrate bone loss.[29–31] In a cadaveric study comparing the diagnostic accuracy of CT with MRI in the measurement of glenoid bone loss, Gyftopoulos and colleagues[32] showed that the MRI quantification of gle-noid bone loss compared favorably with measurements obtained using CT. However, a learning curve was identified by the authors and the accuracy of the measurements correlated with the level of training.

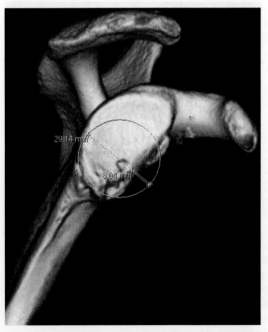

Fig. 2. Three-dimensional computed tomography sagittal view demonstrating circle tech-nique for identifying anterior glenoid bone loss. (*Courtesy of* Columbia University Center for Shoulder, Elbow, and Sports Medicine, New York, NY; with permission.)

In addition to imaging evaluation, diagnostic arthroscopy may be helpful for the quantification of glenoid bony defects. Burkhart and colleagues[33] proposed a unique method of quantifying glenoid bone loss arthroscopically using the glenoid bare spot as the center of the inferior circle of the glenoid. A calibrated probe can be used to measure the distance from the bare spot to the posterior margin and anterior margin of the glenoid. The percentage of bone loss can then be calculated by dividing the measured anterior distance by the posterior distance from the bare spot. Other authors have questioned the validity and reliability of the glenoid bare spot method. Kralinger[34] and colleagues used CT to show that the glenoid bare spot is approximately 1.4 mm anterior to the true center point of the glenoid. This technique can, therefore, lead to an overestimation of glenoid bone loss.[22,34]

Having an accurate understanding of the extent of glenoid bone loss is crucial to making an informed surgical decision. Many surgeons recognize that significant glenoid bone loss can be a cause of recurrence even after proper soft tissue surgical stabilization.[24,35] Bone loss leading to an "inverted-pear glenoid" and engagement of the Hill-Sachs lesion have been associated with failure after arthroscopic soft tissue stabilization.[36] Burkhart and De Beer[35] defined glenoid bone loss of greater than 25% or an engaging Hill-Sachs lesion as significant, with a recurrence of dislocation after arthroscopic soft tissue stabilization in 67% of patients. In such cases, open surgical procedures, including Latarjet coracoid transfer, will portend a better outcome. Shoulders with less than 25% bone loss demonstrated only 4% recurrent dislocation.[35]

The importance of humeral-sided bone loss is best determined using the concept of the glenoid track.[37,38] Yamamoto and colleagues[38] defined "off-track" lesions as a Hill-Sachs defect that engaged the glenoid rim. Using cadaveric specimens and 3-dimensional imaging, "off-track" Hill-Sachs lesions frequently occurred if the distance between the medial margin of the rotator cuff footprint and the Hill-Sachs lesions was less than 84% of the glenoid width. In our practice, we apply the glenoid track model to humeral lesions that are medial, wide, or when there is significant glenoid bone loss that decreases the glenoid track width. If the bone loss is near but not greater than 84% of the glenoid width, we will fill the defect using a remplissage technique (infraspinatus capsulodesis). When anterior glenoid bony augmentation is performed with the Latarjet or bone grafting, we do not routinely perform a remplissage as the glenoid width and track is restored. However, if the Hill-Sachs defect is very large (>35%), we will treat the defect with a fresh size-matched humeral head allograft.

Failure to Appreciate Ligamentous Laxity

Patients with hyperlaxity and instability are more likely to experience episodes of recurrent subluxation than they are to have recurrent dislocation.[39] A history without any significant traumatic episode may direct the physician toward a heightened suspicion for hyperlaxity.[40–42] Poor quality of the soft tissues surrounding the glenohumeral joint, whether caused by multiple previous operations, multiple subluxation or dislocation episodes, or an underlying connective tissue disorder, has the potential to threaten the success of any shoulder stabilization procedure. An accurate diagnosis is critical in guiding treatment, because patients with hyperlaxity require an extended period of nonoperative care.

There are 2 groups of patients with hyperlaxity: patients with congenital ligamentous laxity, and those who subject their shoulder to repetitive microtrauma (eg, overhead throwers and swimmers).[43] Patients with laxity often have subjective instability during daily activities. Bilateral symptoms, feelings of instability with the arm adducted, or difficulty with carrying heavy objects raise the possibility of hyperlaxity.[44]

There may also be a family history of shoulder instability and hyperlaxity, and this must not be missed by the physician. Heritable connective tissue disorders will predispose the patient to hyperlaxity, not only in the shoulder, but elsewhere in the body (hip, ankle, knee, wrist, thumb, and elbow).[45,46] Any history of ocular or cardiovascular pathology must also be ascertained.

Upon initial inspection, a gynecoid morphology, as well as the presence of skin striae, can be subtle yet helpful clues that can lead the clinician to suspect an underlying global soft tissue laxity. Anterior shoulder hyperlaxity should be presumed if the humeral head subluxates over the glenoid rim with little force on anterior drawer or load and shift testing. Additionally, if there is greater than 85° of passive external rotation with the arm at the side on examination, this factor may be suggestive of anterior hyperlaxity.[47] A positive sulcus sign or hyperabduction test of Gagey (considered positive with asymmetry >20° compared with the contralateral shoulder) will likely correlate with inferior shoulder hyperlaxity.[12,48] The Beighton hypermobility score, which focuses on hypermobility in the small finger, wrist, elbow, knee, and spine must be calculated. A score of greater than 4 (out of total of 9 possible points) is diagnostic of generalized joint laxity.[46,49,50]

Plain radiographs will usually be normal in the patient with hyperlaxity. Although osseous abnormalities are rare, the clinician must still be aware of osseous abnormalities that may be evident on plain radiographic views, such as glenoid dysplasia, glenoid rim defects or fractures, or humeral head lesions.[51] CT scans and MRI, especially involving arthrography, are helpful in assessing for capsulolabral or osseous structural abnormalities that may be contributing to instability.[52] Capsular distention or disappearance of the capsule, as well as labral lesions are identified with MR arthrography.

A common error with stabilization surgery includes failure to recognize capsular laxity during repair.[4,53] Bigliani and colleagues[54] demonstrated that anterior capsular stretching and attenuation could occur with or without labral detachment. Even after Bankart repair, persistently lax capsular tissue may be responsible for failure. In this case, capsular plication in the setting of an intact labrum may be required.

In hyperlax patients, the clinician must expand the differential diagnosis beyond labral and bony causes because other pathologies may coexist. Underappreciation of humeral avulsions of the glenohumeral ligament, appearing in approximately 9% of anterior instability cases, can also be responsible for persistent postoperative instability.[55] Young patients with hyperlaxity and accompanying pain may also have concomitant shoulder pathology, including a superior labral tear, anterior and posterior labral tears, impingement, or rotator cuff dysfunction.

Volunatry dislocators need to be identified before any contemplation of surgical intervention, given the high failure rate in this surgical cohort.[56] Warren and colleagues divided voluntary dislocators into 2 distinct groups: positional and muscular types. Positional voluntary dislocators can demonstrate shoulder instability in specific arm positions, and are often emotionally stable. Muscular type dislocators use selective muscular activation. Although voluntary dislocators may not necessarily exhibit psychiatric disorders, it has been shown that successful results are more predictable after treatment of emotionally stable voluntary dislocators.[57,58]

INTRAOPERATIVE PHASE

Shoulder instability surgery requires meticulous planning and technical expertise, and involves an intensive operative workflow. Once the surgeon has sufficiently assessed the patient and identified the soft tissue or osseous lesions, the subsequent selection of the individual treatment plan is just as important as the surgical procedure itself.

This section addresses the more frequent complications of shoulder instability surgery occurring in the intraoperative period.

Suture Anchor Positioning and Properties

Arthroscopic shoulder stabilization is often used in the younger patient with relatively good bone quality. However, subtle differences in the glenoid rim may make solid anchor purchase difficult. Additionally, postoperative immobilization can be highly variable, depending on the surgeon, which can lead to early stresses applied to the repair.

Glenoid anchors at the 6 o'clock position are often required to address laxity within the inferior capsule and posterior band of the inferior glenohumeral ligament.[59,60] Visualization from the anterosuperior portal is critical to allow proper identification of the pathology and to allow instrumentation and maneuvering in the lower quadrant (**Fig. 3**).

Suture anchors must be placed on the glenoid articular surface during shoulder stabilization surgery to recreate the capsulolabral anatomy. The inherent size and shape of the glenoid will dictate that successfully placed anchors remain below the articular margin with firm purchase in the subchondral bone. Anchors that are best suited for the glenoid rim have a smaller footprint averaging 2 to 3 mm, which is useful in preserving bone stock in the case of future revision surgeries (**Fig. 4**). In addition, a solely suture-based anchor has been developed, constructed with a single suture strand that passes through a sleeve of braided polyester in a "V" configuration. This anchoring mechanism seems to be promising, although long-term studies are still pending.[61]

Anchors placed at 2 mm onto the articular rim, at an angle of 45° relative to the surface of the glenoid will minimize articular penetration and minimize the risk of inadvertent medial placement along the scapular neck.[62,63] The angle of insertion is critical to avoid too shallow a trajectory and articular cartilage breaching (**Fig. 5**). Failed arthroscopic instability repair can also be a result of too few points of fixation with modern

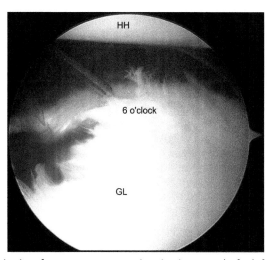

Fig. 3. Arthroscopic view from an anterosuperior viewing portal of a left shoulder. The spinal needle is percutaneously placed from a posterolateral position at the 6 o'clock position. GL, glenoid; HH, humeral head. (*Courtesy of* Columbia University Center for Shoulder, Elbow, and Sports Medicine, New York, NY; with permission.)

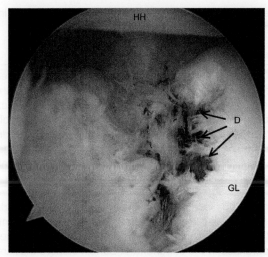

Fig. 1. Arthroscopic view from an anterosuperior viewing portal of a right shoulder in a 19-year-old right-hand dominant male who had three 3.0-mm anchors placed too close together leading to bone loss and recurrent instability. D with arrows indicates significant defect in anteroinferior glenoid. GL, glenoid; HH, humeral head. (*Courtesy of* Columbia University Center for Shoulder, Elbow, and Sports Medicine, New York, NY; with permission.)

suture anchors.[6] To secure the repair, a minimum of 3 anchors should be placed in the anteroinferior quadrant (3'oclock to 6 o'clock right shoulder).[62,64]

Overtightening

Overtightening of the repair during surgery can lead to a nonanatomic repair and loss of external rotation. This factor is especially critical in the overhead athlete, where range of motion is pivotal in generating velocity during the throwing motion. Moreover, posterior instability and late glenohumeral arthritis are potential outcomes of overtightening.

The rotator interval is important in maintaining both the inferior and posterior stability of the glenohumeral joint and has been a source of controversy surrounding shoulder stabilization surgery. Although clinical and biomechanical studies have shown that arthroscopic rotator interval closure augments anterior stability, the effects on posterior and inferior stability remain controversial. Based on work from Provencher et al and other investigators,[65–67] closure of the rotator interval can decrease external rotation with the arm at the side. Patients with multidirectional instability, poor anterior capsular tissue, or revision surgery for failed instability repair are candidates for possible rotator interval closure at the time of repair.

Historical procedures including the Putti-Platt, reverse Putti-Platt, and Magnuson-Stack were deliberately intended to tighten the anterior shoulder structures, including the capsule and subscapularis. The subscapularis is subsequently attenuated and scarred down, limiting external rotation and leading to postcapsulorrhaphy arthritis, which has largely led to the abandonment of such procedures.[13,68,69]

Failure to Address Hill-Sachs Lesions

It is crucial to the success of the repair that the surgeon recognizes concomitant pathology, such as and engaging Hill-Sachs lesion as mentioned. Although this lesion will

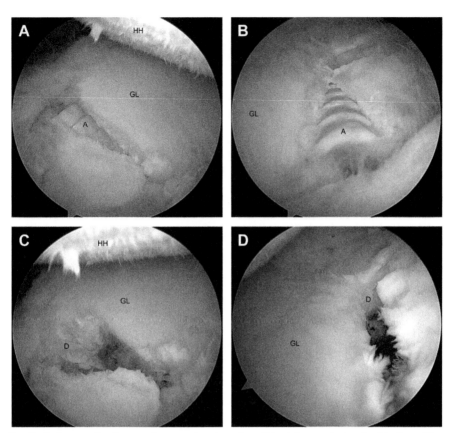

Fig. 5. Arthroscopic photos of a prominent anchor (A) at the posterior 2 o'clock position (left shoulder) in a 21-year-old male football player presenting 1 year after the index position with severe pain and squeaking. (*A*) Anterosuperior viewing portal demonstrating prominent anchor at the 2 o'clock position. (*B*) posterior viewing portal demonstrating prominent anchor (A). (*C*) Anterosuperior viewing portal after implant removal with resultant defect. (*D*) Posterior viewing portal after implant removal with resultant defect. D, defect; GL, glenoid; HH, humeral head. (*Courtesy of* Columbia University Center for Shoulder, Elbow, and Sports Medicine, New York, NY; with permission.)

likely be recognized preoperatively, it can also be evaluated intraoperatively during arthroscopy. Arthroscopic Hill-Sachs remplissage can be used to fill the posterosuperior osseous humeral head defect (**Fig. 6**). Contact athletes have a significantly higher chance of failure after arthroscopic labral repair with or without remplissage or additional procedures.[70,71] Burkhart and deBeer[35] reported that contact athletes who had "significant" bony involvement had an 89% failure rate after arthroscopic labral repair. This study highlights the concept that collision athletes with any appreciable bone loss may need to have their Hill-Sachs lesion addressed, glenoid bony augmentation, or in extreme cases both sides addressed.

Failures with Coracoid Transfer and Latarjet

Despite the reported success of coracoid transfer for management of patients with recurrent anterior glenohumeral instability, recent studies and large reviews reported

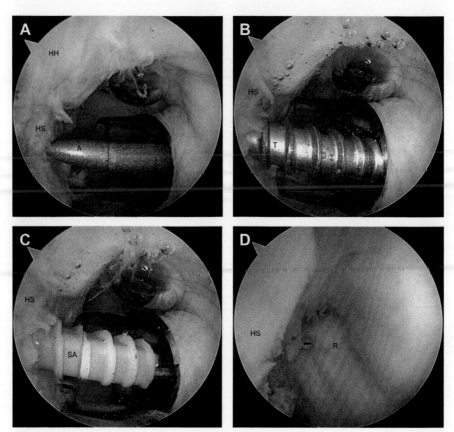

Fig. 6. Arthroscopic photos of the same patient from **Fig. 4** who failed a primary instability repair owing to inappropriate anchor placement with resultant bone loss and failure to address a significant "off-track" Hill-Sachs deformity. (*A*) Anterosuperior view of the awl in the Hill-Sachs defect. (*B*) Anterosuperior view of the tap in the tunnel created by the awl (we recommend use of an awl in young patients to avoid anchor breakage owing to dense cortical bone). (*C*) Anterosuperior view of a double-loaded suture anchor in the tunnel. (*D*) Anterosuperior view of the completed remplissage procedure. A, awl; HH, humeral head; HS, Hill-Sachs defect; SA, suture anchor; T, tap. (*Courtesy of* Columbia University Center for Shoulder, Elbow, and Sports Medicine, New York, NY; with permission.)

an overall complication rate in the open Latarjet procedure of up to 30%.[72] However, the published recurrence rate of instability after Latarjet procedure can be as low as 1% to 3%, and this success can be attributed in part to optimal positioning of the graft.[73,74] Ideally, the graft sits flush with the articular surface in the axial plane and below the equator of the glenoid in the sagittal plane. In the case of significant bone block osteolysis leading to recurrence after a Latarjet procedure, a modified Eden-Hybinette procedure or distal tibia allograft can be used.

To reduce the risk of neurovascular injury, the surgeon must always know where the musculocutaneous and axillary nerves are, but routine exploration is not typically necessary. Neurovascular injury is a devastating complication with a reported 1% rate of neurovascular injury across open and arthroscopic techniques, and as high as 20% in some series.[73,75,76] The management of nerve injuries is expectant with regular follow-up visits and appropriate investigation with referral and electromyography at 3 months if there is no improvement.

Loss of terminal external rotation is typically 5° after the Latarjet procedure.[77] However, other studies have reported significant loss of external rotation after the Latarjet technique.[78] To avoid stiffness postoperatively, it is important to use a subscapularis-splitting approach and repair the coracoaromial stump to the capsule with the arm in near-maximal external rotation.

Pseudarthrosis of the coracoid process can occur in 1.5% to 9.0% of cases and is usually related to unicortical or single screw fixation.[73] Patients with uncontrolled seizure disorders represent a cohort who should not undergo stabilization attempts until the seizures are controlled (this is an example of a preoperative phase error leading to a postoperative complication). Screw bending and breakage are not infrequent occurrences in these patients (**Fig. 7**). Malpositioned grafts placed too low may predispose to fibrous nonunion owing to insufficient bone in the glenoid.

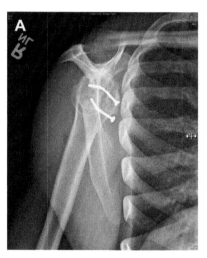
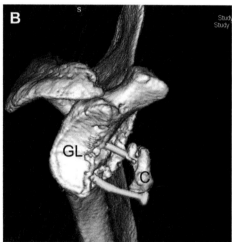
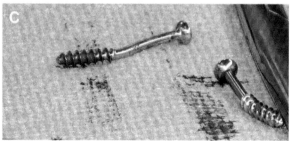

Fig. 7. A 40-y-year-old right hand dominant male who underwent a revision open Latarjet procedure for recurrent anterior instability in conjunction with uncontrolled seizure disorders. He continued to have seizures and ultimately went on to nonunion and screw bending and breakage. (*A*) Scapular Y view demonstrating bent screws. (*B*) Three-dimensional computed tomography scan demonstrating coracoid nonunion and bent screws. (*C*) Intraoperative photo demonstrating the 4.5-mm solid malleolar screws have bent and are broken. C, coracoid; GL, glenoid. (*Courtesy of* Columbia University Center for Shoulder, Elbow, and Sports Medicine, New York, NY; with permission.)

Fracture of the coracoid process occurs in 1.5% of cases and usually within 3 months of surgery. This complication is often as a result of intraoperative overtightening of the screws. Older age and excessive decortication of the undersurface of the coracoid weakens the graft and may predispose to iatrogenic graft fracture. This complication can be minimized by using a "2-finger" tightening technique, drilling with a drill bit 3.2 mm or smaller and leaving an adequate bone bridge between the 2 drill holes.

Osteoarthritis can also develop in patients with shoulder instability after Latarjet procedures about 20% to 25% of the time.[79,80] Preexisting osteoarthritis, older age at the time of the first dislocation and at the time of the surgery, longer postoperative delay, preoperative fracture of the anterior glenoid rim, severe Hill-Sachs lesions, and high-demand sports contribute to the development of postoperative osteoarthritis. To prevent a laterally overhanging coracoid process, the surgeon should check the final position of the coracoid by visualization and palpation.

POSTOPERATIVE PHASE

Postoperative rehabilitation programs should be adapted to the pathology and the repair that was performed. Noncompliance with immobilization, rehabilitation regimens, or return to activity restrictions makes up a significant proportion of complications and failures after shoulder stabilization surgery.[81] Repairs are significantly weaker than the normal capsulolabral complex, so it is important to convey to the patient that a necessary period of immobilization is required. Trauma in the postoperative period, either accidental or as a consequence of noncompliance with return-to-sport restrictions, can also lead to failure in the postoperative period. Delaying return to sports for approximately 6 months postoperatively has been suggested as a means for decreasing recurrence rates.[82]

Immediately after surgery, unrestricted range of the hand, wrist, and elbow is encouraged. Cole and Romeo[62] have suggested active forward elevation be restricted to 120° the first 2 to 3 weeks to decrease the stresses on the capsulolabral repair. At 8 to 10 weeks, resistive exercises are instituted into the rehabilitation regimen.[62] Wall and Warren[58] proposed that, by 10 to 12 weeks postoperatively, nonthrowing athletes should regain normal motion. In throwing athletes, this goal is hoped to be achieved by 6 to 8 weeks postoperatively. In those patients who are recovering from capsular shifts or Bankart repair, motion may remain restricted. If this persists at 4 months postoperatively, it is reasonable to consider a gentle manipulation under anesthesia.[58]

SUMMARY

Although shoulder instability is a common problem, it remains a complicated and challenging issue for orthopedic surgeons, even amid the rapidly expanding advancement in techniques. Failures of shoulder instability surgery can result from inadequate assessment of the patient in the preoperative, intraoperative, or postoperative phase. To prevent complications, the surgeon must identify structural lesions and recognize patient factors that may contribute to glenohumeral instability. In the postoperative period, the rehabilitation regimen must be tailored to each individual patient. An understanding of potential complications and failures that can arise throughout the chronology of the unstable shoulder is critical to maximize patient outcomes.

REFERENCES

1. Uhorchak JM, Arciero RA, Huggard D, et al. Recurrent shoulder instability after open reconstruction in athletes involved in collision and contact sports. Am J Sports Med 2000;28(6):794–9.
2. Owens BD, Harrast JJ, Hurwitz SR, et al. Surgical trends in Bankart repair: an analysis of data from the American Board of Orthopaedic Surgery certification examination. Am J Sports Med 2011;39(9):1865–9.
3. Bessiere C, Trojani C, Pelegri C, et al. Coracoid bone block versus arthroscopic Bankart repair: a comparative paired study with 5-year follow-up. Orthop Traumatol Surg Res 2013;99(2):123–30.
4. Tauber M, Resch H, Forstner R, et al. Reasons for failure after surgical repair of anterior shoulder instability. J Shoulder Elbow Surg 2004;13(3):279–85.
5. Arciero RA, Spang JT. Complications in arthroscopic anterior shoulder stabilization: pearls and pitfalls. Instr Course Lect 2008;57:113–24.
6. Boileau P, Villalba M, Hery JY, et al. Risk factors for recurrence of shoulder instability after arthroscopic Bankart repair. J Bone Joint Surg Am 2006;88(8): 1755–63.
7. Provencher MT, Bhatia S, Ghodadra NS, et al. Recurrent shoulder instability: current concepts for evaluation and management of glenoid bone loss. J Bone Joint Surg Am 2010;92(Suppl 2):133–51.
8. Barron OA, Biglliani LU. Revision instability surgery. Clin Sports Med 1995;14(4): 955–72.
9. Sugaya H. Instability with bone loss. In: Angelo RL, Esch JC, Ryu RK, editors. AANA advanced arthroscopy: the shoulder. Philadelphia: Elsevier; 2010. p. 136–46.
10. Mascarenhas R, Rusen J, Saltzman BM, et al. Management of humeral and glenoid bone loss in recurrent glenohumeral instability. Adv Orthop 2014;2014: 640952.
11. Jobe FW, Kvitne RS, Giangarra CE. Shoulder pain in the overhand or throwing athlete. The relationship of anterior instability and rotator cuff impingement. Orthop Rev 1989;18(9):963–75.
12. Gagey OJ, Gagey N. The hyperabduction test. J Bone Joint Surg Br 2001;83(1): 69–74.
13. Neer CS 2nd, Foster CR. Inferior capsular shift for involuntary inferior and multidirectional instability of the shoulder. A preliminary report. J Bone Joint Surg Am 1980;62(6):897–908.
14. Kim SH, Park JC, Park JS, et al. Painful jerk test: a predictor of success in nonoperative treatment of posteroinferior instability of the shoulder. Am J Sports Med 2004;32(8):1849–55.
15. Rokous JR, Feagin JA, Abbott HG. Modified axillary roentgenogram. A useful adjunct in the diagnosis of recurrent instability of the shoulder. Clin Orthop Relat Res 1972;82:84–6.
16. Danzig LA, Greenway G, Resnick D. The Hill-Sachs lesion. An experimental study. Am J Sports Med 1980;8(5):328–32.
17. Rozing PM, de Bakker HM, Obermann WR. Radiographic views in recurrent anterior shoulder dislocation. Comparison of six methods for identification of typical lesions. Acta Orthop Scand 1986;57(4):328–30.
18. Provencher MT, Romeo AA, Ebrary I. Shoulder instability a comprehensive approach. In: Provencher M, Romeo A, editors. Expert consult. 1st edition.

Philadelphia: Elsevier/Saunders; 2012. p. 67–259. Available at: http://www.columbia.edu/cgi-bin/cul/resolve?clio9447627.

19. Kwon YW, Powell KA, Yum JK, et al. Use of three-dimensional computed tomography for the analysis of the glenoid anatomy. J Shoulder Elbow Surg 2005;14(1):85–90.

20. Sugaya H, Moriishi J, Dohi M, et al. Glenoid rim morphology in recurrent anterior glenohumeral instability. J Bone Joint Surg Am 2003;85-A(5):878–84.

21. Mologne TS, Provencher MT, Menzel KA, et al. Arthroscopic stabilization in patients with an inverted pear glenoid: results in patients with bone loss of the anterior glenoid. Am J Sports Med 2007;35(8):1276–83.

22. Huysmans PE, Haen PS, Kidd M, et al. The shape of the inferior part of the glenoid: a cadaveric study. J Shoulder Elbow Surg 2006;15(6):759–63.

23. Huijsmans PE, Haen PS, Kidd M, et al. Quantification of a glenoid defect with three-dimensional computed tomography and magnetic resonance imaging: a cadaveric study. J Shoulder Elbow Surg 2007;16(6):803–9.

24. Bigliani LU, Newton PM, Steinmann SP, et al. Glenoid rim lesions associated with recurrent anterior dislocation of the shoulder. Am J Sports Med 1998;26(1):41–5.

25. Chuang TY, Adams CR, Burkhart SS. Use of preoperative three-dimensional computed tomography to quantify glenoid bone loss in shoulder instability. Arthroscopy 2008;24(4):376–82.

26. Baudi P, Righi P, Bolognesi D, et al. How to identify and calculate glenoid bone deficit. La Chirurgia degli organi di movimento 2005;90(2):145–52.

27. Sugaya H, Kon Y, Tsuchiya A. Arthroscopic repair of glenoid fractures using suture anchors. Arthroscopy 2005;21(5):635.

28. Piasecki DP, Verma NN, Romeo AA, et al. Glenoid bone deficiency in recurrent anterior shoulder instability: diagnosis and management. J Am Acad Orthop Surg 2009;17(8):482–93.

29. Palmer WE, Brown JH, Rosenthal DI. Labral-ligamentous complex of the shoulder: evaluation with MR arthrography. Radiology 1994;190(3):645–51.

30. Gusmer PB, Potter HG, Schatz JA, et al. Labral injuries: accuracy of detection with unenhanced MR imaging of the shoulder. Radiology 1996;200(2):519–24.

31. Beltran J, Bencardino J, Mellado J, et al. MR arthrography of the shoulder: variants and pitfalls. Radiographics 1997;17(6):1403–12 [discussion: 1412-5].

32. Gyftopoulos S, Hasan S, Bencardino J, et al. Diagnostic accuracy of MRI in the measurement of glenoid bone loss. AJR Am J Roentgenol 2012;199(4):873–8.

33. Burkhart SS, Debeer JF, Tehrany AM, et al. Quantifying glenoid bone loss arthroscopically in shoulder instability. Arthroscopy 2002;18(5):488–91.

34. Kralinger F, Aigner F, Longato S, et al. Is the bare spot a consistent landmark for shoulder arthroscopy? A study of 20 embalmed glenoids with 3-dimensional computed tomographic reconstruction. Arthroscopy 2006;22(4):428–32.

35. Burkhart SS, De Beer JF. Traumatic glenohumeral bone defects and their relationship to failure of arthroscopic Bankart repairs: significance of the inverted-pear glenoid and the humeral engaging Hill-Sachs lesion. Arthroscopy 2000;16(7):677–94.

36. Lo IK, Parten PM, Burkhart SS. The inverted pear glenoid: an indicator of significant glenoid bone loss. Arthroscopy 2004;20(2):169–74.

37. Yamamoto N, Itoi E, Abe H, et al. Contact between the glenoid and the humeral head in abduction, external rotation, and horizontal extension: a new concept of glenoid track. J Shoulder Elbow Surg 2007;16(5):649–56.

38. Di Giacomo G, Itoi E, Burkhart SS. Evolving concept of bipolar bone loss and the Hill-Sachs lesion: from "engaging/non-engaging" lesion to "on-track/off-track" lesion. Arthroscopy 2014;30(1):90–8.
39. Johnson SM, Robinson CM. Shoulder instability in patients with joint hyperlaxity. J Bone Joint Surg Am 2010;92(6):1545–57.
40. Smith R, Damodaran AK, Swaminathan S, et al. Hypermobility and sports injuries in junior netball players. Br J Sports Med 2005;39(9):628–31.
41. Levine WN, Prickett WD, Prymka M, et al. Treatment of the athlete with multidirectional shoulder instability. Orthop Clin North Am 2001;32(3):475–84.
42. Mahaffey BL, Smith PA. Shoulder instability in young athletes. Am Fam Physician 1999;59(10):2773–82, 2787.
43. Neer CS 2nd. Involuntary inferior and multidirectional instability of the shoulder: etiology, recognition, and treatment. Instr Course Lect 1985;34:232–8.
44. O'Driscoll SW, Evans DC. Contralateral shoulder instability following anterior repair. An epidemiological investigation. J Bone Joint Surg Br 1991;73(6):941–6.
45. Grahame R. Heritable disorders of connective tissue. Baillieres Best Pract Res Clin Rheumatol 2000;14(2):345–61.
46. Beighton P, De Paepe A, Steinmann B, et al. Ehlers-Danlos syndromes: revised nosology, Villefranche, 1997. Ehlers-Danlos National Foundation (USA) and Ehlers-Danlos Support Group (UK). Am J Med Genet 1998;77(1):31–7.
47. Coudane H, Walch G, Sebesta A. Chronic anterior instability of the shoulder in adults. Methodology. Rev Chir Orthop Reparatrice Appar Mot 2000;86(Suppl 1):94–5 [in French].
48. Coste JS, Jund S, Lemaire M. Evaluation prospective arthroscopique du test de laxité du ligament gléno-huméral inférieur. Revue De Chirurgie Orthopedique 1999.
49. Beighton P, Horan F. Orthopaedic aspects of the Ehlers-Danlos syndrome. J Bone Joint Surg Br 1969;51(3):444–53.
50. Grahame R, Bird HA, Child A. The revised (Brighton 1998) criteria for the diagnosis of benign joint hypermobility syndrome (BJHS). J Rheumatol 2000;27(7): 1777–9.
51. Schenk TJ, Brems JJ. Multidirectional instability of the shoulder: pathophysiology, diagnosis, and management. J Am Acad Orthop Surg 1998;6(1):65–72.
52. Craig EV. Clinical orthopaedics. In: Warren RF, Carson EW, editors. Multidirectional instability: diagnosis and management. Philadelphia: Lippincott Williams and Wilkins; 1999. p. 203–12.
53. Hawkins RH, Hawkins RJ. Failed anterior reconstruction for shoulder instability. J Bone Joint Surg Br 1985;67(5):709–14.
54. Bigliani LU, Pollock RG, Soslowsky LJ, et al. Tensile properties of the inferior glenohumeral ligament. J Orthop Res 1992;10(2):187–97.
55. Wolf EM, Cheng JC, Dickson K. Humeral avulsion of glenohumeral ligaments as a cause of anterior shoulder instability. Arthroscopy 1995;11(5):600–7.
56. Rowe CR, Pierce DS, Clark JG. Voluntary dislocation of the shoulder. A preliminary report on a clinical, electromyographic, and psychiatric study of twenty-six patients. J Bone Joint Surg Am 1973;55(3):445–60.
57. Fronek J, Warren RF, Bowen M. Posterior subluxation of the glenohumeral joint. J Bone Joint Surg Am 1989;71(2):205–16.
58. Wall MS, Warren RF. Complications of shoulder instability surgery. Clin Sports Med 1995;14(4):973–1000.
59. Bartl C, Schumann K, Paul J, et al. Arthroscopic capsulolabral revision repair for recurrent anterior shoulder instability. Am J Sports Med 2011;39(3):511–8.

60. Shin JJ, Mascarenhas R, Patel AV, et al. Clinical outcomes following revision anterior shoulder arthroscopic capsulolabral stabilization. Arch Orthop Trauma Surg 2015;135(11):1553–9.
61. Nagra NS, Zargar N, Smith RD, et al. Mechanical properties of all-suture anchors for rotator cuff repair. Bone Joint Res 2017;6(2):82–9.
62. Cole BJ, Romeo AA. Arthroscopic shoulder stabilization with suture anchors: technique, technology, and pitfalls. Clin Orthop Relat Res 2001;(390):17–30.
63. Kang RW, Frank RM, Nho SJ, et al. Complications associated with anterior shoulder instability repair. Arthroscopy 2009;25(8):909–20.
64. Mazzocca AD, Brown FM Jr, Carreira DS, et al. Arthroscopic anterior shoulder stabilization of collision and contact athletes. Am J Sports Med 2005;33(1):52–60.
65. Provencher MT, Mologne TS, Hongo M, et al. Arthroscopic versus open rotator interval closure: biomechanical evaluation of stability and motion. Arthroscopy 2007;23(6):583–92.
66. Mologne TS, Zhao K, Hongo M, et al. The addition of rotator interval closure after arthroscopic repair of either anterior or posterior shoulder instability: effect on glenohumeral translation and range of motion. Am J Sports Med 2008;36(6):1123–31.
67. Plausinis D, Bravman JT, Heywood C, et al. Arthroscopic rotator interval closure: effect of sutures on glenohumeral motion and anterior-posterior translation. Am J Sports Med 2006;34(10):1656–61.
68. Regan WD Jr, Webster-Bogaert S, Hawkins RJ, et al. Comparative functional analysis of the Bristow, Magnuson-Stack, and Putti-Platt procedures for recurrent dislocation of the shoulder. Am J Sports Med 1989;17(1):42–8.
69. Bigliani LU, Kurzweil PR, Schwartzbach CC, et al. Inferior capsular shift procedure for anterior-inferior shoulder instability in athletes. Am J Sports Med 1994;22(5):578–84.
70. Rhee YG, Ha JH, Cho NS. Anterior shoulder stabilization in collision athletes: arthroscopic versus open Bankart repair. Am J Sports Med 2006;34(6):979–85.
71. Hubbell JD, Ahmad S, Bezenoff LS, et al. Comparison of shoulder stabilization using arthroscopic transglenoid sutures versus open capsulolabral repairs: a 5-year minimum follow-up. Am J Sports Med 2004;32(3):650–4.
72. Griesser MJ, Harris JD, McCoy BW, et al. Complications and re-operations after Bristow-Latarjet shoulder stabilization: a systematic review. J Shoulder Elbow Surg 2013;22(2):286–92.
73. Bhatia S, Frank RM, Ghodadra NS, et al. The outcomes and surgical techniques of the latarjet procedure. Arthroscopy 2014;30(2):227–35.
74. Schmid SL, Farshad M, Catanzaro S, et al. The Latarjet procedure for the treatment of recurrence of anterior instability of the shoulder after operative repair: a retrospective case series of forty-nine consecutive patients. J Bone Joint Surg Am 2012;94(11):e75.
75. Shah AA, Butler RB, Romanowski J, et al. Short-term complications of the Latarjet procedure. J Bone Joint Surg Am 2012;94(6):495–501.
76. Gupta A, Delaney R, Petkin K, et al. Complications of the Latarjet procedure. Curr Rev Musculoskelet Med 2015;8(1):59–66.
77. Degen RM, Giles JW, Johnson JA, et al. Remplissage versus latarjet for engaging Hill-Sachs defects without substantial glenoid bone loss: a biomechanical comparison. Clin Orthop Relat Res 2014;472(8):2363–71.
78. Giles JW, Degen RM, Johnson JA, et al. The Bristow and Latarjet procedures: why these techniques should not be considered synonymous. J Bone Joint Surg Am 2014;96(16):1340–8.

79. Mizuno N, Denard PJ, Raiss P, et al. Long-term results of the Latarjet procedure for anterior instability of the shoulder. J Shoulder Elbow Surg 2014;23(11):1691–9.
80. Allain J, Goutallier D, Glorion C. Long-term results of the Latarjet procedure for the treatment of anterior instability of the shoulder. J Bone Joint Surg Am 1998; 80(6):841–52.
81. Green MR, Christensen KP. Arthroscopic Bankart procedure: two- to five-year followup with clinical correlation to severity of glenoid labral lesion. Am J Sports Med 1995;23(3):276–81.
82. Snyder SJ, Strafford BB. Arthroscopic management of instability of the shoulder. Orthopedics 1993;16(9):993–1002.

Shoulder Rotator Cuff Pathology

Common Problems and Solutions

Harrison S. Mahon, MD, James E. Christensen, MD,
Stephen F. Brockmeier, MD*

KEYWORDS

- Rotator cuff repair • Retear • Stiffness • Adhesive capsulitis • SLAP lesion
- Biceps tendinitis • Septic arthritis

KEY POINTS

- There are many patient factors and technical factors which may increase the risk for retear.
- Dermal allograft augmentation or reverse total shoulder arthroplasty provide options for irreparable failed rotator cuff repairs.
- Always consider other sources of shoulder pain when evaluating a rotator cuff tear in order to rule out other pathology
- Infection should be considered in patients who have persistent pain postoperatively with no obvious source.

INTRODUCTION

Rotator cuff repair is one of the most common orthopedic procedures performed, with an estimated 200,000 to 300,000 cases worldwide each year.[1] An aging population and advancements in arthroscopic technique have led to a steady increase in the number of repairs performed annually. Although rotator cuff repair generally improves pain and function, studies have estimated a complication rate as high as 14%.[2] This review aims to outline the most common complications associated with arthroscopic rotator cuff repair, including retear, failure to heal, stiffness, failure to recognize concomitant pathology, and infection.

There are no personal conflicts of interests to disclose in the writing or publishing of this article.
Department of Orthopaedic Surgery, University of Virginia, 400 Ray C. Hunt Drive, Suite 330, Charlottesville, VA 22903, USA
* Corresponding author.
E-mail address: SFB2E@hscmail.mcc.virginia.edu

Clin Sports Med 37 (2018) 179–196
https://doi.org/10.1016/j.csm.2017.12.013
sportsmed.theclinics.com

RETEAR
Case Example

A 63-year-old right-hand-dominant man presented to clinic with 1 year of right shoulder pain after no inciting incident. His examination was notable for limited forward flexion and reduced strength on both supraspinatus and infraspinatus testing. MRI showed a full-thickness supraspinatus tear with retraction to the level of the acromion and mild fatty atrophy and a partial thickness subscapularis tear (**Fig. 1**A). He subsequently underwent arthroscopic repair of both the supraspinatus and subscapularis using a linked dual-row transosseous equivalent–type repair with knotless tape sutures (**Fig. 1**B). The patient was kept in a sling for 6 weeks total after surgery, with physical therapy beginning at 2 weeks postoperatively. He made excellent progress and was cleared to slowly resume work as a maintenance worker at 3 months after surgery. Four months after surgery, he felt a pop in his operative shoulder while lifting something at work. The examination was notable for reduced strength in both supraspinatus and infraspinatus testing. MRI showed a medially ruptured supraspinatus tendon with a healed footprint (type 2 failure) as well as interval development of a full-thickness infraspinatus tear. The anterior aspect of the supraspinatus and the subscapularis repair appeared to be intact (**Fig. 1**C). A revision rotator cuff repair was carried out using a single-row technique medialized to the margin of the footprint with margin convergence sutures (**Fig. 1**D).

One of the most important and potentially challenging complications after rotator cuff repair is retear of the repaired cuff. Historically, retear rates have been reported between 11% and 94%. The highest retear rate (94%) was found in a series of 18 patients who underwent arthroscopic repair of a massive rotator cuff tear.[3] The lowest retear rate (11%) was found in a prospective series of 105 consecutive shoulders undergoing arthroscopic double-row repair of the supraspinatus or supraspinatus and infraspinatus.[4] More recent studies have suggested that retear rates may actually be lower than previously thought, between 11% and 57%.[5] At any rate, retear of rotator cuff repair is a common complication.

Interestingly, many studies have suggested that rotator cuff repair provides a benefit to patients regardless of the repair integrity. For example, in the previously cited study with a 94% retear rate, patients had significant increases in pain and function at 12 months despite retear. At the 2-year follow-up, pain and function had deteriorated from the 12-month mark but were still higher than preoperative levels.[3] Several other studies have found similar results, both finding that postoperative cuff integrity has no significant effect on outcomes and that those with retear still show improvements in satisfaction, pain, and clinical function scores.[6,7]

Although data have failed to indicate that a retear of cuff repair leaves patients worse off than before surgery, most recent studies agree that intact repairs lead to better outcomes, especially over the longer-term. Kim and colleagues[8] found that among patients in their cohort with retears, all age groups had poorer satisfaction and American Shoulder and Elbow Surgeons' and Simple Shoulder Test scores compared with patients with no retear. In addition, they found that several demographic factors among patients with retears were associated with poorer outcomes. These factors included younger age, lower education level, and workers' compensation claim. Intact repairs have been correlated with more durable subjective and objective outcomes in other studies as well.[5]

A significant amount of research has been devoted to determining which patient factors and surgical techniques predispose one to a rotator cuff retear. Perhaps the most frequently implicated patient factor is advanced age. Although some studies have shown that age does correlate with higher retear rates, univariate analyses in other studies have failed to show significance. Other implicated patient factors have

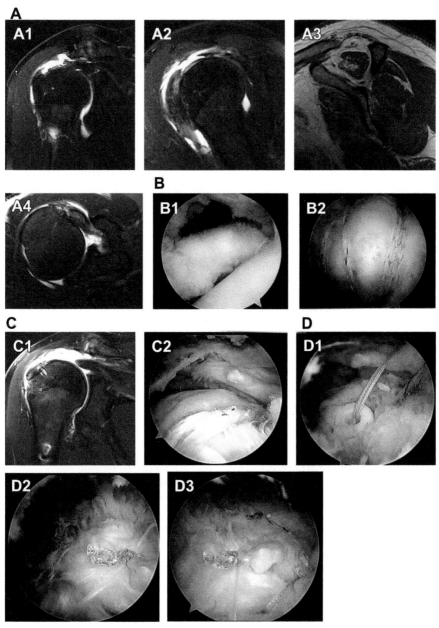

Fig. 1. (A) Coronal (A1) and sagittal (A2) T1 imaging of the retracted supraspinatus and in-fraspinatus tear in a 63-year-old man. There was mild fatty atrophy present in the supraspi-natus muscle (A3). Axial imaging shows partial-thickness subscapularis tearing (A4). (B1) Arthroscopic imaging of a large crescent-shaped supraspinatus and infraspinatus tear. (B2) Final repair construct with 2 medial and 2 lateral row anchors. (C) Coronal T1 MRI demon-strating type II retear of the tendon. Note that the greater tuberosity still has a significant amount of cuff tissue, which appears well fixed to the footprint (C1). Arthroscopic photo of the large recurrent rotator cuff tear (C2). (D) Arthroscopic photo showing the 8.0-mm an-chor and 5.5-mm anchor placed in the debrided footprint (D1). Three margin convergence sutures were placed to repair the superior cuff (D2). Final photo showing the lateralized and repaired rotator cuff (D3).

included fatty infiltration and larger tear size. Some studies have used biceps and acromioclavicular (AC) joint lesions as surrogate markers of tendon quality and found that these factors are associated with a higher retear rate.[1,5]

Any step in surgical repair of the rotator cuff has the potential to affect integrity of the repair. In general, the wide variety of suture and anchor configurations can be grouped into one of the following: traditional transosseous, single row, double row, and transosseous equivalent. Traditional transosseous repair is a knotless repair that must be done using open or mini-open technique. This technique was initially described as the gold standard because it created superior contact area and pressure across the footprint compared with simple anchor techniques.[9] The sutures are passed through the tendon and then through transosseous tunnels which pass from the cuff footprint to the lateral aspect of the proximal humerus. Single-row repairs use one row of laterally based anchors. Double-row repairs use one row of medially based anchors and one row of laterally based anchors. In 2006, Park and colleagues[10] initially described the transosseous equivalent repair. In this repair method, 2 suture anchors are used to secure the medial side of the tendon. The sutures are then passed through the tendon but are not cut. The free ends are instead brought through a knotless anchor, which is placed laterally and then tensioned over the cuff. This, in theory, recreates the footprint and pressure mechanics of a transosseous repair.[10,11] This repair method has also been called the suture bridge technique.

Many studies have been performed in an effort to determine which suture and anchor configuration leads to the best outcomes. In general, biomechanical studies have shown that the transosseous equivalent technique results in higher load to failure, greater resistance to shear and rotational forces, and more consistent recreation of the cuff footprint with minimal gap formation compared with single- and double-row repair techniques.[11] Clinical comparisons between single-row, double-row, and suture bridge techniques have also been performed. Hein and colleagues[12] performed a systematic review of 32 studies on patients with imaging at a minimum of 1 year of follow-up. They found that double-row and suture bridge repairs had lower retear rates than single-row repairs in most tear size categories. However, there was no difference in retear rates between double-row and suture bridge repairs.

As transosseous equivalent repair has become more popular, the location and method of fixation in the medial row has drawn some attention. Although passing sutures through the tendon as medial as possible maximizes the footprint of the repair, biomechanical studies have shown that passage directly through the musculotendinous junction leads to higher rates of medial row failure.[13] The medial row suture can be tied in horizontal or vertical mattress fashion or not tied at all and simply brought down to the lateral knotless anchors. Cadaveric studies have shown that the vertical mattress technique demonstrated a higher load to failure than the horizontal mattress technique but no difference in tendon gapping.[14] By not tying the medial row, there is some thought that this maximizes compression when the tendon is placed under tension. A sheep model demonstrated this to be true; however, it did not translate into differences in stiffness, ultimate failure load, or total energy to failure.[15]

Biomechanical studies have also examined the anchor type and placement in terms of failure strength. Interestingly, the size of the anchor has not demonstrated a statistically significant effect on failure load.[16] Studies have indicated that anchors have higher pullout strength in areas with higher bone densities. In other words, placement of the lateral row anchors within the proximal part of the tuberosity may lead to lower failure rates.[17] Most of the studies regarding construct variables are biomechanical studies, and it is generally unclear how clinically relevant these results truly are.

In order to prevent rotator cuff retears, it is important to understand how suture anchor constructs usually fail. Early studies suggested that retears commonly occur at the suture-tendon interface.[18] More recent studies on arthroscopic repair with the suture bridge technique found a higher incidence of failures medial to the repair and created a classification system for failure types. A type 1 failure occurs when none of the repaired cuff tissue remains on the tuberosity. A type 2 failure occurs when there is intact repaired tendon on the tuberosity.[19,20] Some biomechanical studies indicate that the bone-anchor interface may be an important site of failure as well.[21]

When a retear does occur after rotator cuff repair, most instances occur in the early postoperative period. In a prospective study of patients followed by ultrasound, Miller and colleagues[22] found that most retears occurred within 3 months of surgery. No retears occurred after 6 months. Other studies have confirmed this finding and found that retears occurring 2 to 5 years postoperatively were related to sports or direct trauma.[23,24]

FAILURE TO HEAL
Case Example

A 54-year-old woman presented to the clinic with years of right shoulder pain. She had positive impingement and empty can signs on examination with mildly reduced cuff strength. MRI showed a full-thickness supraspinatus tear measuring 15 mm in the antoroposterior (AP) plane with minimal retraction. She subsequently underwent a knotless suture bridge repair with 2 medial and 2 lateral anchors (**Fig. 2**A and B).

The patient regained full motion postoperatively but had continued pain and subjective weakness. An MRI was done at 7 months postoperatively, which showed a recurrent defect with degenerative tissue at the footprint, representing a failure to heal. She elected to proceed with revision cuff repair. Diagnostic arthroscopy confirmed a 2 × 2-cm area of degenerative tissue near the footprint, which was then debrided (**Fig. 2**C). The footprint was also vented to promote healing. The authors elected to use a 3 × 3-cm decellularized dermal allograft to augment their repair. Two 5.5-mm double-loaded anchors were placed for the medial row. One suture from each anchor was then passed through the medial corners of the dermal allograft, and it was secured into place. Two more 5.5-mm anchors were used to create the lateral row and secure the lateral edge of the graft (**Fig. 2**D).

Dermal allograft augmentation represents a fairly novel technique in the management of large to massive rotator cuff tears. Although the indications for reverse total shoulder arthroplasty have increased in recent years, there remains a younger and more active patient population that would be better served by delaying joint replacement. Surgeons have tried many different autograft, allograft, and xenograft options for the treatment of larger rotator cuff tears. A systematic review demonstrated promising results for human dermal allografts with significantly improved function and structural outcomes compared with conventional primary repair.[25]

Some may question whether the tendon ever healed at all when rotator cuff repair fails. In reality, it is difficult to discern which patients constitute a failure to heal and which ones truly sustained a retear of the tendon. Patients who retear may describe a traumatic incident that they think caused the reinjury, but often times this is not the case. Boileau and colleagues[26] followed 65 patients after arthroscopic repair of a chronic full-thickness supraspinatus tear and reimaged them with either a computed tomography scan or MRI. They found that 71% of the patients completely healed the rotator cuff. Patients who did not heal their repair were older on average and had higher rates of associated delamination of the subscapularis and/or infraspinatus. Most studies seem to agree with these findings and implicate age, tear size, and fatty infiltration as

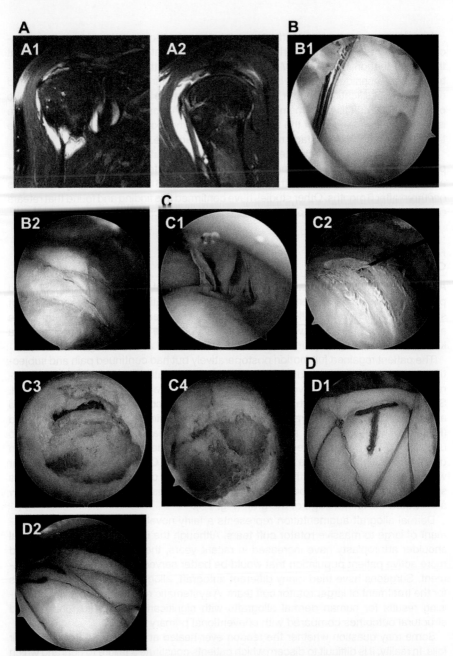

Fig. 2. (A) Coronal (A1) and sagittal (A2) T1 MRI showing a small supraspinatus tear in a 54-year-old woman. (B) Arthroscopic photo showing an arthroscopic probe in the supraspinatus tear (B1). Final repair construct with 2 medial and 2 lateral row anchor (B2). (C) Degenerative tissue at the rotator cuff footprint with failure of the suture anchor (C1). PDS suture was passed through the tear in order to facilitate finding the tear with the arthroscope once outside the joint (C2). The degenerative cuff tissue was debrided as was the cuff footprint (C3). The authors elected to vent the footprint in order to facilitate healing (C4). (D) The medial edge of the dermal allograft was brought down over 2 medial anchors (D1). Final allograft construct demonstrating appropriate coverage and recreation of the superior capsule (D2).

negative predictive factors in terms of healing. Interestingly, a systematic review of studies on healing after rotator cuff repair found that arthroscopic repair, double-row repair, performing a concomitant acromioplasty, and the use of platelet-rich plasma do not demonstrate increased healing rates compared with their alternatives.[27,28]

Traditionally, rotator cuff repair is followed by 4 to 6 weeks of sling immobilization with gradual initiation of range of motion and strengthening exercises. Logically this would seem to help prevent retear, but data have not consistently shown this to be the case. A meta-analysis comparing early mobilization with delayed mobilization found no significant difference in retear rates. In this case, early mobilization was defined as passive range of motion within 2 weeks of surgery. Delayed mobilization consisted of 4 weeks of immobilization but did allow pendulum exercises during this period.[29] Other reviews have also failed to demonstrate a difference between the two.[28] In practice, patient factors and the quality of the repair achieved are likely the best guides for determining when and how to initiate rehabilitation.

POSTOPERATIVE STIFFNESS/ADHESIVE CAPSULITIS
Case Example

A 52-year-old woman presented to the authors' clinic with several years of worsening right shoulder pain. Imaging showed a full-thickness supraspinatus tear with minimal retraction. She subsequently underwent arthroscopic repair with 2 medial and 2 lateral row anchors. Her initial postoperative course was uncomplicated, but she failed to make progress with range of motion. At the 6-month follow-up, her active and passive forward flexion was limited to 90°. This flexion was significantly worse than her preoperative forward flexion of 160°. She elected to proceed with an arthroscopic lysis of adhesions and manipulation under anesthesia (**Fig. 3**A and B). At the time of this procedure, her rotator cuff repair was noted to have healed. After immediate institution of postoperative physical therapy and progression over the course of 3 months, the patient was pain free and had symmetric range of motion to her contralateral shoulder at the final follow-up.

Another common complication after rotator cuff repair is stiffness. As most surgeons recommend at least a short period of immobilization after surgery, a certain degree of postoperative stiffness is to be expected and usually resolves with physical therapy. However, some patients may develop stiffness, which fails to improve with

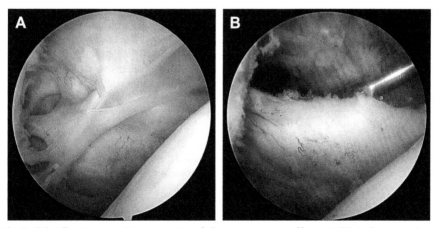

Fig. 3. (*A*) Adhesive capsulitis in a patient following rotator cuff repair. (*B*) Arthroscopic lysis of adhesions.

conservative measures. The prevention and management of this complication is an important aspect of rotator cuff repair.

The incidence of stiffness after arthroscopic rotator cuff repair has been reported between 4.9% and 8.7%. Of course, stiffness is difficult to define and can be somewhat subjective. Huberty and colleagues[30] found a 4.9% incidence of patients who were dissatisfied with the result of their repair because of the development of stiffness. Workers' compensation, age less than 50 years, calcific tendinitis, adhesive capsulitis, single tendon cuff repair, partial articular-sided supraspinatus tendon avulsion (PASTA) repair, and concomitant labral repair were all statistically significant risk factors for developing postoperative stiffness. This study also found that patients with concomitant coracoplasty and large tears were less likely to develop stiffness. Chung and colleagues[31] defined stiffness objectively in a cohort of patients undergoing arthroscopic repair and reported findings at different time points postoperatively. They found that 18.6% of patients at 3 months, 2.8% at 6 months, and 6.6% at the final follow-up had stiffness defined as reduced forward elevation, external rotation, or internal rotation. Older patients were more likely to be stiff at all time points. Preoperative stiffness was a risk factor for postoperative stiffness only at the 3-month time mark. Larger tear size, fatty infiltration, and open surgery were risk factors for stiffness only at the final follow-up. The study also found that late postoperative stiffness was a significant risk factor for retear. It must be noted that these studies defined stiffness differently. Younger patients may not be objectively stiff but may be more likely to have higher functional demands and report subjective stiffness.

Some studies have suggested that the development of some stiffness after surgery may actually promote healing. A large study of 1533 consecutive patients found that stiffness at 6 weeks and 12 weeks postoperatively, but not 24 weeks, correlated with higher rates of rotator cuff integrity at 6 weeks postoperatively. Patients in this study with more than 20° of external rotation at 6 weeks had a 15% retear rate.[32] This finding may support the idea that stiffness after surgery is not necessarily a cause for concern and that overly aggressive physical therapy can risk repair integrity.

The American Society of Shoulder and Elbow Therapists recommend a 2-week period of immobilization followed by gradual and progressive passive range of motion between weeks 2 and 6. This period is followed by initiation of active range of motion and then finally progressive strengthening starting at week 12.[33] Many of the studies comparing rehabilitation protocols have failed to demonstrate significant clinical differences in outcomes. The meta-analysis by Denard and colleagues[34] found an overall stiffness rate of 1.5% for patients enrolled in an immediate passive range of motion protocol and a rate of 4.5% for patients in a 6-week sling immobilization protocol. Koo and colleagues[35] suggested a modified protocol for patients at high risk of developing stiffness and did not see any cases of stiffness in their cohort. This protocol adds immediate closed-chain passive forward flexion exercises to a standard protocol consisting of sling immobilization without overhead shoulder motion for 6 weeks.[35]

MISSED CONCOMITANT PATHOLOGY
Case Example

A 33-year-old woman presented to the clinic after a motor vehicle accident with anterior and lateral shoulder pain. An MRI at that time showed a high-grade supraspinatus articular-sided tear; she underwent arthroscopy with PASTA repair, with the rotator cuff tear and subsequent repair seen in **Fig. 4**A, B, respectively. The long head biceps tendon at that time did not show any pathology (**Fig. 4**C). She was recovering and regaining her strength but continued to have anterior shoulder pain after 3 months. Because of the continued pain, an MRI was performed, which demonstrated severe

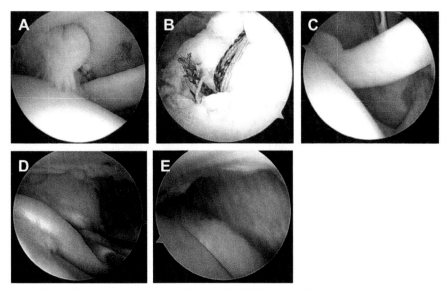

Fig. 4. (*A*) Partial, articular rotator cuff tear. (*B*) PASTA repair. Biceps during second arthroscopy with noted tear. (*C*) Biceps at time of initial arthroscopy. (*D*) Biceps during second arthroscopy with noted tear. (*E*) Biceps during second arthroscopy with erythema along the tendon.

biceps tendinopathy with progression from the previous MRI. A corticosteroid injection is an option for patients if they elect conservative therapy, but the patient elected an open biceps tenodesis. At the time of arthroscopy, there was erythema along the tendon and significant adhesions within the biceps groove (**Fig. 4**D, E). She underwent open subpectoral biceps tenodesis whereby these adhesions had to be released. She went on to have complete resolution of her pain and a return to her activities.

Rotator cuff pathology is also commonly seen with other concomitant pathology. This other pathology often involves the biceps,[36,37] labrum/SLAP (superior labral tear from anterior to posterior) tears,[38–40] and AC joint arthrosis.[41] Often this can be realized before surgery or at the time of surgery, but it can also be missed in these instances. Moreover, additional pathology can develop or become more pronounced in the postoperative period. Although patients recover at different rates based on patient factors and the surgery performed, persistent pain in patients should be explored. Pathology often exists within the shoulder girdle itself, but it is also important to evaluate causes outside the shoulder. Internal derangements can include biceps pathology, labral pathology and possible associated instability, AC arthrosis, subacromial bursitis, and glenohumeral arthrosis as well as postoperative stiffness. In addition to internal derangements of the shoulder, patients can also have persistent pain due to more external causes, such as neuropathic pain. Persistent pain can lead to poor outcomes in patients after rotator cuff repair; in the face of persistent pain, it is important to maintain vigilance for other areas that can be addressed that lead to better outcomes in function as well as subjective patient scoring.

When it comes to addressing concomitant pathology in patients with continued pain, there are many sources that may be contributing to the pain; it is important to be thorough in the assessment of the causes. As mentioned previously, there are causes within the shoulder girdle as well as outside it that may contribute to persistent pain after surgery. In a review looking at painful shoulders after rotator cuff repair,

Williams[42] divided causes of persistent pain into extrinsic and intrinsic causes. Extrinsic causes are primarily related to neuropathic conditions, such as brachial plexopathy, cervical radiculopathy, reflex sympathetic dystrophy or chronic regional pain syndrome, suprascapular neuropathy, and thoracic outlet syndrome as well neoplasms. Cervical radiculopathy most commonly manifests as a fifth or sixth cervical root pathology. Radiographs of the neck may show cervical spondylosis, and MRI and electromyography (EMG) may confirm the diagnosis. Long thoracic and spinal accessory neuropathies that lead to scapular winging, but a true scapular winging diagnosis can be difficult as patients can have scapular dyskinesis during their normal recovery from surgery. EMG can be useful in cases when this is suspected.

Suprascapular neuropathy can also be present in patients preoperatively or postoperatively. It can be associated with paralabral cysts at the suprascapular or spinoglenoid notch as well as massive rotator cuff tears, as retraction of the tendons can cause medialization of the tendons and ultimately traction on the nerve. Some studies have shown improvement in suprascapular neuropathy after surgery, as it can relieve traction on the nerve[43,44]; but Collin and colleagues[45] did not suggest routine decompression of the suprascapular nerve because, based on preoperative EMGs in their study, the incidence of suprascapular neuropathy in massive rotator cuff tears was rare, only 1 out of 49 shoulders. If postoperative neuropathy is suspected, EMG can be helpful; if that is negative or equivocal, a guided anesthetic injection at the suprascapular or spinoglenoid notch can aid the diagnosis. If either of these are positive and patients have not improved, decompression can be performed either arthroscopically or open. Another very rare entity that Williams[42] discusses in his review is the consideration given to a Pancoast tumor (apical lung tumor) that can cause compression or infiltration of the brachial plexus or cervical roots and subsequently persistent pain.

Intrinsic causes of pain were further divided by Williams[42] into intra-articular and extra-articular causes. Extra-articular causes of persistent pain include AC joint arthrosis and subacromial bursitis or impingement. Because AC joint arthrosis develops in most of the population after 30 years of age, and often remains asymptomatic,[46] the utility of distal clavicle resection has been questioned as a routine procedure in all patients. In relation to rotator cuff pathology, it has been thought that it can contribute to impingement on the rotator cuff[41,47]; but there has been movement only to address more symptomatic patients rather than radiographic AC joint arthrosis.[48] Park and colleagues[49] suggests that there may not be utility in addressing it in patients who have symptoms of AC joint arthrosis with concurrent rotator cuff repair. They found no difference at 2 years in patients who were randomized to either isolated rotator cuff repair or rotator cuff repair with distal clavicle excision. Razmjou and colleagues,[50] though, did find that those who did not undergo distal clavicle excision, even with mild arthroscopic findings of arthritis, had lower postoperative scores than those who did undergo excision. The AC joint can be left untreated based on a patient-by-patient basis; but in those patients who have persistent pain after rotator cuff repair, it may be prudent to explore the AC joint as a source of pain with clinical examination and possible intervention, such as an injection or surgery if necessary.

Postoperative subacromial bursitis or impingement can also cause persistent pain. Although decompression with acromioplasty was more prevalently performed, there has been movement toward less of an acromioplasty or no acromioplasty after recent studies have questioned its necessity.[51–53] Still, patients can present with impingement signs after the normal convalescence period. Although revision decompression may not necessarily be warranted, an injection may be beneficial for patients who continue to struggle with impingement symptoms after surgery. Shin and colleagues[54] performed corticosteroid injections in patients who still had severe persistent pain 1 month after rotator cuff repair and found no increase in retear rates.

In terms of intra-articular issues, persistent pain can commonly be caused by biceps pathology or labral pathology, especially SLAP lesions. Whether it is tendinitis, subluxation, dislocation from the groove, or frank tearing, long head biceps tendon pathology is commonly present with rotator cuff tears[36,55,56] and in up to 96% of massive rotator cuff tears.[37] Pathology can be present at the time of surgery and can be missed, especially if most of the intra-articular portion appears relatively benign if the portion in the groove is not pulled into the joint at the time of arthroscopy. Biceps pathology can also develop or become more pronounced postoperatively. Persistent pain in the anterior shoulder after surgery coupled with positive tests like the Yergason and Speed tests can aid the diagnosis; ultrasound-guided biceps sheath injection can also be helpful diagnostically and therapeutically. Anterior shoulder pain after surgery can also be caused by unaddressed SLAP pathology. Similar to biceps pathology, SLAP lesions, especially types I and II tears, are associated with rotator cuff tears.[57] Their symptoms can be similar to biceps lesions but can also be variable; their cause can also coincide with rotator cuff injury mechanisms, such as traction on the arm.[58] MRI can be helpful in diagnosis, but its accuracy in determining pathologic tears from anatomic variants is variable.[59] Nonetheless, SLAP tears should be queried at the time of surgery. If an SLAP tear is noted postoperatively to be causing persistent pain, and patients have failed conservative treatment, there are multiple treatment options. SLAP repair in the older population (older than 40 years) has become less commonly performed, even in isolated lesions, as it can lead to increased stiffness and a higher reoperation rate.[60] Ji and colleagues[60] also found that biceps tenotomy or SLAP debridement was favored over SLAP repair with concurrent rotator cuff repair. Kim and colleagues,[57] likewise, found that those who underwent biceps tenotomy did better than those who underwent SLAP repair with rotator cuff repair. Biceps tenotomy or tenodesis can be performed in those patients with persistent biceps pathology or SLAP pathology, with the decision for either tenotomy or tenodesis depending on a combination of factors, such as cosmesis, age, and demand.

INFECTION
Case Example

A 62-year-old right-hand-dominant man presented to the authors' clinic with left shoulder pain and dysfunction after a mini-open rotator cuff repair 3 months prior. His medical history was notable for congestive heart failure (CHF) and hypertension. After his cuff repair, he was hospitalized for CHF exacerbation. He then noticed redness and warmth over the anterior portal site, which improved with 10 days of cephalexin. The redness then returned with chronic drainage (**Fig. 5**A). His examination was notable for limited range of motion but intact cuff strength. Radiographic imaging showed acromial and humeral head osteolysis concerning for osteomyelitis (**Fig. 5**B). MRI was then obtained, which was suggestive of septic glenohumeral arthritis, AC joint septic arthritis, and recurrent rotator cuff tear (**Fig. 5**C).

Given these findings, the patient was taken for left shoulder irrigation and debridement with placement of an antibiotic hemiarthroplasty spacer. A deltopectoral approach with subscapularis peel was used with excision of the sinus tracts. Glenoid exposure was achieved. A size 12 antibiotic cement spacer (Biomet, Warsaw, Indiana) was then reamed for and placed in the humerus (**Fig. 5**D). The subscapularis was repaired, and a drain was placed. Intraoperative cultures were taken and grew methicillin-susceptible *Staphylococcus aureus*. He was treated with 6 weeks of

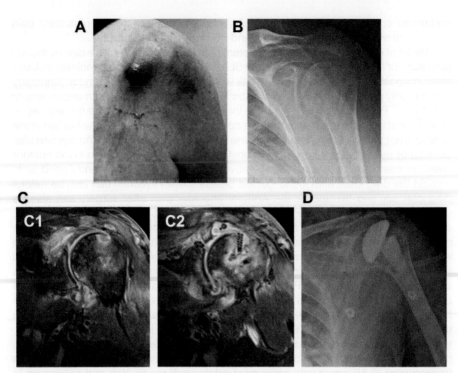

Fig. 5. (*A*) Infection after mini-open rotator cuff. (*B*) AP shoulder radiograph demonstrating humeral head and acromion osteolysis. (*C*) Coronal MRI showing recurrent rotator cuff tear, septic glenohumeral arthritis, and septic AC joint arthritis (*C1*). Note the loose suture anchor and completely detached anchor within the rotator interval (*C2*). (*D*) Implanted hemiarthroplasty with antibiotic cement spacer.

intravenous nafcillin and is to remain in a sling for most of that time. Further follow-up is pending.

Infection in arthroscopic rotator cuff surgery, as well as open or mini-open rotator cuff repair, is a rare entity. But a postoperative infection can have significant morbidity and lead to poorer patient outcomes.[61] Infection rates after open rotator cuff repair have been shown to be relatively low, from 1.9% to less than 1.0%[62]; but arthroscopic repair seems to portend an even lower risk of infection with most studies less than 1.0%.[63] Although infections are rare, there are risk factors that may predispose patients for a higher risk of infection; these risk factors include male sex, age more than 60 years, and surgery length more than 90 minutes.[63] Infections after rotator cuff repair tend to be low grade and tend to present with an insidious onset with pain as the primary complaint; because of this, their diagnosis may be delayed. Therefore, in patients with persistent pain without other likely causes, infection should be considered as a possible cause.

An infection after rotator cuff surgery is rare,; but when it occurs, it can have significant morbidity for patients. Infections rates range from 1.9% to 0.1%.[2,62,64] There are risk factors that may make patients more likely to be affected by infection. These risk factors include male sex, age more than 60 years, and surgery length more than 90 minutes.[63] Although functional outcomes tend to be similar between open and arthroscopic procedures for rotator cuff repairs,[60,65,66] there does seem to be a difference between infection rates between open rotator cuff repair and arthroscopic repair. The infection rate in mini-open repairs ranges from 1.9%[66] to 0.27%.[67] In their retrospective review, Vopat and colleagues[68] suggested that nonarthroscopic surgery was a risk factor for infection after rotator cuff repair. Owens and colleagues[64] also showed similar findings with superficial infection (1.0% vs 0.1%) and deep infection (0.3% vs 0.1%) being significantly greater in the open group than the arthroscopic group. Similarly, Hughes and colleagues[69] showed a greater infection rate in open versus arthroscopic repair, though their rate for open surgery was higher than most reported rates (2.45%). The arthroscopic rate was 0.44%. The most commonly isolated organisms in both arthroscopic and open infections are *Propionibacterium acnes*, *Staphylococcus epidermidis*, and *Staphylococcus aureus*.[63,67,70]

Infections can present insidiously after shoulder surgery, as the most common, but nonspecific, presenting symptom is pain; but in multiple studies on open rotator cuff repair, in addition to pain, other common presenting symptoms were local erythema, wound drainage, and swelling.[61,67,68,70] The average presentation with infection was about 3 to 4 weeks postoperatively in most studies.[67,70,71] Patients often had elevated C-reactive protein (CRP) and erythrocyte sedimentation rate. Although, in Athwal and colleagues,[71] only half had an elevated CRP at presentation; but the average presentation time was more extended at 49 days and may have caused more insidious symptoms. After infection in open rotator cuff repair, most shoulders required more than one debridement, with some studies averaging more than 3 debridements.[61,67] With debridement, most studies left the cuff intact if it was intact with the initial debridement; but most had at least a partial defect, if not complete disruption, at the time of initial debridement. The necrotic material and any loose suture should be removed during debridement; in Kwon and colleagues,[71] loose sutures were debrided but anchors were retained.

Variable outcomes resulted when there was disruption of the rotator cuff at the initial debridement. After the final debridement, Kwon and colleagues[71] had a cuff defect remaining in all patients; Herrera and colleagues[70] were only able to repair about one-third of the complete disruptions. However, in the study by Settecerri and colleagues,[67] about two-thirds of patients either had their initial repair intact after their final debridement or they were able to have rerepair of their defect. Most patients did not have a full return of range of motion, with 110° and 120° of active range of motion in Settecerri and colleagues[67] and Athwal and colleagues,[61] respectively. As may be expected, outcomes after infection tended to be poor, with Settecerri and colleagues[67] reporting only half of patients having a satisfactory outcome and Kwon and colleagues[71] reporting two-thirds of patients were dissatisfied. Those who did have an intact rotator cuff did have better clinical scores.[71]

In arthroscopic rotator cuff infection, pain was the most common symptom; but patients did present with local signs of infection (erythema, swelling, drainage) in two-thirds of patients.[63] Patients who did receive preoperative antibiotics had a significantly lower risk of infection than those who did not. The time to presentation was similar to open surgery, with the average about 29 days. *P acnes* did show a significantly longer time to presentation with 41 days versus 24 days. Most were treated with open debridement (93%) versus arthroscopic debridement, and most (86%) were able to be treated with just one debridement. All anchors and sutures were removed during debridement.

When an infection is encountered, preoperative work-up can include an MRI to look for any pockets that may not be easily visualized during surgery; but it also may be reserved for refractory cases of infection that have not responded to initial debridement. Irrigation and debridement can be undertaken arthroscopically initially, but there should be a low threshold for performing an open debridement for a thorough debridement of necrotic tissue. Eradication of the infection is the most important goal, but trying repair if adequate tissue remains can be attempted. If the cuff becomes irreparable after adequate debridement, and the infection has been eradicated, the patients and surgeon may also elect to undertake arthroplasty to improve function and pain. The risk, though, of periprosthetic infection would presumably be higher in this patient population; the risks and benefits of this should be weighed heavily before undertaking.

SUMMARY

Rotator cuff repair is perhaps the most common shoulder surgery performed today. Despite advances in technique, complications are not infrequent and continue to limit the success of this procedure. There are many patient and technical factors that increase the risk for retear or failure to heal. Most of the time, revision repair can be performed for smaller retears. Larger-sized retears may require allograft augmentation or even reverse total shoulder arthroplasty. Stiffness is perhaps the most common complication after rotator cuff repair. If therapy fails to improve motion, lysis of adhesions and manipulation under anesthesia has been successful.

In those patients with persistent pain after rotator cuff repair, it is important to rule out other pain generators that may exist, including causes extrinsic and intrinsic to the shoulder, including neuropathy, AC joint arthrosis, and biceps pathology. Infection can also be a cause of persistent pain and rotator cuff failure. Although infections are rare, they can lead to significant morbidity for patients and expectedly poorer outcomes.

REFERENCES

1. McElvany MD, McGoldrick E, Gee AO, et al. Rotator cuff repair: published evidence on factors associated with repair integrity and clinical outcome. Am J Sports Med 2015;43(2):491–500.
2. Randelli P, Spennacchio P, Ragone V, et al. Complications associated with arthroscopic rotator cuff repair: a literature review. Musculoskelet Surg 2012;96(1): 9–16.
3. Galatz LM, Ball CM, Teefey SA, et al. The outcome and repair integrity of completely arthroscopically repaired large and massive rotator cuff tears. J Bone Joint Surg Am 2004;86-A(2):219–24.
4. Lafosse L, Brozska R, Toussaint B, et al. The outcome and structural integrity of arthroscopic rotator cuff repair with use of the double-row suture anchor technique. J Bone Joint Surg Am 2007;89(7):1533–41.
5. Le BTN, Wu XL, Lam PH, et al. Factors predicting rotator cuff retears: an analysis of 1000 consecutive rotator cuff repairs. Am J Sports Med 2014;42(5):1134–42.
6. Harryman DT, Mack LA, Wang KY, et al. Repairs of the rotator cuff. Correlation of functional results with integrity of the cuff. J Bone Joint Surg Am 1991;73(7): 982–9.
7. Klepps S, Bishop J, Lin J, et al. Prospective evaluation of the effect of rotator cuff integrity on the outcome of open rotator cuff repairs. Am J Sports Med 2004; 32(7):1716–22.
8. Kim HM, Caldwell J-ME, Buza JA, et al. Factors affecting satisfaction and shoulder function in patients with a recurrent rotator cuff tear. J Bone Joint Surg Am 2014;96(2):106–12.

9. Park MC, Cadet ER, Levine WN, et al. Tendon-to-bone pressure distributions at a repaired rotator cuff footprint using transosseous suture and suture anchor fixation techniques. Am J Sports Med 2005;33(8):1154–9.

10. Park MC, ElAttrache NS, Ahmad CS, et al. "Transosseous-equivalent" rotator cuff repair technique. Arthroscopy 2006;22(12):1360.e1–5.

11. Cole BJ, ElAttrache NS, Anbari A. Arthroscopic rotator cuff repairs: an anatomic and biomechanical rationale for different suture-anchor repair configurations. Arthroscopy 2007;23(6):662–9.

12. Hein J, Reilly JM, Chae J, et al. Retear rates after arthroscopic single-row, double-row, and suture bridge rotator cuff repair at a minimum of 1 year of imaging follow-up: a systematic review. Arthroscopy 2015;31(11):2274–81.

13. Virk MS, Bruce B, Hussey KE, et al. Biomechanical performance of medial row suture placement relative to the musculotendinous junction in transosseous equivalent suture bridge double-row rotator cuff repair. Arthroscopy 2017;33(2): 242–50.

14. Montanez A, Makarewich CA, Burks RT, et al. The medial stitch in transosseous-equivalent rotator cuff repair: vertical or horizontal mattress? Am J Sports Med 2016;44(9):2225–30.

15. Smith GCS, Bouwmeester TM, Lam PH. Knotless double-row SutureBridge rotator cuff repairs have improved self-reinforcement compared with double-row SutureBridge repairs with tied medial knots: a biomechanical study using an ovine model. J Shoulder Elbow Surg 2017;26(12):2206–12.

16. Barber FA, Herbert MA. Cyclic loading biomechanical analysis of the pullout strengths of rotator cuff and glenoid anchors: 2013 update. Arthroscopy 2013; 29(5):832–44.

17. Tingart MJ, Apreleva M, Zurakowski D, et al. Pullout strength of suture anchors used in rotator cuff repair. J Bone Joint Surg Am 2003;85-A(11):2190–8.

18. Cummins CA, Murrell GAC. Mode of failure for rotator cuff repair with suture anchors identified at revision surgery. J Shoulder Elbow Surg 2003;12(2):128–33.

19. Cho NS, Yi JW, Lee BG, et al. Retear patterns after arthroscopic rotator cuff repair: single-row versus suture bridge technique. Am J Sports Med 2010; 38(4):664–71.

20. Kim KC, Shin HD, Cha SM, et al. Comparisons of retear patterns for 3 arthroscopic rotator cuff repair methods. Am J Sports Med 2014;42(3):558–65.

21. Zheng N, Harris HW, Andrews JR. Failure analysis of rotator cuff repair: a comparison of three double-row techniques. J Bone Joint Surg Am 2008;90(5):1034–42.

22. Miller BS, Downie BK, Kohen RB, et al. When do rotator cuff repairs fail? Serial ultrasound examination after arthroscopic repair of large and massive rotator cuff tears. Am J Sports Med 2011;39(10):2064–70.

23. Kim JH, Hong IT, Ryu KJ, et al. Retear rate in the late postoperative period after arthroscopic rotator cuff repair. Am J Sports Med 2014;42(11):2606–13.

24. Kluger R, Bock P, Mittlböck M, et al. Long-term survivorship of rotator cuff repairs using ultrasound and magnetic resonance imaging analysis. Am J Sports Med 2011;39(10):2071–81.

25. Ferguson DP, Lewington MR, Smith TD, et al. Graft utilization in the augmentation of large-to-massive rotator cuff repairs: a systematic review. Am J Sports Med 2016;44(11):2984–92.

26. Boileau P, Brassart N, Watkinson DJ, et al. Arthroscopic repair of full-thickness tears of the supraspinatus: does the tendon really heal? J Bone Joint Surg Am 2005;87(6):1229–40.

27. Charousset C, Duranthon LD, Grimberg J, et al. [Arthro-C-scan analysis of rotator cuff tears healing after arthroscopic repair: analysis of predictive factors in a consecutive series of 167 arthroscopic repairs]. Rev Chir Orthop Reparatrice Appar Mot 2006;92(3):223–33.

28. Mall NA, Tanaka MJ, Choi LS, et al. Factors affecting rotator cuff healing. J Bone Joint Surg Am 2014;96(9):778–88.

29. Chan K, MacDermid JC, Hoppe DJ, et al. Delayed versus early motion after arthroscopic rotator cuff repair: a meta-analysis. J Shoulder Elbow Surg 2014; 23(11):1631–9.

30. Huberty DP, Schoolfield JD, Brady PC, et al. Incidence and treatment of postoperative stiffness following arthroscopic rotator cuff repair. Arthroscopy 2009;25(8): 880–90.

31. Chung SW, Huong CB, Kim SH, et al. Shoulder stiffness after rotator cuff repair: risk factors and Influence on outcome. Arthrosc J Arthrosc Relat Surg 2013;29(2): 290–300.

32. McNamara WJ, Lam PH, Murrell GAC. The relationship between shoulder stiffness and rotator cuff healing: a study of 1,533 consecutive arthroscopic rotator cuff repairs. J Bone Joint Surg Am 2016;98(22):1879–80.

33. Thigpen CA, Shaffer MA, Gaunt BW, et al. The American Society of Shoulder and Elbow Therapists' consensus statement on rehabilitation following arthroscopic rotator cuff repair. J Shoulder Elbow Surg 2016;25(4):521–35.

34. Denard PJ, Lädermann A, Burkhart SS. Prevention and management of stiffness after arthroscopic rotator cuff repair: systematic review and implications for rotator cuff healing. Arthroscopy 2011;27(6):842–8.

35. Koo SS, Parsley BK, Burkhart SS, et al. Reduction of postoperative stiffness after arthroscopic rotator cuff repair: results of a customized physical therapy regimen based on risk factors for stiffness. Arthroscopy 2011;27(2):155–60.

36. Redondo-Alonso L, Chamorro-Moriana G, Jiménez-Rejano JJ, et al. Relationship between chronic pathologies of the supraspinatus tendon and the long head of the biceps tendon: systematic review. BMC Musculoskelet Disord 2014;15:377.

37. Chen C-H, Hsu K-Y, Chen W-J, et al. Incidence and severity of biceps long head tendon lesion in patients with complete rotator cuff tears. J Trauma 2005;58: 1189–93.

38. Seo J-B, Yoo J-S, Lee J-Y, et al. What are the anatomical predictive factors of degenerative superior labrum anterior to posterior lesion in rotator cuff tear? J Orthop 2017;14:425–9.

39. Kim S-J, Lee I-S, Kim S-H, et al. Arthroscopic repair of concomitant type II SLAP lesions in large to massive rotator cuff tears: comparison with biceps tenotomy. Am J Sports Med 2012;40:2786–93.

40. Oh JH, Lee YH, Kim SH. Comparison of treatments for superior labrum-biceps complex lesions with concomitant rotator cuff repair: a prospective, randomized, comparative analysis of debridement, biceps tenotomy, and biceps tenodesis. Arthroscopy 2016;32:958–67.

41. Cuomo F, Kummer FJ, Zuckerman JD, et al. The influence of acromioclavicular joint morphology on rotator cuff tears. J Shoulder Elbow Surg 1998;7:555–9.

42. Williams GR Jr. Painful shoulder after surgery for rotator cuff disease. J Am Acad Orthop Surg 1997;5:97–108.

43. Mallon WJ, Wilson RJ, Basamania CJ. The association of suprascapular neuropathy with massive rotator cuff tears: a preliminary report. J Shoulder Elbow Surg 2006;15:395–8.

44. Costouros JG, Porramatikul M, Lie DT, et al. Reversal of suprascapular neuropathy following arthroscopic repair of massive supraspinatus and infraspinatus rotator cuff tears. Arthroscopy 2007;23:1152–61.
45. Collin P, Treseder T, Lädermann A. Neuropathy of the suprascapular nerve and massive rotator cuff tears: a prospective electromyographic study. J Shoulder Elbow Surg 2014;23:28–34.
46. Stein BE, Wiater JM, Pfaff HC, et al. Detection of acromioclavicular joint pathology in asymptomatic shoulders with magnetic resonance imaging. J Shoulder Elbow Surg 2001;10:204–8.
47. Petersson CJ, Gentz CF. Ruptures of the supraspinatus tendon. The significance of distally pointing acromioclavicular osteophytes. Clin Orthop Relat Res 1983;(174):143–8.
48. Oh JH, Kim JY, Choi JH, et al. Is arthroscopic distal clavicle resection necessary for patients with radiological acromioclavicular joint arthritis and rotator cuff tears? A prospective randomized comparative study. Am J Sports Med 2014; 42:2567–73.
49. Park YB, Koh KH, Shon MS, et al. Arthroscopic distal clavicle resection in symptomatic acromioclavicular joint arthritis combined with rotator cuff tear: a prospective randomized trial. Am J Sports Med 2015;43:985–90.
50. Razmjou H, ElMaraghy A, Dwyer T, et al. Outcome of distal clavicle resection in patients with acromioclavicular joint osteoarthritis and full-thickness rotator cuff tear. Knee Surg Sports Traumatol Arthrosc 2015;23:585–90.
51. MacDonald P, McRae S, Leiter J, et al. Arthroscopic rotator cuff repair with and without acromioplasty in the treatment of full-thickness rotator cuff tears: a multicenter, randomized controlled trial. J Bone Joint Surg Am 2011;93:1953–60.
52. Abrams GD, Gupta AK, Hussey KE. Arthroscopic repair of full-thickness rotator cuff tears with and without acromioplasty: randomized prospective trial with 2-year follow-up. Am J Sports Med 2014;42:1296–303.
53. Shin S-J, Oh JH, Chung SW, et al. The efficacy of acromioplasty in the arthroscopic repair of small- to medium-sized rotator cuff tears without acromial spur: prospective comparative study. Arthroscopy 2012;28:628–35.
54. Shin S-J, Do N-H, Lee J, et al. Efficacy of a subacromial corticosteroid injection for persistent pain after arthroscopic rotator cuff repair. Am J Sports Med 2016; 44:2231–6.
55. Beall DP, Williamson EE, Ly JQ. Association of biceps tendon tears with rotator cuff abnormalities: degree of correlation with tears of the anterior and superior portions of the rotator cuff. AJR Am J Roentgenol 2003;180:633–9.
56. Koh KH, Ahn JH, Kim SM, et al. Treatment of biceps tendon lesions in the setting of rotator cuff tears: prospective cohort study of tenotomy versus tenodesis. Am J Sports Med 2010;38:1584–90.
57. Kim TK, Queale WS, Cosgarea AJ, et al. Clinical features of the different types of SLAP lesions: an analysis of one hundred and thirty-nine cases. J Bone Joint Surg Am 2003;85-A(1):66–71.
58. Strauss EJ, McCormack RA, Onyekwelu I, et al. Management of failed arthroscopic rotator cuff repair. J Am Acad Orthop Surg 2012;20(5):301–9.
59. Keener JD, Brophy RH. Superior labral tears of the shoulder: pathogenesis, evaluation, and treatment. J Am Acad Orthop Surg 2009;17:627–37.
60. Ji X, Bi C, Wang F, et al. Arthroscopic versus mini-open rotator cuff repair: an up-to-date meta-analysis of randomized controlled trials. Arthroscopy 2015;31: 118–24.

61. Athwal GS, Sperling JW, Rispoli DM, et al. Deep infection after rotator cuff repair. J Shoulder Elbow Surg 2007;16:306–11.
62. Mirzayan R, Itamura JM, Vangsness CT, et al. Management of chronic deep infection following rotator cuff repair. J Bone Joint Surg Am 2000;82-A(8):1115–21.
63. Pauzenberger L, Grieb A, Hexel M, et al. Infections following arthroscopic rotator cuff repair: incidence, risk factors, and prophylaxis. Knee Surg Sports Traumatol Arthrosc 2017;25:595–601.
64. Owens BD, Williams AE, Wolf JM. Risk factors for surgical complications in rotator cuff repair in a veteran population. J Shoulder Elbow Surg 2015;24:1707–12.
65. Morse K, Davis AD, Afra R, et al. Arthroscopic versus mini-open rotator cuff repair: a comprehensive review and meta-analysis. Am J Sports Med 2008;36:1824–8.
66. Nho SJ, Shindle MK, Sherman SL, et al. Systematic review of arthroscopic rotator cuff repair and mini-open rotator cuff repair. J Bone Joint Surg Am 2007;89(Suppl 3):127–36.
67. Settecerri JJ, Pitner MA, Rock MG, et al. Infection after rotator cuff repair. J Shoulder Elbow Surg 1999;8:1–5.
68. Vopat BG, Lee BJ, DeStefano S. Risk factors for infection after rotator cuff repair. Arthroscopy 2016;32:428–34.
69. Hughes JD, Hughes JL, Bartley JH, et al. Infection rates in arthroscopic versus open rotator cuff repair. Orthop J Sports Med 2017;(5):2325967117715416.
70. Herrera MF, Bauer G, Reynolds F, et al. Infection after mini-open rotator cuff repair. J Shoulder Elbow Surg 2002;11:605–8.
71. Kwon YW, Kalainov DM, Rose HA, et al. Management of early deep infection after rotator cuff repair surgery. J Shoulder Elbow Surg 2005;14:1–5.

Shoulder Acromioclavicular and Coracoclavicular Ligament Injuries
Common Problems and Solutions

James D. Wylie, MD, MHS[a], Jeremiah D. Johnson, MD[b],
Jessica DiVenere, BS[b], Augustus D. Mazzocca, MD, MS[b],*

KEYWORDS

- Coracoclavicular ligaments • Reconstruction • Repair • Weaver-Dunn
- Acromioclavicular ligaments • Acromioclavicular joint • Complications • Problems

KEY POINTS

- Acromioclavicular and coracoclavicular repair and/or reconstructions have high complication rates, even in expert hands.
- Anatomic placement of repair or reconstruction grafts or devices may help to prevent many of the common problems encountered.
- Most common problems and complications have revision or salvage treatment options.

INTRODUCTION

Acromioclavicular (AC) joint and coracoclavicular (CC) ligament injuries are common in active individuals and commonly occur with a fall on the affected acromion with the shoulder in an adducted position.[1] AC joint injuries are most commonly graded based on the Rockwood classification.[2] Treatment of grade I and II injuries involves nonoperative management and progressive return to activities.[3] Most orthopedists agree that treatment of grade IV, V, and VI injuries generally require surgical intervention, either in the acute setting or after continued pain and dysfunction after attempted nonoperative management.[3] The treatment of grade III injuries is

Disclosure Statement: Dr J.D. Wylie has received research funding from Arthrex, Inc. Dr A.D. Mazzocca receives research funding and is a paid consultant for Arthrex, Inc, and is a paid consultant for Orthofix, Inc. J. DiVenere and Dr J.D. Johnson have nothing to disclose.
[a] Department of Orthopedic Surgery, Boston Children's Hospital, 300 Longwood Avenue, Boston, MA 02115, USA; [b] Department of Orthopedic Surgery, University of Connecticut, 263 Farmington Avenue, Farmington, CT 06030, USA
* Corresponding author.
E-mail address: mazzocca@uchc.edu

Clin Sports Med 37 (2018) 197–207
https://doi.org/10.1016/j.csm.2017.12.002
0278-5919/18/© 2018 Elsevier Inc. All rights reserved.

sportsmed.theclinics.com

more controversial, with some providers advocating for operative and some for nonoperative management.[3]

In the higher grade injuries, the goals of surgical treatment include anatomic reduction of the clavicle in relation to the scapula and recreation of proper scapulothoracic biomechanics.[4] This procedure can be performed in either the acute or the chronic setting. More commonly, reconstructions with tendon grafts are performed in the chronic setting, whereas repairs are performed acutely.[4] Historical and contemporary surgical options fall into 4 different groups:

- Primary AC and CC repair and fixation;
- The Weaver-Dunn procedure;
- Anatomic CC reconstruction; and
- Arthroscopic reconstruction techniques.

PROBLEMS ENCOUNTERED IN ACROMIOCLAVICULAR JOINT AND CORACOCLAVICULAR LIGAMENTS REPAIR AND RECONSTRUCTION TECHNIQUES

A recent database study showed an 11% reoperation rate in the first 6 months after undergoing AC joint reconstruction.[5] This study investigated reoperations after AC joint surgery by Current Procedural Terminology codes and, therefore, was unable to discern the technique used. The investigators reported the following revision surgery rates in 2106 patients: 2.8% irrigation and debridement, 1.3% manipulation under anesthesia, 4.2% revision reconstruction, 2.8% distal clavicle excision, and 6.2% removal of hardware.[5] Common problems and complications included clavicle and coracoid fractures, loss of fixation or graft failure, hardware irritation, wound healing problems and infection, adhesive capsulitis of the shoulder, and subacromial impingement.[5–7] The specific complications encountered are related to the technique and fixation construct chosen.

First-Generation Fixation and Reconstruction Options

Older fixation and repair constructs included cerclage wire around the clavicle and the coracoid, a lag screw (Bosworth screw) from the clavicle to the coracoid, and screws, or pins across the AC joint from the acromial side. Initial reports on these procedures demonstrated good clinical outcomes.[8] More recently, the biomechanical fixation properties of these constructs have been questioned,[9] and the potential for pin migration into the thoracic cavity or spinal canal has made pin fixation less popular in clinical use.[10,11] Problems encountered with these fixation methods included fracture, hardware breakage, loss of reduction, and, in the setting of pins, could lead to pin migration in the chest with potentially devastating complications. We do not currently perform these procedures; however, if these fixation techniques are attempted, then frequent radiographic follow-up and hardware removal is encouraged to prevent hardware breakage and/or migration.

The Weaver-Dunn procedure involved detachment of the coracoacromial ligament from the acromion and fixation to the clavicle with a distal clavicle resection.[12] Similar to the older repair constructs, initial reports portrayed good clinical outcomes.[12] However, further follow-up was fraught with loss of reduction and continued patient pain and shoulder dysfunction.[13] Both clinical comparative studies[13–15] and biomechanical studies revealed inferiority in comparison with the anatomic CC reconstruction.[16] Failure of the Weaver-Dunn procedure can be rectified with revision using an anatomic CC reconstruction technique (**Fig. 1**).

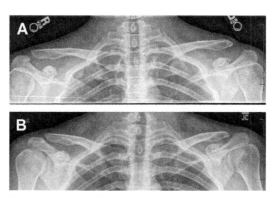

Fig. 1. A 22-year-old male college golfer who sustained a left type III acromioclavicular joint separation 4 years prior presented after undergoing treatment at an outside hospital. He was initially treated nonoperatively, but after 1 year of ongoing pain he underwent an arthroscopic subacromial decompression and distal clavicle excision. His symptoms did not resolve and a Weaver-Dunn procedure was performed. He did well afterward and returned to golfing, but unfortunately his pain returned, impeding his ability to play golf. On examination, he had pain with instability and radiographs after his failed Weaver-Dunn revision had an increased coracoclavicular (CC) distance (*A*). He underwent an anatomic CC reconstruction (*B*) and did well postoperatively.

Anatomic Coracoclavicular Reconstruction

Given the poor patient-reported outcomes and biomechanical inferiority of historical techniques, we recommend performing AC and CC operations using anatomic CC reconstructions or arthroscopic assisted reconstruction techniques.[4,17] These anatomic reconstructions with biologic grafts have gained significant popularity over the last 2 decades. Overall, most studies describe good to excellent patient-reported outcomes.[14,17–19] Arthroscopic or arthroscopic-assisted reconstruction techniques with biologic grafts show similar improvements in patient reported outcome measures to their open counterparts.[20,21] The exception to this rule is the GraftRope system (Arthrex, Naples, FL), which has been plagued by reports of early failures.[21–23] Despite improvement in patient-reported symptoms, complication and reoperation rates are still higher than desired for most fixation and reconstruction constructs. In the chronic setting, complications have been reported in between 27% and 52% of cases.[6,7] Patients who experience complications demonstrate lower satisfaction with their surgery and in some series lower shoulder-specific scores.[7,24]

In anatomic CC ligament reconstructions, clavicular and coracoid bone tunnels lead to a risk of fracture in both of these locations. Reported rates of clavicle fracture have ranged up to 18% in patients with tunnels drilled in the clavicle.[6,7] In patients with coracoid tunnel drilling, fracture rates have been reported in up to 20%.[6] Similarly, suture button constructs in the acute and chronic setting are at risk for clavicle and coracoid fractures owing to tunnel drilling.[25] Loss of fixation and graft failure outside of fracture includes loss of fixation owing to suture button failure, interference screw failure, graft rupture, or graft elongation leading to loss of reduction. Using a single strand construct with 1 clavicle and coracoid tunnel, Milewski and colleagues[6] reported a 50% loss of reduction rate and concomitantly reported a much lower rate with a double clavicular tunnel and coracoid loop technique (6% loss of reduction). Similarly, Martetschlager and colleagues[7] reported a 9% graft failure rate in patients undergoing reconstruction with a tendon graft looped around the coracoid with 2 bone tunnels in the clavicle. Spencer and colleagues[13] examined the radiographic failure rate in patients undergoing CC reconstruction and found a 47% failure rate with clavicle and coracoid tunnels, a 22% failure with looped coracoid fixation, and a 5% failure rate if allograft reconstruction was combined with suture buttons in a load-sharing construct.

Given the minimal soft tissue envelope over the clavicle, a meticulous dissection with open techniques is needed to avoid wound complications. Postoperative surgical site infections can have devastating complications. Infections have been reported in 4% to 6% of CC reconstructions.[6,19] Adhesive capsulitis of the shoulder has been described in multiple techniques for CC reconstruction, and this likely is due to prolonged immobilization postoperatively to protect graft healing. Spencer and colleagues[13] reported 2 out of 206 patients undergoing manipulation under anesthesia for shoulder stiffness. Similarly, Martetschlager and colleagues[7] and Milewski and colleagues[6] reported adhesive capsulitis in 1 of 59 and 1 of 27 cases, respectively. Patients' stiffness resolved with either aggressive physical therapy and/or manipulation under anesthesia.

Acute Reduction and Fixation Constructs

In the acute setting, fixation with hook plates or suture button devices reduce the joint and theoretically allow healing of the native ligaments.[17,26] The strength of these fixation constructs are similar to the native ligaments and function as an internal splint while the native tissues heal in the appropriate position.[27] These acute fixation techniques have evolved to primarily involve single or double suture button constructs and hook plates. Biomechanically, double suture button constructs provide the best suture construct compared with the intact CC ligaments.[27,28]

Good to excellent patient-reported outcomes are reported with acute repair using double suture buttons and hook plates.[29,30] A recent metaanalysis revealed patient-reported outcomes were better when suture or suspensory devices were used, but these patients were at a greater risk of developing a complication compared with those who received hook plates.[31] The complications reported included wound problems, loss of reduction, implant migration, and osteolysis.[31] However, it is important to note that these injuries need to be recognized and treated expeditiously to take advantage of the biologic healing window and thus allow acute repair to be a viable treatment option. The biologic window of repair explains why the hook plate construct has led to worse outcomes when used in the chronic setting.[32] Similar to reconstruction in the chronic setting, there is a high degree of complications and loss of reduction when injuries are treated acutely.[33]

Suture button techniques have a complication rate ranging from 20% to 44%.[25,34] These complications includes infection, hardware migration, clavicle fracture, coracoid fracture, and hardware irritation.[25,34] Hook plate fixation holds the reduction in place, but 12% of patients lose reduction after plate removal.[30] The hook plate has unique complications, given that part of the plate resides in the subacromial space. Lin and colleagues[35] reported that 15 of 40 patients had subacromial impingement after plate fixation and 6 patients were noted to have partial or full-thickness rotator cuff tears. The impingement patients had poorer patient-reported outcomes compared with those without impingement. In addition, 50% of patients had some degree of acromial erosion caused by hook pressure.[35] Owing to these hardware complications, most surgeons advocate for hook plate removal after soft tissue healing. Therefore, choosing this treatment option necessitates a second operative procedure for hardware removal. A recent randomized study showed no difference in quality of life comparing acute hook plate fixation with nonoperative treatment of complete AC joint dislocations, questioning the need for acute repair versus waiting for chronic reconstruction of symptomatic patients.

PREVENTION AND TREATMENT STRATEGIES FOR COMMON PROBLEMS
Clavicle Fracture

Clavicle fracture has been reported with multiple techniques of AC repair and reconstruction. Any technique involving drilling the clavicle increases the risk of fracture. This applies to anatomic ligament reconstructions and suture button repair constructs. Spiegl and colleagues[36] also found smaller drill holes in the clavicle create a higher load to failure and therefore a lower fracture risk. Many authors advocate for placing the smallest possible drill holes in the clavicle in an effort to prevent clavicle fractures postoperatively. The clavicle bone mineral density is lowest at the most lateral aspect of the clavicle and, therefore, we advocate for anatomically placed clavicular tunnels at 25 and 45 mm from the distal aspect of the clavicle.[37] A biomechanical evaluation by Geaney and colleagues[37] found more laterally based tunnels had a lower load to failure owing to weaker bone in the lateral clavicle. Therefore, more laterally based tunnels will be at greater risk of fracture owing to the lower bone mineral density. We use a 5.0-mm drill followed by a 5.5-mm tap and placement of a 5.5-mm tenodesis screws for graft fixation after passage.

Clavicle fractures after reconstruction can commonly be treated with nonoperative treatment if there is minimal displacement (**Fig. 2**).[11] In the setting of marked displacement, open reduction and internal fixation with plate fixation may be advantageous. If the fracture is lateral and involves the loss of reduction of the AC joint, then hook plating can be another option for fixation of these fractures and reduction of the AC joint.

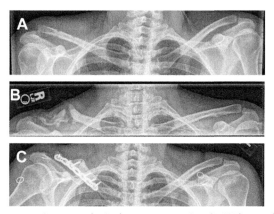

Fig. 2. Case of an anatomic coracoclavicular reconstruction (ACCR) complicated by a postoperative clavicle fracture through the medial tunnel. Patient is a 44-year-old woman with a grade III acromioclavicular (AC) separation who underwent reconstruction. Postoperative radiograph (A) shows a well-positioned ACCR. Four months postoperatively, she had acute pain in the clavicle that was treated nonoperatively by an outside physician. She presented at 1 year postoperatively with a hypertrophic nonunion at the medial tunnel (B). She elected to undergo revision with a clavicle open reduction and internal fixation with autologous iliac crest bone grafting, and has resolution of her symptoms after healing (C).

Coracoid Fracture

Coracoid fractures follow similar principles to clavicle fractures. They occur after tunnel placement in the coracoid. There have been multiple reports of coracoid fractures after treatment with ligamentous or suture button reconstruction.[6,38] Similar to clavicle fractures, the risk seems to depend on size of tunnel and location of the tunnel within the coracoid. Ferreira and colleagues[39] investigated this phenomenon biomechanically and found a 6-mm drill tunnel had a variable fracture risk based on its orientation. The tunnel placed in a superior to inferior direction was best oriented from a center to the center or medial to the center of the coracoid to avoid clavicle fracture in mechanical testing. These constructs failed through suture failure rather than coracoid fracture. Trajectories violating the lateral coracoid or directed from the center of the superior aspect of the coracoid through the medial aspect of the inferior coracoid failed by coracoid fracture.[39]

Using smaller dill holes, drilling in the trajectory as noted, or using looped tendon grafts around the base of the coracoid help to prevent this complication. Multiple studies comparing coracoid tunnels with looped grafts have demonstrated coracoid fractures only occurred when a coracoid tunnel was placed.[6,40] After a coracoid fracture is diagnosed, there are multiple treatment options. These include nonoperative treatment if nondisplaced and asymptomatic. In the symptomatic displaced coracoid fracture, a tunnel can be placed in the scapula at the base of the coracoid. This tunnel is used to place a looped tendon graft through the scapula.[11,38]

Fixation or Graft Failure

In addition to patients who fracture their coracoid or clavicle, many patients experience fixation or graft failure. These instances likely account for the majority of the patients with radiographic failure of their repairs or reconstructions. Fixation or graft failure may be due to many different reasons. In the setting of suture button fixation, radiographic studies have reported button failure into the tunnel on both the coracoid and clavicle sides.[7,34,40] Failure on the coracoid side is more commonly reported. Coracoid button failure can potentially be prevented with arthroscopic assistance because this technique allows the button to be visualized on the inferior cortex of the clavicle. In addition to button failure, suture button devices can fail at the suture's midsubstance. Bracing the patient with a Lerman shoulder orthosis in the healing phase postoperatively to stress shield the suture construct while the ligament heals may help to prevent this injury.[41] Tendon grafts are commonly fixed with interference screws on the clavicle or tied over the top of a bone bridge.[19] The senior author has experienced graft fixation failure most commonly at the lateral interference screw (**Fig. 3**). This failure may be owing to the lower bone density on the more lateral aspect of the clavicle.[37] In most reported series, graft reconstructions are performed with allograft tissue.[6,13,19] In addition, most failures of fixation with graft reconstruction happen within the first 6 weeks after surgery.[13] For this reason, we advocate for Lerman shoulder orthosis fixation for 6 weeks after reconstruction to support the arm and allow graft healing during the early healing phase and when the graft is weakest.[41]

After graft or fixation failure with loss of reduction of the AC joint, a discussion with the patient is necessary to understand their motivation for undergoing revision surgery. If the patient is asymptomatic and the loss of reduction is purely a radiographic finding in follow-up, then they can be observed to see if symptoms develop. In the setting of symptomatic failure, revision reconstruction is likely needed to alleviate symptoms. Cortical button constructs may have failed owing to poor intrinsic healing of the ligaments, so revision with a tendon graft may be needed to provide a biologic

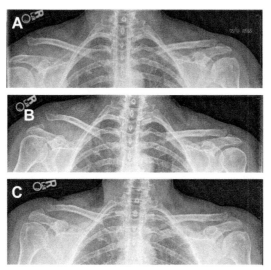

Fig. 3. A 56-year-old woman who sustained a traumatic grade III acromioclavicular separation after falling down stairs (*A*). She failed nonoperative management and elected to undergo an anatomic coracoclavicular reconstruction with 5.5 × 8.0-mm PEEK screws and a semitendinosus allograft. Unfortunately, 2 weeks after surgery she reports a "pop" while trying to wash her hair in the shower and was noted to have loss of reduction on physical examination and radiographs (*B*). During her revision surgery, the lateral screw seemed to have loosened with slippage of the graft through the tunnel. The medial screw was intact. Both screws were revised with 7.0 × 10.0-mm bioabsorbable screws and a new semitendinosus allograft (*C*). The patient did well postoperatively and was able to return to swimming with minimal pain.

graft for healing. With cortical button pull-out in the coracoid, placement of a suture anchor in the coracoid can be used to revise this construct.[11]

Surgical Site Infection

Given the subcutaneous nature of the clavicle and its minimal soft tissue envelope, large reconstructive surgery in this area can be complicated by postoperative infection. Therefore, meticulous surgical dissection with full-thickness skin flaps must be created and a thorough layered closure must be performed to aid in wound healing. In addition, full-thickness flaps both anteriorly and posteriorly of the deep facial tissue of the clavicle is important to allow for a secure layered fascial closure. Infection rates have ranged from 3% to 6% with open reconstruction[6,19,40] and may be lower in less invasive arthroscopically assisted fixation techniques.[21,29,34]

Infections can be divided into superficial and deep, or simple and complicated. Superficial or simple infections can generally be treated with oral antibiotics and observation. Deep or complicated infections generally require surgical treatment, including debridement and removal of hardware and graft tissue. In the setting of deep infection, revision with irrigation and debridement and graft or hardware removal can be performed with primary closure and possible future revision if symptomatic. If tissue debridement in the area of the clavicle is extensive, then the need for free tissue transfer for coverage of the bone is sometimes necessary. In this situation, a latissumus dorsi free tissue transfer can be used to salvage the situation (**Fig. 4**), and sometimes combined with revision ligament reconstruction.

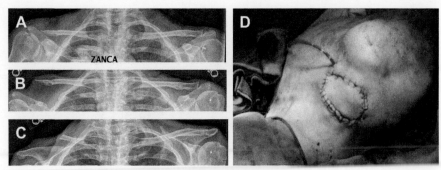

Fig. 4. This 59-year-old woman had a grade V acromioclavicular joint separation 15 years prior treated by an outside physician with distal clavicle excision with chronic pain. She underwent anatomic coracoclavicular reconstruction (*A*) and presented at 6 weeks with concern for deep infection and underwent irrigation and debridement (I & D) with treatment with antibiotics. She did well until 8 months postoperatively, when she developed worsening pain (*B*) and underwent repeat I & D with graft and screw removal and repeat antibiotic treatment. At 10 months postoperatively, she developed a draining sinus and underwent extensive debridement and latissimus dorsi tissue transfer and proceeded to heal her wound (*C, D*).

SUMMARY

AC and CC repair and reconstruction techniques are fraught with problems and complications. The specific complications are linked to the technique and construct used. Operative treatment of acute complete AC dislocations is controversial but may allow for more of a biologic healing response than in the chronic setting where reconstruction with graft tissue is more commonly performed owing to the lack of intrinsic healing potential. Commonly encountered complications include clavicle and coracoid fractures that can be minimized by appropriate tunnel placement and minimizing tunnel

---

Box 1
Clinical pearls on operatively treating symptomatic complete acromioclavicular joint dislocations

- For anatomic coracoclavicular joint reconstruction, keep the lateral clavicular tunnel at least 20 mm from the lateral cortex of the clavicle.
- Increase stability by reconstructing acromioclavicular ligaments, especially in patients with scapular dyskinesia.
- Do not perform a distal clavicle excision, because this increases the instability of the acromioclavicular joint, especially in the horizontal plane.
- Make sure the acromioclavicular joint is reduced anatomically and all the slack is removed from the graft or fixation device. Cycling the graft until taught can accomplish this.
- Ream 5 mm for clavicular and coracoid tunnels to minimize the stress riser.
- For arthroscopic procedures, ream more medial and central through the coracoid process.
- Tap bone tunnels and use PEEK screws in the clavicle.
- Brace and unload the reconstruction for 6 weeks to protect the allograft during the healing phase.
- The bailout procedure for a fractured coracoid is drilling through the scapula at the coracoid base.

diameter. Symptomatic loss of reduction can be due to graft, fixation, or device failure, and is best treated with revision anatomic reconstruction. Techniques and indications continue to evolve owing to high complication rates and less than optimal patient outcomes. **Box 1** contains clinical pearls from the senior authors' practice based on their experience with treating the symptomatic complete AC joint dislocation.

REFERENCES

1. Li X, Ma R, Bedi A, et al. Management of acromioclavicular joint injuries. J Bone Joint Surg Am 2014;96(1):73–84.
2. Rockwood CJ. Injuries to the acromioclavicular joint. In: Rockwood CJ, Green DP, Wilkins KE, et al, editors. Fractures in adults, vol. 1, 2nd edition. Philadelphia: JB Lippincott; 1984. p. 806–10.
3. Simovitch R, Sanders B, Ozbaydar M, et al. Acromioclavicular joint injuries: diagnosis and management. J Am Acad Orthop Surg 2009;17(4):207–19.
4. Beitzel K, Cote MP, Apostolakos J, et al. Current concepts in the treatment of acromioclavicular joint dislocations. Arthroscopy 2013;29(2):387–97.
5. Wang D, Bluth BE, Ishmael CR, et al. Early complications of acromioclavicular joint reconstruction requiring reoperation. Knee Surg Sports Traumatol Arthrosc 2017;25(7):2020–4.
6. Milewski MD, Tompkins M, Giugale JM, et al. Complications related to anatomic reconstruction of the coracoclavicular ligaments. Am J Sports Med 2012;40(7): 1628–34.
7. Martetschlager F, Horan MP, Warth RJ, et al. Complications after anatomic fixation and reconstruction of the coracoclavicular ligaments. Am J Sports Med 2013; 41(12):2896–903.
8. Post M. Current concepts in the diagnosis and management of acromioclavicular dislocations. Clin Orthop Relat Res 1985;(200):234–47.
9. Harris RI, Wallace AL, Harper GD, et al. Structural properties of the intact and the reconstructed coracoclavicular ligament complex. Am J Sports Med 2000;28(1): 103–8.
10. Batin S, Ozan F, Gurbuz K, et al. Case report: migration of a broken Kirschner wire after surgical treatment of acromioclavicular joint dislocation. Case Rep Surg 2016;1–3.
11. Geaney LE, Miller MD, Ticker JB, et al. Management of the failed AC joint reconstruction: causation and treatment. Sports Med Arthrosc 2010;18(3):167–72.
12. Weaver JK, Dunn HK. Treatment of acromioclavicular injuries, especially complete acromioclavicular separation. J Bone Joint Surg Am 1972;54(6):1187–94.
13. Spencer HT, Hsu L, Sodl J, et al. Radiographic failure and rates of re-operation after acromioclavicular joint reconstruction: a comparison of surgical techniques. Bone Joint J 2016;98-B(4):512–8.
14. Tauber M, Gordon K, Koller H, et al. Semitendinosus tendon graft versus a modified Weaver-Dunn procedure for acromioclavicular joint reconstruction in chronic cases: a prospective comparative study. Am J Sports Med 2009;37(1):181–90.
15. Hegazy G, Safwat H, Seddik M, et al. Modified Weaver-Dunn procedure the use of semitendinosus autogenous tendon graft for acromioclavicular joint reconstruction. Open Orthop J 2016;10(1):166–78.
16. Mazzocca AD, Santangelo SA, Johnson ST, et al. A biomechanical evaluation of an anatomical coracoclavicular ligament reconstruction. Am J Sports Med 2016; 34(2):236–46.

17. Lee S, Bedi A. Shoulder acromioclavicular joint reconstruction options and outcomes. Curr Rev Musculoskelet Med 2016;9(4):368–77.

18. Millett PJ, Horan MP, Warth RJ. Two-year outcomes after primary anatomic coracoclavicular ligament reconstruction. Arthroscopy 2015;31(10):1962–73.

19. Carofino BC, Mazzocca AD. The anatomic coracoclavicular ligament reconstruction: surgical technique and indications. J Shoulder Elbow Surg 2010; 19(Supplement):37–46.

20. Parnes N, Friedman D, Phillips C, et al. Outcome after arthroscopic reconstruction of the coracoclavicular ligaments using a double-bundle coracoid cerclage technique. Arthroscopy 2015;31(10):1933–40.

21. Tauber M, Valler D, Lichtenberg S, et al. Arthroscopic stabilization of chronic acromioclavicular joint dislocations. Am J Sports Med 2016;44(3):482–9.

22. Cook JB, Shaha JS, Rowles DJ, et al. Early failures with single clavicular transosseous coracoclavicular ligament reconstruction. J Shoulder Elbow Surg 2012; 21(12):1746–52.

23. Singh B, Mohanlal P, Bawale R. Early failure of coracoclavicular ligament reconstruction using tightrope system. Acta Orthop Belg 2016;82(1):119–23.

24. Choi NH, Lim SM, Lee SY, et al. Loss of reduction and complications of coracoclavicular ligament reconstruction with autogenous tendon graft in acute acromioclavicular dislocations. J Shoulder Elbow Surg 2017;26:692–8.

25. Clavert P, Meyer A, Boyer P, et al. Complication rates and types of failure after arthroscopic acute acromioclavicular dislocation fixation. Prospective multicenter study of 116 cases. Orthop Traumatol Surg Res 2015;101(8):S313–6.

26. Cisneros LN, Reiriz JS. Management of acute unstable acromioclavicular joint injuries. Eur J Orthop Surg Traumatol 2016;26(8):817–30.

27. Beitzel K, Obopilwe E, Chowaniec DM, et al. Biomechanical comparison of arthroscopic repairs for acromioclavicular joint instability. Am J Sports Med 2011;39(10):2218–25.

28. Walz L, Salzmann GM, Fabbro T, et al. The anatomic reconstruction of acromioclavicular joint dislocations using 2 tightrope devices: a biomechanical study. Am J Sports Med 2008;36(12):2398–406.

29. Venjakob AJ, Salzmann GM, Gabel F, et al. Arthroscopically assisted 2-bundle anatomic reduction of acute acromioclavicular joint separations. Am J Sports Med 2013;41(3):615–21.

30. Di Francesco A, Zoccali C, Colafarina O, et al. The use of hook plate in type III and V acromio-clavicular Rockwood dislocations: clinical and radiological midterm results and MRI evaluation in 42 patients. Injury 2012;43(2):147–52.

31. Arirachakaran A, Boonard M, Piyapittayanun P, et al. Post-operative outcomes and complications of suspensory loop fixation device versus hook plate in acute unstable acromioclavicular joint dislocation: a systematic review and meta-analysis. J Orthop Traumatol 2017;18(4):293–304.

32. Heideken JV, Windhamre HB, Une-Larsson V, et al. Acute surgical treatment of acromioclavicular dislocation type V with a hook plate: superiority to late reconstruction. J Shoulder Elbow Surg 2013;22(1):9–17.

33. Woodmass JM, Esposito JG, Ono Y, et al. Complications following arthroscopic fixation of acromioclavicular separations: a systematic review of the literature. Open Access J Sports Med 2015;6:97–107.

34. Shin SJ, Kim NK. Complications after arthroscopic coracoclavicular reconstruction using a single adjustable. Arthroscopy 2015;31(5):816–24.

35. Lin HY, Won PK, Ho WP, et al. Clavicular hook plate may induce subacromial shoulder impingement and rotator cuff lesion - dynamic sonographic evaluation. J Orthop Surg Res 2014;9(6):1–9.
36. Spiegl UJ, Smith SD, Euler SA, et al. Biomechanical consequences of coracoclavicular reconstruction techniques on clavicle strength. Am J Sports Med 2014; 42(7):1724–30.
37. Geaney LE, Beitzel K, Chowaniec DM, et al. Graft fixation is highest with anatomic tunnel positioning in acromioclavicular reconstruction. Arthroscopy 2013;29(3): 434–9.
38. Virk MS, Lederman E, Stevens C, et al. Coracoid bypass procedure: surgical technique for coracoclavicular reconstruction with coracoid insufficiency. J Shoulder Elbow Surg 2017;26:679–86.
39. Ferreira JV, Chowaniec D, Obopilwe E, et al. Biomechanical evaluation of effect of coracoid tunnel placement on load to failure of fixation during repair of acromioclavicular joint dislocations. Arthroscopy 2012;28(9):1230–6.
40. Rush LN, Lake N, Stiefel EC, et al. Comparison of short-term complications between 2 methods of coracoclavicular ligament reconstruction. Orthop J Sports Med 2016;4(7). 232596711665841.
41. Cote MP, Wojcik KE, Gomlinski G, et al. Rehabilitation of acromioclavicular joint separations: operative and nonoperative considerations. Clin Sports Med 2010; 29(2):213–28.

Elbow Injuries
Common Problems and Solutions

Felix H. Savoie, MD

KEYWORDS

- Elbow • Arthroscopy • Arthrofibrosis

KEY POINTS

- The elbow is one of the more difficult joints in which to obtain good results.
- Common issues include placement of correct portals, neuropraxia, ankylosis, heterotopic bone formation, and simple failure of the procedure.
- Common solutions include portal placement safeguards, nerve protection, early motion and cryocompression, oral or injectable steroids, radiation therapy, secure stabilization, and postoperative protection and rehabilitation based on available evidence and imaging.

INTRODUCTION

Many issues may occur when managing disorders of the elbow. This article presents common issues based on access, fixation, initial postoperative issues, and late onset issues. In each of these periods, there are specific problems that often occur that could be prevented or managed in a way to allow a more satisfactory outcome.

ACCESS ISSUES: ARTHROSCOPY
Arthroscopic Portals

In placing anterior medial or lateral portals, the more anterior the portals are, the more the safety margin increases in terms of neurovascular injury (**Fig. 1**). In addition to increasing the safety margin, an anterior location also allows the surgeon to enter the elbow in a safer location.[1]

In the past, the author has performed multiple anatomic studies regarding portal safety. Recently, the author's institution has undertaken a systematic review of all portals and has done anatomic dissections to correlate, confirm, or in some cases change the current literature regarding portal placement and safety.[1–3]

Medial Access

The proximal anterior medial portal, originally described by Poehling and Whipple, is the safest area in which to access the elbow.[4] Originally described as 2 cm proximal and 1 to

Department of Orthopaedics, Tulane University, 1430 Tulane Avenue, New Orleans, LA 70112, USA
E-mail address: Fsavoie@Tulane.edu

Clin Sports Med 37 (2018) 209–215
https://doi.org/10.1016/j.csm.2017.12.003
sportsmed.theclinics.com
0278-5919/18/© 2018 Published by Elsevier Inc. This is an open access article under the CC BY-NC-ND license (http://creativecommons.org/licenses/by-nc-nd/4.0/).

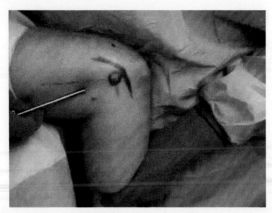

Fig. 1. A more anterior location of the medial and lateral portals increases the safety margin for arthroscopy and improves visualization.

2 cm anterior to the tip of the epicondyle, the author has found that moving it to 2 cm proximal and 3 cm anterior, into a palpable soft spot between the flexor-pronator muscles, increases the safety margin from the ulnar nerve. The skin puncture in this area allows the cannula to be directed in a more anterior to posterior direction, entering the joint on the most medial and superior area of the anterior capsule. This redirection actually increases the safety margin between the median nerve and the cannula, as well as allows a full view, even of the medial side of the elbow (**Fig. 2**). Proper access here makes anterior arthroscopic surgery, which is usually limited to the lateral side in the anterior compartment (except in ankylosis and arthritis) a relatively simple (and safer) procedure.

Lateral Access

These portals are best established outside-in by testing with a spinal needle under direct visualization. The only area to avoid is the distal anterior lateral portal because of its proximity to the posterior interosseous nerve.

Posterior Portals

These are all relatively safe and effective. The surgeon must always mark and remember the location of the ulnar nerve. In the stiff elbow, resection of the posterior band of the ulnar collateral ligament may be performed arthroscopically only if the ulnar nerve is identified and protected. Alternatively, the proximal cubital tunnel may be opened superficially at the beginning of a case and then, on conclusion, the nerve retracted and the posterior band released via an open approach.

The more distal posterior lateral portals allow easy access to the lateral gutter and posterior radiocapitellar joint. The author favors keeping the arthroscope superior and changing to a 70° arthroscope to use the soft spot, straight lateral and distal posterior lateral (Steinman portal) for instrumentation (**Fig. 3**).

Key points

1. A more anterior location of the skin incision increases both visualization and the margin of safety.

2. Liberal use of a 70° arthroscope is useful for visualization while allowing more instrument portals.

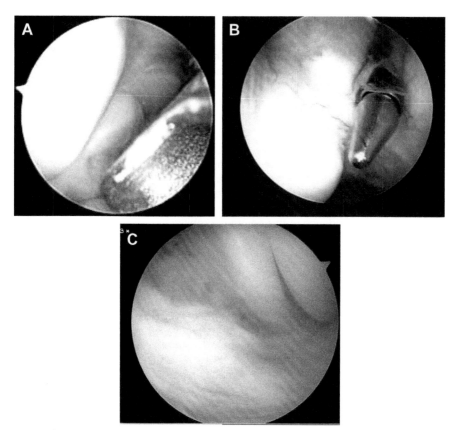

Fig. 2. (*A*) The incorrect entry point on the medial side prevents full visualization and actually increases the risk to the more anterior neurovascular structures. (*B*) The correct entry point, located more medially, allows full visualization of the anterior compartment of the elbow. (*C*) Medial anterior gutter from proximal anterior medial portal.

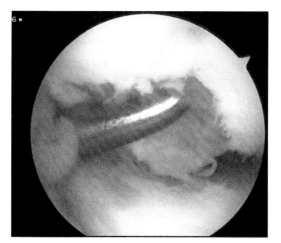

Fig. 3. View of the capitellum using a 70° arthroscope, with instrumentation from a distal posterior lateral (Steinman) portal.

ARTHROFIBROSIS, ANKYLOSIS, AND HETEROTOPIC OSSIFICATION: THE STIFF ELBOW

One of the most dreaded, and unfortunately common, problems in the elbow is postoperative stiffness. Unfortunately, there has not been much progress in identifying the source of the problem. Arthritic patients seem to have increased risk of this complication, including those who require extensive procedures with high use of electrocautery and open procedures that are especially bloody.[5]

Prevention

Interestingly, a recent presentation on complications from the Barnes group in St Louis, IL, seemed to show that intraarticular injection of steroids at the end of the procedure might decrease the risk of this dreaded complication (Yamaguichi K, personal communication, 2015). In addition, the use of cryocompression and oral steroids may also decrease the incidence of this common problem.

Management

In cases in which it has already occurred, arthroscopic intervention, even in cases of heterotopic bone formation, may be useful. The initial management of early arthrofibrosis should center on a preservative-free intraarticular steroid injection; oral steroids or antiinflammatory medications; cryocompression; gentle, pain-free mobilization; and turnbuckle orthoses. If ineffective after a few weeks, or if the condition worsens, then early arthroscopic treatment should be considered. In these cases, the operative surgeon needs to be an experienced elbow arthroscopist. The surgery should be as atraumatic as possible, using the more anterior portals for the anterior release and excision of heterotopic bone, and the posterior and posterior central portals for posterior release and bone excision. The decision whether or not to release or transpose the ulnar nerve is individualized depending on the specific areas of involvement.

Key points

1. Prevention is easier than occurrence, but the problem may occur anyway.

2. Once it starts to occur, early intervention is aggressive by both nonoperative and operative measures.

LIGAMENT REPAIR OR RECONSTRUCTION
Medial Ulnar Collateral Ligament

Injuries to the medial ligament are common in the overhead athlete, wrestlers, and gymnasts. Nonoperative management in the nonprofessional athlete can be quite successful. Two recent reports documenting the efficacy of nonoperative treatment allowed 90% of players to return to sport at the same level of play. Surgery may consist of repair, repair with augmentation, or grafting. The most common problem with repair centers on patient choice. Not all ligaments are amenable to repair, only those that are normal except for a proximal or distal avulsion. In repair with augmentation with an internal brace, the key is to not over-tension the brace. If too tight, the brace will limit motion. Prevention of this problem involves adding 15 to 16 mm to the area of tape going through the second anchor and placing a hemostat under the tape before final tensioning. Checking for full range of motion before cutting the tape also is a good technical tip.

Medial ulnar collateral ligament (MUCL) reconstruction has several areas of potential problems. The first involves graft harvest. A recent paper from Leslie and colleagues[6] presented the results of a survey of the Hand Society and detailed 24 incidences of harvest of the median nerve, rather than the palmaris, for use in MUCL. A simple test of touching the thumb and forefinger together while slightly flexing the wrist can demonstrate the presence or absence of the palmaris longus and prevent this catastrophic problem (**Fig. 4**).

Fracture of the tunnels placed under the sublime tubercle can be prevented by the use of an endobutton or interference screw. Using the docking technique, described by Altchek, proximally can prevent medial condyle fractures.[7] Fractures should be managed by standard fixation techniques.

Lateral Ligament Repair and Reconstruction

The main complication associated with radial ulnohumeral ligament (RUHL) repair and reconstruction is loss of flexion. In most cases, this is simply due to over-tensioning of the ligament or graft. This can be avoided by tensioning the ligament or graft in 90° to 100° of flexion. If stiffness occurs postoperatively, injection and therapy, or even surgical release, are needed.

Key points

1. Avoid over-tensioning of the ligaments on each side.

2. Anatomic placement of the proximal and distal attachment is critical to success.

3. If harvesting the palmaris, check for its presence or absence preoperatively and ensure all members of the operating room team know the results.

TENDON REPAIRS
Tennis Elbow

Excision of Nirchl lesion is a straightforward procedure done both open and arthroscopically. The main problem is damage to the radial collateral portion of the RUHL complex. This can be easily avoided by keeping the dissection anterior to the tip of the lateral epicondyle. If damaged, repair is the only option to solve this problem.

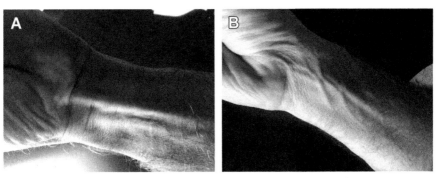

Fig. 4. The test to show the presence (*A*), left hand, or absence (*B*), right hand, of the palmaris longus tendon.

Golfer's Elbow

Medial epicondylitis, which is different from lateral epicondylitis, requires an evaluation of the ulnar nerve. The most common problem is persistent pain, and the solution is usually to release the fascia over the ulnar nerve and excise the small sensory branch that is located in the medial intermuscular septum.

Biceps Tendon Repair

Repair of the distal biceps has been a subject of much interest. Problems with the single-incision repair include damage to the lateral antebrachial cutaneous nerve or posterior interosseous nerve. Fortunately, almost all recover spontaneously. Avoidance of aggressive retraction is the most common solution. Double incision repair, popularized by the Mayo clinic, follows the Boyd-Anderson technique and is associated with increased risk of heterotopic ossification. Prevention centers on hemostasis, irrigation, and minimizing the trauma to the interval between the radius and ulna. Treatment is by surgical excision, with radiation therapy to prevent recurrence.[8]

Triceps Tendon Repair

Triceps injuries occur in 2 age ranges: young patients with high trauma or older patients with degeneration. In the younger, high-trauma group, the main issues are stiffness and heterotopic bone. Prevention centers on the same techniques (previously described) as treatment. However, heterotopic ossification in the triceps seems to be relatively well tolerated compared with other areas of the elbow and may often be ignored.

In the older group, the tears are usually partial, and the main issue is skin breakdown. The author has switched to an all-arthroscopic technique, which has eliminated this problem. If it occurs, irrigation and debridement with use of a negative pressure device can work, or a rotational flap may be needed.

Key points

1. Remain anterior to the tip of the epicondyle to avoid detaching the RUHL when performing tennis elbow surgery.

2. Carefully evaluate and treat concurrent neuropathy when managing medial epicondylitis.

3. When performing biceps tendon repairs, limit retraction on the lateral antebrachial and posterior interosseous nerves.

4. Minimize dissection between the radius and ulnar during 2 incision techniques to decrease the risk of synostosis.

SUMMARY

The elbow is often associated with complications with all surgical procedures. This article has presented a series of these common problems with thoughts on both prevention and treatment.

REFERENCES

1. Thon S, Gold P, Rush L, et al. Modified anterolateral portals in elbow arthroscopy: a cadaveric study on safety. Arthroscopy 2017. https://doi.org/10.1016/j.arthro.2017.06.012.

2. Desai MJ, Mothani SK, Lodha SJ, et al. Major peripheral nerve injuries after elbow arthroscopy. Arthroscopy 2016;32(6):999–1002.

3. Hilgerson NF, Oh LS, Flipsen M, et al. Tips to avoid nerve injure in elbow arthroscopy. World J Orthop 2017;18(8):99–106.
4. Poehling GG, Whipple TL, Sisco L, et al. Elbow arthroscopy: a new technique. Arthroscopy 1989;(5):222–4.
5. Andrachuk JS, Scillia AJ, Aune KT, et al. Symptomatic heterotopic ossification after ulnar collateral ligament reconstruction: clinical significance and treatment outcome. Am J Sports Med 2016;44:1324–8.
6. Leslie BM, Osterman AL, Wolfe SL. Inadvertent harvest of the median nerve instead of the Palmaris Longus tendon. J Bone Joint Surg Am 2017;99(14): 1173–82.
7. Dodson CC, Thomas A, Dines JS, et al. Medial ulnar collateral ligament reconstruction of the elbow in throwing athletes. AM J Sports Med 2006;34(12):1926–32.
8. Dunphy TR, Hudson J, Batech M, et al. Surgical treatment of distal biceps tendon ruptures: an analysis of complications in 784 surgical repairs. Am J Sports Med 2017. https://doi.org/10.1177/063546517720200.

Hand and Wrist Injuries
Common Problems and Solutions

Nicholas Pulos, MD, Sanjeev Kakar, MD, MBA*

KEYWORDS

- Wrist arthroscopy • Scaphoid • Hook of hamate • Scapholunate ligament • TFCC

KEY POINTS

- Sports injuries of the hand and wrist may involve acute or chronic trauma to several tissue types, including bones, tendons, and ligaments.
- Accurate and timely diagnosis guides treatment and can avoid prolonged time away for sport and/or permanent disability.
- Many procedures for the treatment of sports injuries of the hand and wrist can be performed with an arthroscope.

INTRODUCTION

Injuries to the hands and wrist are common among athletes, accounting for 3% to 9% of all sporting injuries.[1] Acute traumatic injuries include fractures, dislocations, ligament, and tendon injuries to the hand and wrist, and are more commonly seen in contact sports. In contrast, overuse conditions often present as sprains and strains as a result of repetitive loading, as seen in gymnastics and racquet sports.

Complications in the treatment of sports injuries of the hand and wrist may be divided into 2 categories. The first is incorrect or delayed diagnosis, leading to functional sequelae to the hand and wrist. The second is errors in treatment both surgical and nonsurgical, leading to iatrogenic injury. Both types of complications may require prolonged time away from sport, if not permanent disability.

For the physician treating athletes, knowledge of the anatomy of the hand and wrist, as well as common patterns of injury, aids in proper diagnosis. This article highlights common sports injuries of the hand and wrist and their complications, and provides tips for successful management.

Department of Orthopedic Surgery, Mayo Clinic, 200 1st Street SW, Rochester, MN 55905, USA
* Corresponding author.
E-mail address: kakar.sanjeev@mayo.edu

Clin Sports Med 37 (2018) 217–243
https://doi.org/10.1016/j.csm.2017.12.004
0278-5919/18/© 2017 Elsevier Inc. All rights reserved.

FRACTURES
Distal Radius Fractures

Although distal radius fractures are less commonly seen in young adults than in the pediatric or elderly population, athletics is among the most common causes of injury for this age group.[2] Fractures to the distal radius most frequently occur as a result of a fall on an outstretched hand. In addition to a good physical examination of the extremity, the initial workup always includes orthogonal radiographs of the wrist to assess radial height, radial inclination, volar tilt, and intraarticular involvement. Indications for a computed tomography (CT) scan vary amongst surgeons, but the patient should certainly be considered for fractures with intraarticular involvement, as is commonly seen in this demographic.

Initial closed reduction is performed to restore anatomic length, alignment, and rotation, followed by immobilization in a long arm sugar-tong type splint to prevent pronosupination. Postreduction radiographs are evaluated before determining final treatment recommendations. Radiographic parameters suggesting operative treatment include greater than 5 mm of radial shortening, greater than 5° of dorsal angulation, or greater than 2 mm articular step-off.[3] For fractures that are initially well reduced, several investigators have postulated factors associated with loss of reduction, including initial fracture displacement, age, metaphyseal comminution, and ulnar variance[4,5] (**Fig. 1**).

Even in minimally displaced or well reduced fractures, complications may occur, including skin compromise from improper cast application and extensor pollicis longus (EPL) rupture (**Fig. 2**). One series of nondisplaced distal radius fractures demonstrated a 5% risk of EPL rupture.[6] A high index of suspicion and discussion with the athlete regarding concerning signs and symptoms of tenosynovitis may allow the surgeon to release the third extensor compartment before rupture. A rupture of the EPL tendon may be treated with either tendon grafting or transfer of the extensor indicis proprius because the attritional rupture is generally not amenable to primary repair.

Volar locked plating has become the workhorse for operative treatment of distal radius fractures.[7] This method alleviates many of the concerns that prior operative fixation strategies entailed, including irritation of extensor tendons from dorsal plates, pin site infections, and patient dissatisfaction from external fixators. A modified Henry flexor carpi radialis (FCR) approach is most frequently used, and care must be taken to avoid injury to the palmar cutaneous branch of the median nerve. In more difficult cases, the extended FCR approach releases the radial septum, allowing wide exposure of the fracture surfaces through pronation of the proximal radial fragment.[8]

Even with modern volar locked plating systems, malreduction can occur and irritation to both flexor and extensor tendons has been reported[9] (**Fig. 3**). A skyline view can be used to ensure that distal locking screws do not penetrate the dorsal cortex[10] (**Fig. 4**). A biomechanical study demonstrated that locked unicortical screws of at least 75% length produce similar stiffness to bicortical screws.[11] Symptomatic prominent hardware warrants removal after fracture healing has been confirmed. Malreduction may require a corrective osteotomy after a thorough discussion with the patient regarding their pain and functional limitations.

Technical pearls

- Accurately reduce the fracture before volar locked plate placement.
- The extended FCR approach uses the fracture plane for exposure, improving visualization of fracture fragments.
- A skyline view helps evaluate dorsal screw prominence.

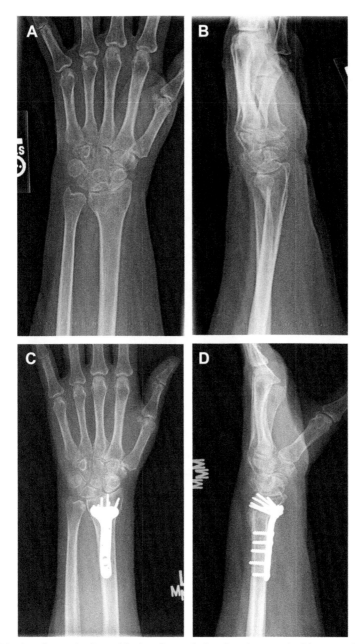

Fig. 1. Distal radius malunion with dorsal angulation (*A, B*) treated with corrective osteotomy (*C, D*).

Scaphoid Fractures

Scaphoid fractures may be seen more commonly in active, younger men.[12] Similar
to distal radius fractures, scaphoid fractures occur because of a fall on the outstretched hand. In an active population, Bond and colleagues[13] demonstrated
that percutaneous cannulated screw fixation for nondisplaced fractures of the

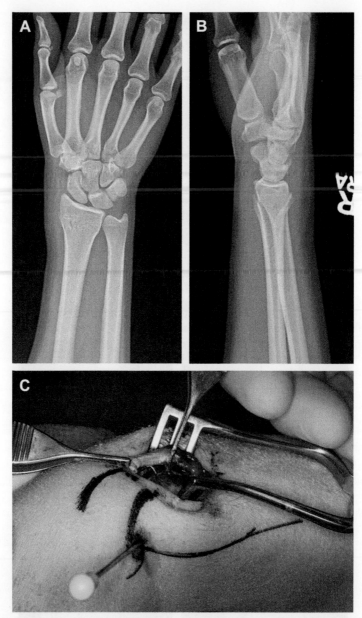

Fig. 2. Minimally displaced distal radius fracture (*A*, *B*) with EPL tendon rupture (*C*).

scaphoid waist resulted in faster radiographic union and return to activity compared with cast immobilization. Thus, the preferred treatment for elite athletes has shifted from cast immobilization to operative fixation of both displaced and nondisplaced fractures.[14]

Although scaphoid fracture healing rates after surgical fixation approach 100%,[15] nonunions continue to be problematic. Risk factors for nonunion include displacement greater than 1 mm, proximal pole fractures, and a missed occult fracture.[16] Typically,

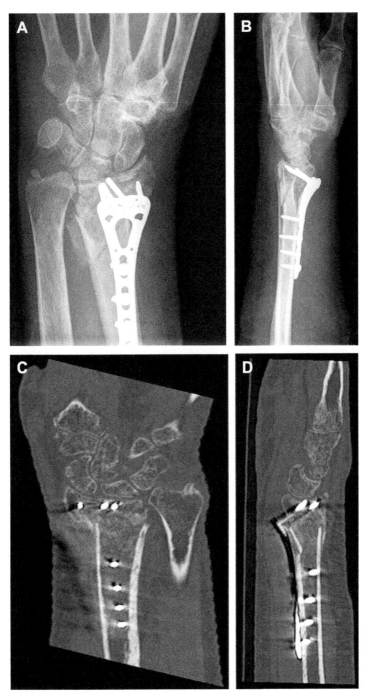

Fig. 3. Radiographs (*A*, *B*) and CT scans (*C*, *D*) of a distal radius fracture treated with volar locked plating with malreduction and symptomatic intraarticular hardware.

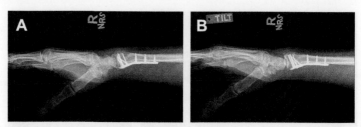

Fig. 4. Lateral (*A*) and skyline radiographs (*B*) demonstrating extraarticular placement of distal locking screws.

patients with an acute scaphoid fracture present with snuffbox tenderness on clinical examination. Although displaced fractures may be seen on anteroposterior (AP), lateral, and scaphoid view radiographs, nondisplaced fractures may not be appreciated at the time of injury. Failure to adequately identify and immobilize a nondisplaced scaphoid fracture early may lead to delayed union, malunion, or even nonunion.[17] MRI can diagnose occult scaphoid fractures with 100% sensitivity and specificity.[18] Therefore, MRI is the preferred imaging modality for the athlete with a suspected occult scaphoid fracture (**Fig. 5**).

Minimally displaced scaphoid fractures may be fixed percutaneously or with a mini-open incision through either a dorsal or volar approach. The dorsal antegrade approach is indicated for proximal pole fractures. Arthroscopically assisted fixation allows not only assessment of the fracture and necessary debridement but also precise placement along the central axis of the scaphoid.[19] Placing the screw through the central axis of the scaphoid maximizes the screw length, which has been shown to be biomechanically superior to shorter screw fixation[20] (**Fig. 6**).

Scaphoid fracture nonunions following surgical fixation may be more common than previously reported.[21] Failure for scaphoid fractures to unite following surgical fixation may be due to poor technique, failure to restore vascularity,[22] or carpal malalignment.[23] Several vascularized and nonvascularized bone grafts have been described. Results of revision surgery for scaphoid nonunion are guarded and success is predicated on matching the type of bone graft procedure to the unique features of the patient's nonunion.[24]

Technical pearls

- Nondisplaced scaphoid fractures may not be initially seen on standard radiographs and an MRI may be warranted in suspected cases.
- Arthroscopically assisted fixation allows for direct visualization of proximal entry site for screw fixation along the central axis of the scaphoid.
- A derotation K-wire prevents fracture fragment rotation during fixation.

Hook of Hamate and Pisiform Fractures

Though less common than scaphoid fractures, fractures of the hamate and pisiform are seen in athletes who handle a club, racquet, or bat, and may be similarly missed on initial radiographic imaging. Hook of the hamate fractures can occur either with repetitive activity or a sudden impaction and present with pain over the hypothenar eminence (**Fig. 7**). It occurs almost exclusively in the leading hand,[25] with patients having difficulty grasping a club or bat, or with pain on impact. Patients are tender over the hook of the hamate, which can be palpated by placing the thumb interphalangeal joint on the pisiform and aiming 45° toward the index finger metacarpophalangeal (MCP) joint. The hook of hamate pull test may be used to diagnose a hook of hamate fracture.

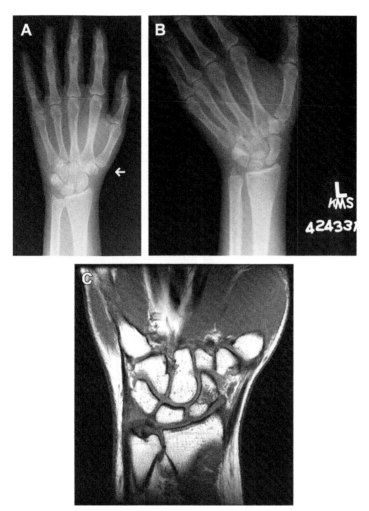

Fig. 5. Initial injury AP and lateral radiographs of suspected scaphoid fracture (*A*, *B*) and MRI (*C*) performed on the same day in a skier. *Arrow* indicates site of pain.

With the patients wrist held in full ulnar deviation, resisted flexion of the ring and small finger elicits pain in the hypothenar eminence as the flexor digitorum profundus (FDP) tendons are pulled across the hook of hamate as a pulley.[26] Standard AP and lateral radiographs often do not show the fracture but a carpal tunnel view should be performed if suspected. A CT scan increases the sensitivity to 100% and specificity to 94.4%.[27] There is limited evidence to guide treatment in elite athletes but excision has become the gold standard for displaced fractures owing to the complications associated with open reduction, internal fixation including nonunion, symptomatic hardware,[28] and prolonged immobilization, though it may lead to decreased power grip.[29]

FDP tendinopathy or rupture of the small and ring fingers may be seen in 15% to 25% of patients with nonunion of the hook of hamate.[28,30] Further, in a series by Yamazaki and colleagues,[30] only half of the subjects with a ruptured flexor tendon secondary to nonunion of fractures of the hook of hamate had antecedent symptoms.

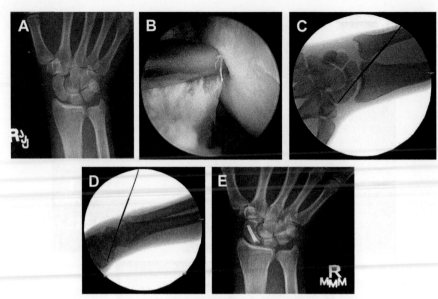

Fig. 6. Scaphoid wrist fracture (*A*) treated with arthroscopically assisted fixation (*B-E*).

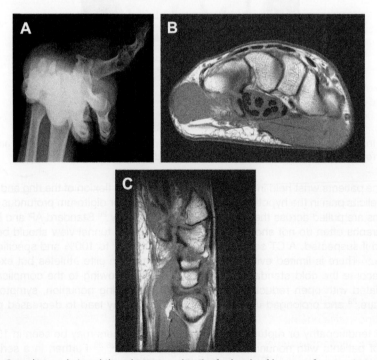

Fig. 7. Carpal tunnel view (*A*) and MRI cuts (*B, C*) of a hook of hamate fracture in a college basketball player.

If this occurs, the physician can perform tendon reconstruction with grafting or tendon transfers,[30] however, adequate treatment requires prolonged time away from sport and lengthy postoperative protocols.

Pisiform fractures are less common than hook of hamate fractures but present similarly with pain in the hypothenar region as a result of a forceful blow. The fracture is frequently missed and a CT scan is helpful in confirming the diagnosis[31] (**Fig. 8**A–D). Although initial treatment usually involves immobilization, complete pisiform excision has been described for patients with displaced fractures, malunions, nonunions, and pisotriquetral joint arthritis.[32]

Ulnar neuropathy may be present with either hook of hamate fractures or pisiform fractures.[33] Compression of the ulnar nerve classically results in numbness and paresthesias in the ulnar 1 and a half digits, and may involve weakness to intrinsic muscles of the hand. As opposed to compression at the elbow (cubital tunnel syndrome), distal compression resulting from a hook of hamate or pisiform fracture will spare sensory innervation to the dorsum of the hand, as well as ulnar innervated extrinsic muscles (FDP to the ring and small fingers). Paradoxically, this distal compression may leads to worse clawing of the digits. Damage to the ulnar nerve may result from either contusion of the nerve, pressure on the nerve from hematoma and edema related to the fracture, or intraneural fibrosis.[34] Due to the anatomy of the ulnar nerve branches at the Guyon canal, the patient may present with pure motor symptoms, pure sensory symptoms, or a mixed motor and sensory deficit. Treatment is aimed at decompression of the nerve and addressing the pathologic cause.

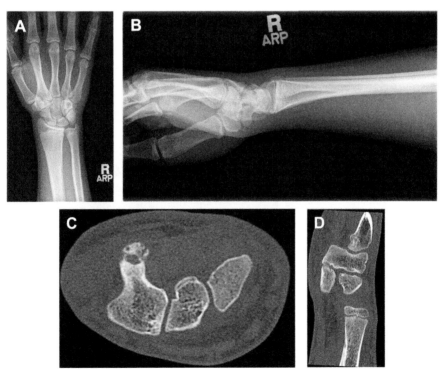

Fig. 8. Radiographs (*A, B*) and CT scans (*C, D*) of a fractured pisohamate coalition in a young tennis player.

Metacarpal Fractures

Metacarpal fractures most commonly occur as a result of a fall on an outstretched hand or direct blow from contact. Plain radiographs in orthogonal and oblique planes are usually sufficient to guide treatment, but CT scans are often indicated for base of the metacarpal fractures to assess the carpometacarpal (CMC) joints (**Fig. 9**). For metacarpal shaft fractures, angulation of 10° to 20° may be accepted in the index and long finger with increasing acceptability of 30° to 40° in the ring and small finger, respectively. Similarly, metacarpal neck angulation of 10° to 15° may be acceptable in the index and long finger, whereas angulation of 40° to 50° may be tolerated in the ring and small finger. In the athlete, operative treatment is indicated for intraarticular fractures of the metacarpal head, unstable or severely angulated fractures of the metacarpal neck and shaft, intraarticular fractures of the CMC joint, or associated CMC instability.[35] In addition to the fracture, other considerations pertaining to nonoperative versus surgical fixation include the time of the season when the injury occurs and whether the patient will tolerate immobilization. Operative treatment may permit earlier return to play.

Options for operative fixation include closed reduction and percutaneous pinning with K-wires, open reduction and internal fixation with plates and/or screws, or intramedullary devices. Complications from percutaneous fixation include damage or irritation to dorsal sensory nerve branches[36] and loss of fixation related to construct stiffness. Although plates and screw fixation adds increased stiffness and rotational stability, meticulous care must be taken to avoid injury to sensory nerve branches and to elevate flaps over hardware to minimize irritation.

Many metacarpal fractures are amenable to nonoperative treatment, provided that the athlete and treating physician are accepting of potential limitations. For every 2 mm of metacarpal shortening an average of 7° of extensor lag was demonstrated

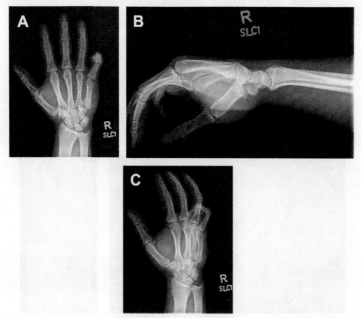

Fig. 9. AP (*A*), lateral (*B*), and oblique (*C*) radiographs of intraarticular fracture of the 5th CMC joint.

in a cadaveric study.[37] Further, with 2 mm of shortening, there is an 8% reduction and grip strength and approximately 55% optimum power at 10 mm of shortening.[38] Up to 10° of malrotation may be tolerated, but appropriate assessment of the deformity requires an end-on view of the finger nails.[39] The prolonged immobilization required with nonoperative treatment increases the risk of stiffness and may require additional procedures to address joint contractures or tenolysis. Further nonoperative treatment and associated deformity may not be acceptable to all athletes. Specifically, apex dorsal angulated fractures of the metacarpal neck and shaft may result in discomfort with grip (eg, in weightlifters).

It is important to counsel patients regarding the long-term sequelae of intraarticular fractures of the metacarpals at the CMC joint. In a study of intraarticular fractures of the base of the fifth metacarpal, 38% of subjects reported some continued pain or dysfunction of their hand despite operative treatment.[40] Instability following intraarticular fractures of the thumb can be particularly problematic for athletes and may necessitate CMC arthrodesis.[35]

Technical pearls

- The use of the fluoroscopy machine as a hand table eases visualization in percutaneous treatment of hand fractures.
- Dorsal sensory nerve branches are at risk with surgical approaches to the metacarpals and should be identified and protected.
- Periosteal flaps closed over thin plates limit irritation to extensor tendons.

LIGAMENTOUS INJURIES
Triangular Fibrocartilage Complex Injuries

There are several potential causes of ulnar-sided wrist pain in the elite athlete. In the diagnostic workup of patients with a suspected distal radioulnar joint (DRUJ) a 4-leaf clover algorithm should be used to assess bony deformity, the articular cartilage surfaces, extensor carpi ulnaris instability, and triangular fibrocartilage complex (TFCC) or ligamentous structures.[41] Chronic and repetitive loading of the TFCC make it particularly susceptible to both acute traumatic injury and degenerative changes (**Fig. 10**). The TFCC is made up of an articular disk (the triangular fibrocartilage proper), dorsal and palmar radioulnar ligaments, meniscal homologue, ulnar capsule, extensor carpi ulnaris subsheath, and ulnolunate and ulnotriquetral ligaments. In addition to stabilizing the DRUJ, the TFCC functions as a shock absorber between the ulnar head and the lunate and triquetrum (**Fig. 11**).

As with other injuries, accurate and timely diagnosis is critical when treating the elite athlete. Patients typically complain of ulnar-sided wrist pain with pronosupination. On physical examination, pain may be elicited with palpation of the fovea between the ulnar styloid and flexor carpi ulnaris tendon. Ulnar or radial deviation of the wrist may elicit pain as the TFCC is compressed or tensioned, respectively. Patients without instability to the DRUJ or ulnocarpal articulation should raise suspicion for an ulnotriquetral split tear[42] (**Fig. 12**). MRI has largely replaced arthrography for the diagnosis of TFCC injuries with 100% sensitivity and 90% specificity.[43] Nevertheless, the gold standard for diagnosing TFCC disorders remains wrist arthroscopy. In addition to larger tears amenable to probing, subtle peripheral tears, which may even have scarred down but not restored proper tension to the TFCC, may be revealed with the suction test arthroscopically.[44] Therefore, wrist arthroscopy should be strongly considered in athletes with a suspected injury because it allows not only diagnosis but also possible treatment.[45]

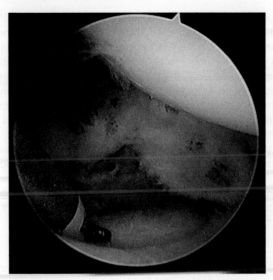

Fig. 10. Large central TFCC degenerative tear seen arthroscopically.

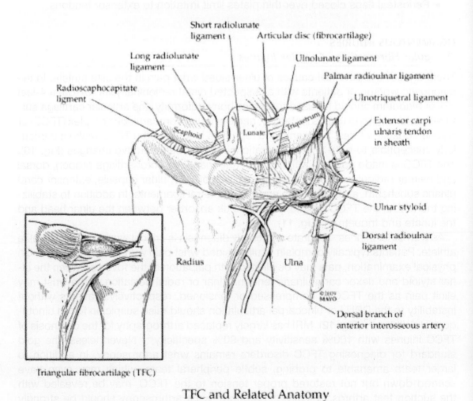

Short radiolunate ligament

Long radiolunate ligament

Articular disc (fibrocartilage)

Ulnolunate ligament

Palmar radioulnar ligament

Radioscaphocapitate ligment

Ulnotriquetral ligament

Extensor carpi ulnaris tendon in sheath

Scaphoid

Lunate

Trapetrum

Ulnar styloid

Dorsal radioulnar ligament

Radius

Ulna

Dorsal branch of anterior interosseous artery

Triangular fibrocartilage (TFC)

TFC and Related Anatomy

Fig. 11. TFCC and related anatomy. (*From* Kakar S, Carlsen BT, Moran SL, et al. The management of chronic distal radioulnar instability. Hand Clin 2010;26(4):519; with permission.)

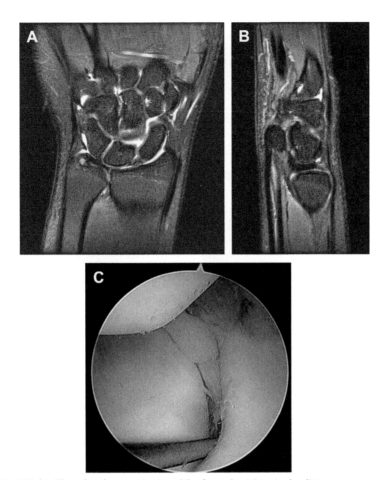

Fig. 12. MRI (*A*, *B*) and arthroscopic view (*C*) of an ulnotriquetral split tear.

For TFCC injuries with central articular disc tears not amenable to repair (see **Fig. 10**), arthroscopic debridement may allow the athlete to return to a high level of play early. In a retrospective review of patients with acute posttraumatic tears, the results of arthroscopic debridement were generally excellent with patients who suffered sports related injuries all returning to unrestricted activity at an average of 6 weeks.[46] However, peripheral tears amenable to surgical fixation may require 3 months before return to sport and this must be discussed with the athlete before commencing treatment. Complications following wrist arthroscopy are likely underreported in the literature.[47] Structures at risk during portal placement include the superficial branch of the radial nerve (1-2 portal), dorsal sensory branch of the ulnar nerve (6R and 6U portals), and extensor tendons (3-4 and 4-5 portals).

For athletes with ulnar positive variance, an arthroscopic wafer procedure or ulnar shortening osteotomy may be indicated (**Fig. 13**). There are several techniques for performing the osteotomy, but all require a prolonged period of immobilization while the osteotomy heals. Delayed union and nonunions of the ulna have been reported and patients may complain of symptomatic hardware necessitating plate removal, with nonunion rates ranging from 0 to 15% and hardware removal rates ranging from 0% to 8% in a retrospectives series.[48]

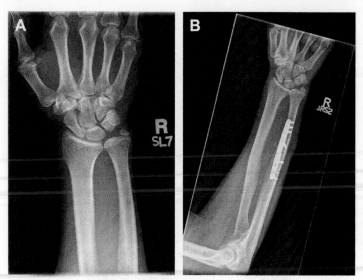

Fig. 13. Ulnar positive variance (*A*) treated with ulnar shortening osteotomy (*B*).

Technical pearls

- The differential diagnosis in athletes with ulnar-sided wrist pain is broad and a systematic approach to evaluation and treatment is imperative.
- The use of a 4-5 working portal decreases risk of injury to dorsal sensory nerve branches of the ulnar nerve.
- A TFCC suction test aids in assessment of TFCC tension and may reveal subtle tears.

Scapholunate Ligament Injuries

The scapholunate interosseous (SLI) ligament is composed of 3 histologically distinct structures, with the dorsal component being the thickest and strongest.[49] A common mechanism of injury is a fall onto the dorsally extended and ulnar deviated wrist with intercarpal supination. Athletes will present with dorsal radial wrist pain and may complain of inability to bear weight with the wrist extended, as in the standard push-up position, or weakness and pain with grip. They may be tender over the SLI, which is just distal and dorsal to the Lister tubercle on dorsum of the wrist (**Fig. 14**). The scaphoid shift test as described by Watson and colleagues[50] should be performed to assess for carpal instability. With the examiner's thumb holding constant pressure on the distal pole of the scaphoid, the wrist is brought from an ulnarly deviated, slightly extended position to radial deviation with slight flexion. In patients with ligamentous injury, thumb pressure will subluxate the scaphoid out of the radial fossa dorsally with radial deviation. Although plain radiographs may be normal, dynamic imaging with a clenched fist view, as well as contralateral wrist views, is often helpful (**Fig. 15**). Signs of instability include widening of the scapholunate interval greater than 3 mm and a signet ring sign, seen with scaphoid flexion. MRI with or without arthrography may be useful in identifying an injury to the SLI ligament when radiographs are normal (**Fig. 16**).

Early diagnosis is particularly important in these injuries because it drives the treatment algorithm. Garcia-Elias and colleagues[51] highlighted 5 prognostic factors that should be considered before deciding on treatment: integrity of the dorsal SLI

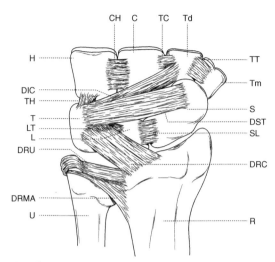

Fig. 14. Fig. 4. The dorsal carpal ligaments from a dorsal perspective. Ligaments: CH, capito-hamate; DIC, dorsal intercarpal; DRC, dorsal radiocarpal; DRMA, dorsal radial metaphyseal arcuate; DRU, dorsal radioulnar; DST, dorsal scaphotriquetral; LT, lunotriquetral; SL, scapho-lunate; TC, trapeziocapitate; TH, triquetrohamate; TT, trapezio trapezoid. Bones: C, capitate; H, hamate; L, lunate; R, radius; S, scaphoid, T, triquetrum; Td, trapezoid; Tm, trapezium; U, ulna. (*From* Berger RA. The ligaments of the wrist. A current overview of anatomy with con-siderations of their potential functions. Hand Clin 1997;13(1):63–82; with permission.)

ligament, healing potential of the disrupted ligaments, status of the secondary stabi-lizers, reducibility of carpal malalignment, and cartilage status.

Acute partial and complete tears may be amenable to arthroscopic debridement or open or arthroscopic primary repair. Darlis and colleagues[52] showed improved pain relief with maintained stability in a series of 16 subjects with partial tears treated with debridement and thermal shrinkage. Complete tears are amenable to direct repair of the SLI ligament with dorsal radioscaphoid capsulodesis.[53] Repair of the SLI liga-ment in patients with static instability does not adequately maintain carpal alignment nor does it provide consistent pain relief.[54]

Chronic or severe tears may require reconstruction, of which several techniques have been described. For patients with reducible deformity in the absence of arthritis, Weiss[55] described the scapholunate reconstruction using bone-retinaculum-bone autograft, which could be harvested locally. In addition to the SLI ligaments, the sca-pholunate articulation is secondarily stabilized by the dorsal intercarpal, dorsal radio-carpal, and the radioscaphocapitate ligaments.[56] Although some surgeons advocate augmenting SLI ligament repair with these secondary stabilizers,[57] the use of a ligament-sparing capsulotomy for open procedures is essential to prevent further car-pal instability.[58] Similarly, Garcia-Elias and colleagues[51] demonstrated good results with the 3-ligament tenodesis procedure, which aims to replicate the action of 3 liga-ments: scaphotrapezial-trapezoidal, dorsal SLI, and dorsal radiotriquetral. The use of these reconstructions in patients with static instability is less predictable.

Untreated SLI ligament injuries may develop a typical pattern of degenerative arthritis called scapholunate advanced collapse (SLAC).[59] O'Meeghan and colleagues[60] re-ported on the natural history of untreated injuries and found that, although patients have ongoing pain and limited range of motion, not all rapidly progress to SLAC wrist. Patients with a malaligned or arthritic carpus may require partial or total wrist fusion.

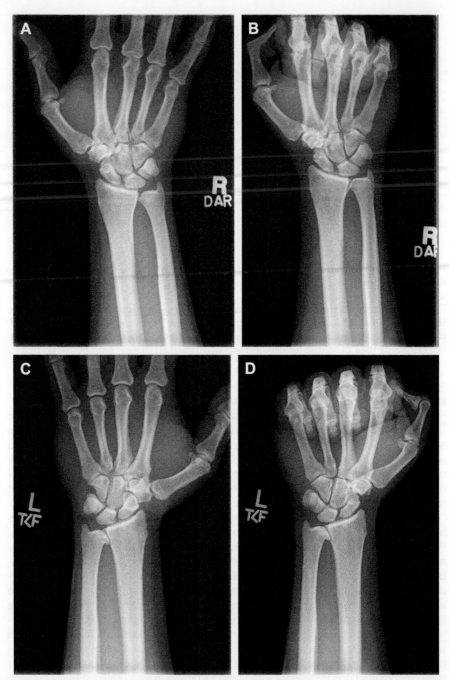

Fig. 15. AP radiograph (*A*) and dynamic clenched fist view (*B*) in patient with SLI ligament injury seen compared with contralateral unaffected side (*C, D*).

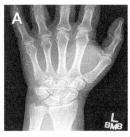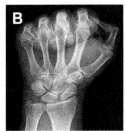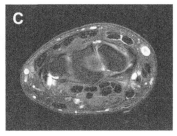

Fig. 16. Radiographs of an SLI ligament injury (*A*, *B*) better visualized on MRI (*C*).

Technical pearls

- A diagnostic algorithm for SLI ligament injuries guides treatment recommendations.
- The 3-lunotriquetral procedure replicates the action of 3 ligaments, including secondary stabilizers of the scapholunate articulation.

Thumb Metacarpophalangeal Joint Injuries

Gamekeeper's thumb was first described by Campbell[61] in 1955 as a mechanism for chronic ulnar thumb MCP ligament instability. An acute injury to the ulnar collateral ligament (UCL) has been described in skiers who sustain forced thumb abduction and hyperextension leading to rupture of the ligament or avulsion from its phalangeal attachment.[62] Patients complain of pain and swelling on the ulnar aspect of the MCP joint, which can be exacerbated when gripping a bat or racquet.

Suspected acute UCL injuries are tested in extension and flexion to assess the accessory and proper collateral ligaments, respectively (**Fig. 17**). Ligamentous laxity is compared with the contralateral side and graded. Rhee and colleagues[63] proposed an algorithm for evaluation and treatment of acute UCL ruptures using stress radiographs or advanced imaging in patients with equivocal examinations (**Fig. 18**). Nonoperative treatment of UCL injuries is generally limited to partial tears and nondisplaced avulsion fractures.[64] Sollerman and colleagues[65] found no difference between immobilization in a plaster thumb spica cast or a functional hinged splint. However, athletic participation may dictate the choice of immobilization used. Operative indications

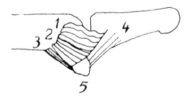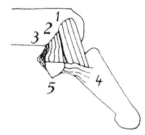

Fig. 17. The UCLs of the thumb MCP joint. In extension (*left*), the accessory collateral ligament (2) and volar plate (3) are taut, whereas the proper collateral ligament (1) is lax. In flexion (*right*), the proper collateral ligament is taut, whereas the accessory collateral ligament and volar plate are lax. The proximal phalanx (4) and sesamoid bone (5) are also shown. (*From* Stener B. Displacement of the ruptured ulnar collateral ligament of the metacarpophalangeal joint of the thumb. J Bone Joint Surg Br 1962;44:870; with permission.)

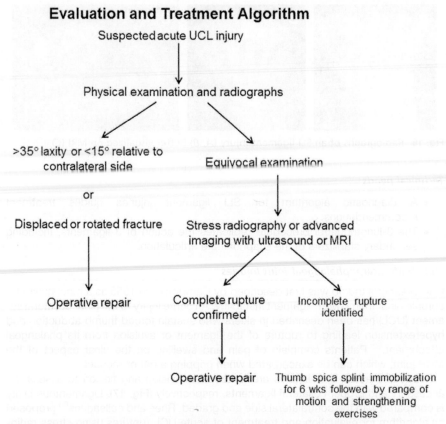

Evaluation and Treatment Algorithm

Suspected acute UCL injury

↓

Physical examination and radiographs

>35° laxity or <15° relative to contralateral side

or

Displaced or rotated fracture

Equivocal examination

↓

Stress radiography or advanced imaging with ultrasound or MRI

Operative repair

Complete rupture confirmed

Incomplete rupture identified

Operative repair

Thumb spica splint immobilization for 6 wks followed by range of motion and strengthening exercises

Fig. 18. Proposed algorithm for the evaluation and treatment of acute UCL ruptures. (*From* Rhee PC, Jones DB, Kakar S. Management of thumb metacarpophalangeal ulnar collateral ligament injuries. J Bone Joint Surg Am 2012;94(21):2008; with permission.)

generally include gross instability, displaced avulsion fractures, and Stener lesions, in which the UCL is displaced superficial to the adductor pollicis aponeurosis (**Fig. 19**). Several surgical options have been described. Those that allow early motion, such as with suture anchors or internal bracing, lead to improved early hand function and return to work. The goal of all operations is to perform an anatomic reduction of the ligament to bone so as not to alter the normal mechanics of the joint.

Chronic injuries are usually defined as being greater than 6 weeks from injury, but the emphasis on this classification should really be whether or not the ligament can be repaired primarily or needs a reconstruction. Static and dynamic stabilization procedures have been described for UCL reconstruction. For patients with chronic UCL injuries and a painful joint, arthrodesis may be recommended.

Technical pearls

- Stress radiographs or advanced imaging in patients suspected of UCL injuries be of value when the examination is equivocal.
- In addition to anatomic repair, augmentation with suture anchor fixation allows earlier motion and return to sport.
- Chronic injuries generally require reconstruction of the UCL.

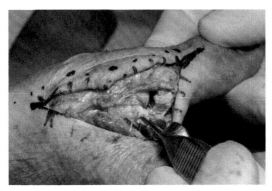

Fig. 19. Intraoperative photograph of a bony Stener lesion with an avulsed fracture fragment displaced superficial to the adductor pollicis aponeurosis.

Proximal Interphalangeal Joint Dislocations

Suboptimal outcomes following proximal interphalangeal (PIP) joint trauma are common owing to the neglect with which many coaches and clinicians approach such injuries. Joint dislocations can be purely ligamentous or associated with fracture, usually of the middle phalanx (**Fig. 20**). Dislocations involve at least one of the collateral ligaments

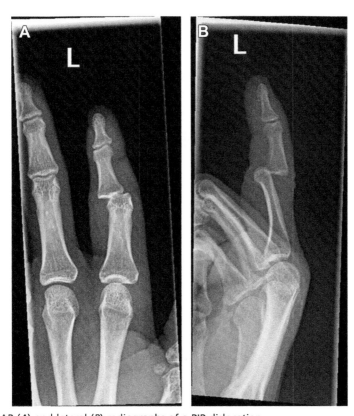

Fig. 20. AP (*A*) and lateral (*B*) radiographs of a PIP dislocation.

and may involve the volar plate or central slip, depending on the direction of displacement. Treatment is based on the stability of the joint. Dorsal dislocations are the most common and biomechanical studies have shown that the volar plate is the primary palmar PIP joint stabilizer. After reduction, it is not uncommon for these patients to be treated by their initial provider with splinting of the PIP joint. This may lead to permanent stiffness and early-protected motion (with buddy taping) is necessary to optimize outcomes. Open reduction of pure ligamentous injuries may be required in cases in which the volar plate is entrapped in the joint, prohibiting reduction of the joint.

For fracture-dislocations of the PIP joint, the primary goal of treatment in the athlete is restoration of middle phalanx rotation around the proximal phalangeal head. Early motion enhances joint function although minimizing contractures. Anatomic restoration of the joint surface is of secondary concern.[66] Eaton and Dray[67] demonstrated that fractures involving more than 40% of the articular surface are unstable and prone to dorsal instability. Extension block splinting allows for early motion because most PIP joints are stable in flexion. Therefore, the surgeon must critically evaluate the joint congruency to maximize motion while adequately constraining the joint to prevent subluxation. Dynamic traction, closed reduction and percutaneous fixation, open reduction, internal fixation, volar plate arthroplasty, interposition arthroplasty, and even arthrodesis have all been advocated for certain fracture dislocations (**Fig. 21**). Lack of appreciation of the seriousness of PIP joint injuries and overtreatment through prolonged immobilization are the common complications of this injury.

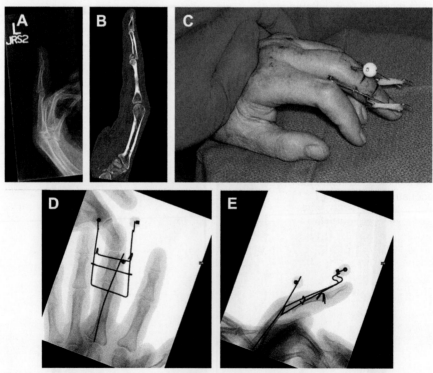

Fig. 21. Lateral radiograph (*A*) and a sagittal CT scan cut (*B*) of a PIP fracture dislocation treated with dynamic external fixation with extension block pinning (*C–E*). The treatment was complicated by a pin site infection.

TENDON INJURIES
Flexor Tendon Ruptures

Flexor tendon injuries are classified as being in 1 of 5 zones as determined by the location of the injury. Zone I injuries are distal to the flexor digitorum superficialis insertion and are termed jersey fingers (**Fig. 22**). The ring finger is most commonly involved because the distal interphalangeal (DIP) is forcibly extended against a maximally contracted FDP tendon (such as an athlete may suffer trying to grab the jersey of a fleeing opponent), resulting in avulsion of the FDP insertion. Patients present with pain and tenderness over the volar distal finger, which may lie in slight extension because the patients have no ability to actively flex the DIP joint. The retracted flexor tendon may be palpable in the proximal tendon sheath. Radiographs are recommended to identify any avulsion fractures.

Treatment of these injuries is operative with either direct repair of the tendon or reduced with the use of suture anchors or a button. The classification system by Leddy and Packer[68] incorporates the level of tendon retraction and the presence or absence of a fracture to guide treatment. Adequate balancing is critical because overtightening of the tendon may result in DIP flexion contracture or quadrigia, leaving the uninjured digits unable to fully flex.

Pulley Ruptures

Five annular and 3 cruciate pulleys reinforce the volar flexor tendon sheath. The A2 and A4 pulleys, which lie over the proximal and middle phalanx, respectively, are most important to maintaining flexor tendon excursion and strength. Rupture of the flexor tendon pulleys in the general population is rare, but may be seen more commonly in the ring fingers of rock climbers using the crimp position.[69] This position involves flexion of the PIP joints with hyperextension of the DIP joints, creating high tension in the flexor tendon pulleys. Most commonly, the A2 pulley is involved.[70] Pulley ruptures in the long finger of the throwing arm in baseball pitchers has also been described, with the A4 being the most commonly injured pulley.[71] Due to the rarity of this diagnosis, the sports physician must maintain a high index of suspicion of these lesions, which may present similar to flexor tenosynovitis on examination with pain and swelling. However, the injury is acute and often patients feel a pop and sudden pain. Bowstringing of the tendons may be evident on examination and the diagnosis is confirmed with MRI. Treatment is generally nonoperative with pulley ring splinting and nonsteroidal antiinflammatory medications. Operative pulley reconstruction is rarely indicated in isolation, but multiple pulley ruptures require reconstruction to prevent functional deficits.[70]

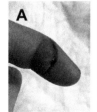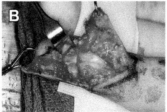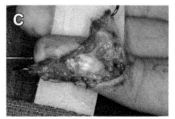

Fig. 22. Sharp flexor tendon laceration in zone 1 (*A*, *B*) treated with suture anchor fixation (*C*).

Extensor Mechanism Injuries

Similar to the flexor tendons, the extensor mechanism has been divided into 9 zones to better classify these injuries (**Fig. 23**). Knowledge of the extensor mechanism anatomy is critical to properly diagnose injuries to extensor mechanism, including central slip and mallet injuries. Zone 1 injuries involve the terminal tendon at the DIP joint and may result in a mallet finger as the joint is forced into flexion during active extension. Closed injuries with no or small fracture fragments may be treated with strict DIP extension splinting for 6 weeks, followed by nighttime extension splinting for another 4 to 6 weeks (**Fig. 24**).

Splinting may also be effective in the delayed (>4 weeks from injury) setting.[72] The goal of treatment is to achieve maximal active extension of the joint (minimizing extensor lag). Many splint options exist, but the key to successful treatment is patient compliance and education about the importance of maintaining DIP joint extension at all times. It may be prudent to see these patients in follow-up before 6 weeks to ensure strict adherence to the protocol, as well as to monitor for any skin changes from an ill-fitting splint. Stern and Kastrup[73] reported a 45% rate of complications in subjects splinted for the treatment of mallet finger. Most complications were skin related and nearly always transient.

Some injuries may require operative treatment, including open injuries or those with associated fracture-dislocations of the DIP joint. Primary repair of the terminal tendon

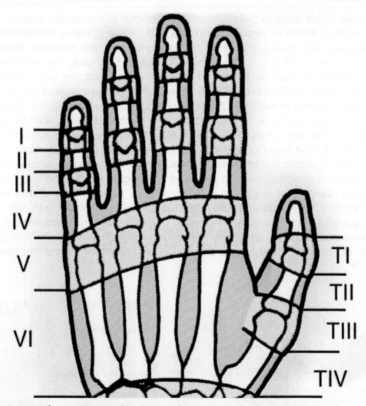

Fig. 23. Zones of extensor tendon injury. (*From* Strauch RJ. Extensor tendon injury. In: Wolfe S, Pederson W, Hotchkiss R, et al, editors. Green's operative hand surgery. 7th edition. Philadelphia: Elsevier; 2017. p. 158; with permission.)

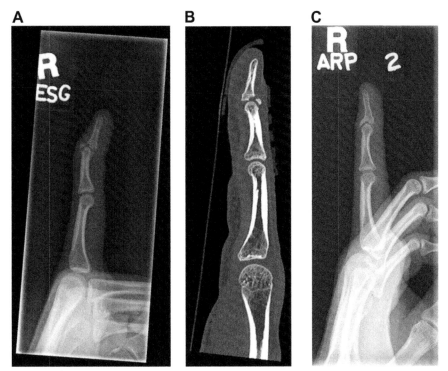

Fig. 24. Lateral radiograph (*A*) and a sagittal CT scan cut (*B*) of a mallet injury with a small bony fragment treated with DIP extension splinting. Four months after injury (*C*).

or repair with a pullout suture, button, or suture anchor is often supplemented with K-wire fixation to protect the repair. Failure to adequately address the terminal tendon may leave the patient with an extensor lag and drooping of the distal phalanx. Later, a swan neck deformity may develop when the imbalance of the PIP and DIP extension forces causes hyperextension of the PIP joint and flexion of the DIP joint.

SUMMARY

Hand and wrist injuries are common in athletes. Complications in the management of these sports injuries may be due to incorrect or delayed diagnosis, or iatrogenic injury related to the treatment itself. Matching the appropriate treatment to the correct diagnosis helps to avoid prolonged time away from sport and/or permanent disability.

REFERENCES

1. Rettig AC. Athletic injuries of the wrist and hand. Part I: traumatic injuries of the wrist. Am J Sports Med 2003;31(6):1038–48.
2. Nellans KW, Kowalski E, Chung KC. The epidemiology of distal radius fractures. Hand Clin 2012;28(2):113–25.
3. Medoff RJ. Essential radiographic evaluation for distal radius fractures. Hand Clin 2005;21(3):279–88.
4. Mackenney PJ, McQueen MM, Elton R. Prediction of instability in distal radial fractures. J Bone Joint Surg Am 2006;88(9):1944–51.

5. Lafontaine M, Hardy D, Delince P. Stability assessment of distal radius fractures. Injury 1989;20(4):208–10.
6. Roth KM, Blazar PE, Earp BE, et al. Incidence of extensor pollicis longus tendon rupture after nondisplaced distal radius fractures. J Hand Surg Am 2012;37(5): 942–7.
7. Orbay JL, Fernandez DL. Volar fixation for dorsally displaced fractures of the distal radius: a preliminary report. J Hand Surg 2002;27(2):205–15.
8. Orbay JL, Badia A, Indriago IR, et al. The extended flexor carpi radialis approach: a new perspective for the distal radius fracture. Tech Hand Up Extrem Surg 2001;5(4):204–11.
9. Soong M, Earp BE, Bishop G, et al. Volar locking plate implant prominence and flexor tendon rupture. J Bone Joint Surg Am 2011;93(4):328–35.
10. Jacob J, Clay N. Re: Pichler et al. Computer tomography aided 3D analysis of the distal dorsal radius surface and the effects on volar plate osteosynthesis. J Hand Surg Eur. 2009, 34: 598-602. J Hand Surg Eur Vol 2010;35(4):335–6.
11. Wall LB, Brodt MD, Silva MJ, et al. The effects of screw length on stability of simulated osteoporotic distal radius fractures fixed with volar locking plates. J Hand Surg Am 2012;37(3):446–53.
12. Van Tassel DC, Owens BD, Wolf JM. Incidence estimates and demographics of scaphoid fracture in the U.S. population. J Hand Surg 2010;35(8):1242–5.
13. Bond CD, Shin AY, McBride MT, et al. Percutaneous screw fixation or cast immobilization for nondisplaced scaphoid fractures. J Bone Joint Surg Am 2001;83(4): 483–8.
14. Belsky MR, Leibman MI, Ruchelsman DE. Scaphoid fracture in the elite athlete. Hand Clin 2012;28(3):269–78.
15. Suh N, Benson EC, Faber KJ, et al. Treatment of acute scaphoid fractures: a systematic review and meta-analysis. Hand (N Y) 2010;5(4):345–53.
16. Buijze GA, Ochtman L, Ring D. Management of scaphoid nonunion. J Hand Surg Am 2012;37(5):1095–100 [quiz: 1101].
17. Langhoff O, Andersen J. Consequences of late immobilization of scaphoid fracture. J Hand Surg Br 1988;13(1):77–9.
18. Gaebler C, Kukla C, Breitenseher M, et al. Magnetic resonance imaging of occult scaphoid fractures. J Trauma Acute Care Surg 1996;41(1):73–6.
19. Slade JF 3rd, Grauer JN, Mahoney JD. Arthroscopic reduction and percutaneous fixation of scaphoid fractures with a novel dorsal technique. Orthop Clin North Am 2001;32(2):247–61.
20. Dodds SD, Panjabi MM, Slade JF 3rd. Screw fixation of scaphoid fractures: a biomechanical assessment of screw length and screw augmentation. J Hand Surg 2006;31(3):405–13.
21. Moon ES, Dy CJ, Derman P, et al. Management of nonunion following surgical management of scaphoid fractures: current concepts. J Am Acad Orthop Surg 2013;21(9):548–57.
22. Kakar S, Bishop AT, Shin AY. Role of vascularized bone grafts in the treatment of scaphoid nonunions associated with proximal pole avascular necrosis and carpal collapse. J Hand Surg 2011;36(4):722–5.
23. Fisk GR. Carpal instability and the fractured scaphoid. Ann R Coll Surg Engl 1970;46(2):63.
24. Smith BS, Cooney WP. Revision of failed bone grafting for nonunion of the scaphoid: treatment options and results. Clin Orthop Relat Res 1996;(327): 98–109.

25. Woo S-H, Lee Y-K, Kim J-M, et al. Hand and wrist injuries in Golfers and their treatment. Hand Clin 2017;33(1):81–96.

26. Wright TW, Moser MW, Sahajpal DT. Hook of hamate pull test. J Hand Surg 2010; 35(11):1887–9.

27. Andresen R, Radmer S, Sparmann M, et al. Imaging of hamate bone fractures in conventional x-rays and high-resolution computed tomography: an in vitro study. Invest Radiol 1999;34(1):46–50.

28. Bishop AT, Beckenbaugh RD. Fracture of the hamate hook. J Hand Surg 1988; 13(1):135–9.

29. Demirkan F, Calandruccio JH, DiAngelo D. Biomechanical evaluation of flexor tendon function after hamate hook excision. J Hand Surg 2003;28(1):138–43.

30. Yamazaki H, Kato H, Nakatsuchi Y, et al. Closed rupture of the flexor tendons of the little finger secondary to non-union of fractures of the hook of the hamate. J Hand Surg Br 2006;31(3):337–41.

31. Fleege MA, Jebson PJ, Renfrew DL, et al. Pisiform fractures. Skeletal Radiol 1991;20(3):169–72.

32. Palmieri TJ. Pisifform area pain treatment by pisiform excision. J Hand Surg 1982; 7(5):477–80.

33. Matsunaga D, Uchiyama S, Nakagawa H, et al. Lower ulnar nerve palsy related to fracture of the pisiform bone in patients with multiple injuries. J Trauma Acute Care Surg 2002;53(2):364–8.

34. Howard FM. Ulnar-nerve palsy in wrist fractures. J Bone Joint Surg Am 1961; 43(8):1197–201.

35. Fufa DT, Goldfarb CA. Fractures of the thumb and finger metacarpals in athletes. Hand Clin 2012;28(3):379–88.

36. Naik AA, Hinds RM, Paksima N, et al. Risk of injury to the dorsal sensory branch of the ulnar nerve with percutaneous pinning of ulnar-sided structures. J Hand Surg 2016;41(7):e159–63.

37. Strauch RJ, Rosenwasser MP, Lunt JG. Metacarpal shaft fractures: the effect of shortening on the extensor tendon mechanism. J Hand Surg 1998;23(3):519–23.

38. Meunier MJ, Hentzen E, Ryan M, et al. Predicted effects of metacarpal shortening on interosseous muscle function. J Hand Surg 2004;29(4):689–93.

39. Royle S. Rotational deformity following metacarpal fracture. J Hand Surg Br 1990; 15(1):124–5.

40. Niechajev I. Dislocated intra-articular fracture of the base of the fifth metacarpal: a clinical study of 23 patients. Plast Reconstr Surg 1985;75(3):406–10.

41. Kakar S, Garcia-Elias M. The "four-leaf clover" treatment algorithm: a practical approach to manage disorders of the distal radioulnar joint. J Hand Surg 2016; 41(4):551–64.

42. Tay SC, Berger RA, Parker WL. Longitudinal split tears of the ulnotriquetral ligament. Hand Clin 2010;26(4):495–501.

43. Potter HG, Asnis-Ernberg L, Weiland AJ, et al. The utility of high-resolution magnetic resonance imaging in the evaluation of the triangular fibrocartilage complex of the wrist. J Bone Joint Surg Am 1997;79(11):1675–84.

44. Greene RM, Kakar S. The suction test: a novel technique to identify and verify successful repair of peripheral triangular fibrocartilage complex tears. J Wrist Surg 2017;6(4):334–5.

45. Ko JH, Wiedrich TA. Triangular fibrocartilage complex injuries in the elite athlete. Hand Clin 2012;28(3):307–21.

46. Minami A, Ishikawa JI, Suenaga N, et al. Clinical results of treatment of triangular fibrocartilage complex tears by arthroscopic debridement. J Hand Surg Am 1996;21(3):406–11.

47. Ahsan ZS, Yao J. Complications of wrist arthroscopy. Arthroscopy 2012;28(6): 855–9.

48. Bernstein MA, Nagle DJ, Martinez A, et al. A comparison of combined arthroscopic triangular fibrocartilage complex debridement and arthroscopic wafer distal ulna resection versus arthroscopic triangular fibrocartilage complex debridement and ulnar shortening osteotomy for ulnocarpal abutment syndrome. Arthroscopy 2004;20(4):392–401.

49. Berger RA. The gross and histologic anatomy of the scapholunate interosseous ligament. J Hand Surg 1996;21(2):170–8.

50. Watson HK, Ashmead D, Makhlouf MV. Examination of the scaphoid. J Hand Surg 1988;13(5):657–60.

51. Garcia-Elias M, Lluch AL, Stanley JK. Three-ligament tenodesis for the treatment of scapholunate dissociation: indications and surgical technique. J Hand Surg 2006;31(1):125–34.

52. Darlis NA, Weiser RW, Sotereanos DG. Partial scapholunate ligament injuries treated with arthroscopic debridement and thermal shrinkage. J Hand Surg 2005;30(5):908–14.

53. Lavernia CJ, Cohen MS, Taleisnik J. Treatment of scapholunate dissociation by ligamentous repair and capsulodesis. J Hand Surg 1992;17(2):354–9.

54. Wyrick JD, Youse BD, Kiefhaber TR. Scapholunate ligament repair and capsulodesis for the treatment of static scapholunate dissociation. J Hand Surg Br 1998; 23(6):776–80.

55. Weiss AP. Scapholunate ligament reconstruction using a bone-retinaculum-bone autograft. J Hand Surg 1998;23(2):205–15.

56. Short WH, Werner FW, Green JK, et al. Biomechanical evaluation of the ligamentous stabilizers of the scaphoid and lunate: part III. J Hand Surg Am 2007;32(3): 297–309.

57. Slater RR Jr, Szabo RM. Scapholunate dissociation: treatment with the dorsal intercarpal ligament capsulodesis. Tech Hand Up Extrem Surg 1999;3(4):222–8.

58. Berger RA, Bishop AT, Bettinger PC. New dorsal capsulotomy for the surgical exposure of the wrist. Ann Plast Surg 1995;35(1):54–9.

59. Watson HK, Ballet FL. The SLAC wrist: scapholunate advanced collapse pattern of degenerative arthritis. J Hand Surg 1984;9(3):358–65.

60. O'Meeghan CJ, Stuart W, Mamo V, et al. The natural history of an untreated isolated scapholunate interosseus ligament injury. J Hand Surg Br 2003;28(4): 307–10.

61. Campbell C. Gamekeeper's thumb. J Bone Joint Surg Br 1955;37(1):148–9.

62. Schultz R, Fox J. Gamekeeper's thumb. Result of skiing injuries. N Y State J Med 1973;73(19):2329–31.

63. Rhee PC, Jones DB, Kakar S. Management of thumb metacarpophalangeal ulnar collateral ligament injuries. J Bone Joint Surg Am 2012;94(21):2005–12.

64. Abrahamsson SO, Sollerman C, Lundborg G, et al. Diagnosis of displaced ulnar collateral ligament of the metacarpophalangeal joint of the thumb. J Hand Surg 1990;15(3):457–60.

65. Sollerman C, Abrahamsson SO, Lundborg G, et al. Functional splinting versus plaster cast for ruptures of the ulnar collateral ligament of the thumb. A prospective randomized study of 63 cases. Acta Orthop Scand 1991;62(6):524–6.

66. Kiefhaber TR, Stern PJ. Fracture dislocations of the proximal interphalangeal joint. J Hand Surg 1998;23(3):368–80.
67. Eaton R, Dray G. Dislocations and ligament injuries in the digits. Operative Hand Surgery 1982;1:637–68.
68. Leddy JP, Packer JW. Avulsion of the profundus tendon insertion in athletes. J Hand Surg Am 1977;2(1):66–9.
69. Bollen SR. Soft tissue injury in extreme rock climbers. Br J Sports Med 1988; 22(4):145–7.
70. Schoffl V, Hochholzer T, Winkelmann HP, et al. Pulley injuries in rock climbers. Wilderness Environ Med 2003;14(2):94–100.
71. Lourie GM, Hamby Z, Raasch WG, et al. Annular flexor pulley injuries in professional baseball pitchers: a case series. Am J Sports Med 2011;39(2):421–4.
72. Garberman SF, Diao E, Peimer CA. Mallet finger: results of early versus delayed closed treatment. J Hand Surg 1994;19(5):850–2.
73. Stern PJ, Kastrup JJ. Complications and prognosis of treatment of mallet finger. J Hand Surg 1988;13(3):329–34.

Hip Arthroscopy
Common Problems and Solutions

Aaron Casp, MD, Frank Winston Gwathmey, MD*

KEYWORDS

- Hip arthroscopy • Femoroacetabular impingement • Labral tear • Femoroplasty
- Capsule

KEY POINTS

- Patient selection is fundamental to ensuring good clinical outcomes after hip arthroscopy.
- Understanding the anatomy around the hip joint, in particular the anatomy of the lateral femoral cutaneous nerve and femoral neurovascular bundle, helps to reduce iatrogenic nerve injury.
- Traction-related complications are unique to hip arthroscopy and careful application and use of traction helps to mitigate potential problems.
- The most common reason for failure of hip arthroscopy for femoroacetabular impingement is inadequate correction of the deformity.
- Recovery after hip arthroscopy is highly variable and a systematic rehabilitation protocol is essential to optimize outcomes.

INTRODUCTION

Hip arthroscopy is becoming more common for an expanding array of indications as surgeons become more comfortable with techniques and instrumentation improves. A recent study showed a 250% increase in hip arthroscopic procedures between 2007 and 2011.[1] The increasing use of this procedure has revealed complications and reasons for poor outcomes. Ultimately, a successful outcome depends on establishing a systematic algorithm for evaluation and treatment of patients and meticulously and efficiently executing the surgical plan. Understanding and avoiding potential pitfalls and complications becomes paramount to optimize clinical outcomes and for the safety of the patient. This article outlines factors that contribute to less-than-favorable outcomes and summarizes potential complications associated with hip arthroscopy.

PREOPERATIVE FACTORS

Successful hip arthroscopy starts in the clinic, and choosing the correct patient as well as the correct surgery are the most important factors affecting surgical outcome.

Disclosure: The authors have nothing to disclose.
Department of Orthopaedic Surgery, University of Virginia, University of Virginia Health System, 400 Ray C. Hunt, Suite 330, Charlottesville, VA 22903, USA
* Corresponding author.
E-mail address: fwg7d@virginia.edu

Ensuring the correct diagnosis is fundamental to planning a successful surgery. It is also important to identify those who are at high risk for failed surgery or complications.

Asymptomatic Radiographic Findings

When working up a patient for hip pain, it is important to keep in mind that there are many pain generators around the hip, and that a broad differential diagnosis should be taken into account. This is especially true if a patient is referred in from an outside provider with radiographic imaging consistent with femoroacetabular impingement (FAI). Radiographic findings of FAI morphology among asymptomatic adults and adolescents are common, with one study showing cam morphology in as many as 14% of asymptomatic volunteers.[2–4] In the preoperative evaluation and work-up, the surgeon should not focus solely on the radiographic findings, because they may not be the source of pain. There can be other disorders as pain generators, and not necessarily the FAI that was identified radiographically. The common asymptomatic radiographic FAI could lead to an operation that not only fails to address the cause of pain but also places the patient at risk for intraoperative and postoperative complications with no clinical benefit. It is critical for surgeons to have a systematic algorithm to ensure that the correct diagnosis is made and the offending disorder is addressed.

Hip Dysplasia

Underlying structural abnormalities that may diminish the efficacy of arthroscopic treatment should be recognized before proceeding with surgery. The most common condition that might contribute to the disorder, as well as being problematic in treating the patient, is developmental dysplasia of the hip (DDH) (**Fig. 1**). In patients with DDH, the labrum may undergo compensatory hypertrophy to increase the relative volume of the hip. This hypertrophy, in combination with the abnormal contact forces in the dysplastic hip, can cause the labrum to degenerate, develop cystic changes, and tear.[5–7] Although hip arthroscopy might be able to address the resultant labral disorder, it is merely indicative of an underlying problem. The underlying structural disorder in DDH cannot be addressed arthroscopically and could potentially be exacerbated by violation of the soft tissue structures around the hip.

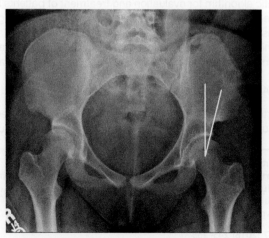

Fig. 1. Lateral center edge angle of less than 20° indicates dysplasia. Hip arthroscopy in the setting of dysplasia is associated with inferior outcomes and increased risk of complications.

Hip arthroscopy outcomes in patients with mild DDH are mixed. Individuals with moderate to severe DDH are not adequately treated with arthroscopy alone, and may require reorientation of the acetabulum to restore normal joint mechanics and forces across the hip.[8,9] An arthroscopic procedure may be able to help correct some of the dynamic impingement or microinstability, but it cannot address the static joint overload that is present in the malformed hip joint. Furthermore, excessive debridement can make these patients worse by causing macroinstability, catastrophic dislocations, or rapid progression of arthritis.[10] Arthroscopic labral debridement in patients with underlying dysplasia is likely to lead to more rapid degradation of the remaining labrum and places greater stress on the articular cartilage, making the patient worse off overall.[11]

Because of the many potential pitfalls of performing hip arthroscopy on patients with underlying hip dysplasia, it is paramount that physicians recognize this preoperatively. The structure of the hip joint can be initially evaluated with plain radiographs, or computed tomography (CT) scan for further evaluation of bony architecture if unsure. Although some of the labral disorder may be addressed arthroscopically, patients are unlikely to get durable relief from an arthroscopic procedure alone, and this may accelerate their joint degeneration. Overall, unrecognized hip dysplasia can lead to failure of clinical improvement and postoperative complications.

Preexisting Osteoarthritis

There is increasing evidence that preoperative joint space narrowing and osteoarthritis are negative predictors of a good clinical outcome after hip arthroscopy, and may predict rates of conversion to a total hip arthroplasty[12–18] (**Fig. 2**). Larson and colleagues[12] stratified clinical outcomes of hip arthroscopy with varying levels of preexisting osteoarthritis and hip disorder, finding a failure rate of 12% with FAI alone, 33% in patients with joint space narrowing, and 82% in patients with advanced preoperative joint space narrowing. Harris and colleagues[18] found total hip arthroplasty as the most common reason for reoperation, whereas others have found that 10-year survivorship of hip arthroscopy was only 12% to 20% for Outerbridge grades III and IV osteoarthritis, compared with 80% for Outerbridge grades 0, I, or II.[17]

All of the existing literature has shown the importance of osteoarthritis on clinical outcomes after hip arthroscopy, and can inform surgeons regarding operative

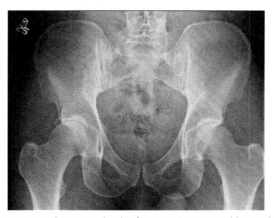

Fig. 2. Inferior outcomes and increased risk of conversion to total hip arthroplasty are seen with hip joint spaces of less than 2 mm.

indications and expectations counseling. Overall, surgeons should be aware of the much higher failure rate of hip arthroscopy in patients with baseline osteoarthritis or joint degeneration before undertaking a hip arthroscopy procedure. This awareness can lead to much better clinical outcomes for the patients and a more satisfied patient population.

Obesity

As the obesity epidemic in the United States continues to grow, it will inevitably influence surgical patients from all fields. Recent literature has shown it to be a well-known risk factor for a host of complications after most orthopedic surgical procedures.[19–21] This can cause particular issues with hip arthroscopy as well, because obese patients may be at greater than 11 times higher odds for developing a complication after hip arthroscopy, despite similar traction and operative times.[22]

This observation is not to say that these patients do not get clinical benefit from the procedure. Gupta and colleagues[23] showed that, although obese patients have lower baseline functional hip scores, their clinical improvement after hip arthroscopy is on par with those patients who are not obese. Therefore, although this patient group has been found to be at greater risk for postoperative complications for all hip arthroscopic procedures and all other orthopedic subspecialties, no high-quality long-term studies exist in the hip arthroscopy realm.

INTRAOPERATIVE FACTORS

Once a patient has been indicated for surgery, the clinical outcome depends on executing the surgical plan meticulously and efficiently. Several intraoperative factors should be considered when performing hip arthroscopy.

Patient positioning is a crucial step to success during surgery. Hip arthroscopy has particular positioning needs that must be considered in order to adequately visualize, navigate, and instrument the hip joint. Careful patient positioning also helps minimize the most common postoperative complications from hip arthroscopy.

Distraction of the hip joint is necessary for access into the central compartment and acetabulum, most commonly using a specialized traction table. This pulling force on the patient's legs can be responsible for many of the common postoperative complications.

Traction-Related Complications

Mechanical traction is needed to separate the femoral head from the acetabulum during hip arthroscopy, which provides adequate working space to introduce arthroscope and instruments. This force is generally applied through a specialized surgical table that is capable of applying traction through the foot or lower leg. This traction can place tension on the soft tissues, leading to traction injuries of the femoral and sciatic nerves, which are the most commonly reported complications in hip arthroscopy, reaching rates of 7% in small series.[24–26] These traction injuries are generally transient neurapraxias caused by the traction that has been applied, especially with prolonged surgical procedures or excessive traction force.

To prevent these traction-type injuries, minimizing the duration of traction and positioning the hip in slight flexion can help relax the anterior capsule and anterior structures. Excessive flexion or extension and traction can endanger the sciatic or femoral nerves.[27] It is generally recommended that traction time not exceed 2 hours, and that intermittent traction be used if a longer time is necessary.[28,29] In order to minimize the traction force necessary and ensure appropriate positioning, a trial of traction has been suggested. This trial involves temporarily applying enough traction to ensure a distractible hip joint before prepping and draping the operative extremity. Once this is confirmed, the traction is released until it is needed during the operation.[27]

Traction neurapraxias are usually benign complications and have generally been found to be transient, resolving within minutes to hours of completion of the procedure.[27,28,30,31] The sciatic and femoral nerves are most at risk for this type of injury, but prolonged sequelae have not been reported.

Another aspect of traction that can cause complications is the use of the perineal post. This post is generally necessary to provide a counterforce to the traction being applied through the limbs, as well as to help provide a traction vector along the femoral neck. Although this aids in visualization, it also applies pressure on the groin, which may put the pudendal nerve at risk. This pressure can also compromise the soft tissues, including scrotal or labial edema, hematoma formation, or even pressure necrosis.[30,32,33] The orthopedic trauma literature has multiple accounts of traction-related complications, such as neurapraxia, pressure necrosis, or even crush syndrome. These complications were attributed to prolonged traction or a malpositioned perineal post.[34] In one study, the pudendal nerve injury was not correlated with duration of traction but with the force of the traction applied.[35]

There are tactics that surgeons can use to avoid these compressive injuries when using a perineal post. These tactics include ensuring that the post is well padded; using a post with a diameter of at least 9 cm to distribute the force over a larger portion of the leg; and to ensure that the pressure is being placed through the medial thigh, and not the groin or genitalia[25,28,36] (**Fig. 3**). Using muscle relaxants as part of anesthesia can be helpful in minimizing the amount of traction force that is needed for articular distraction and adequate visualization intraoperatively, and minimizing traction time with an absolute cutoff time of 2 hours being suggested.[37,38]

Because of the risk of these complications, techniques have been developed to perform the hip arthroscopy without the use of a perineal post. This technique showed no complications in a small group of patients, using alternative methods for securing the patient, and this questioned the notion that a lateralizing force must be applied in the vector of the femoral neck.[37] However, use of a perineal post remains the current standard technique for performing this surgical procedure.

Pressure on the ipsilateral ankle or foot is another potential traction-related complication, especially when using a boot. This site of injury is far from the operative site, often under the surgical drapes, and can easily be overlooked intraoperatively. An overly tight-fitting boot, especially in thin patients, can cause sensation issues in the superficial peroneal nerve distribution, as well as vascular obstruction issues.[39,40]

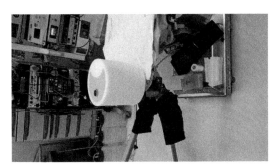

Fig. 3. An oversized perineal post helps to distribute force on the perineum and decrease pressure on the pudendal nerve.

The patient's foot should be well padded, especially around any bony prominences or sites of potential neurovascular compression.

Portal Placement–Related Complications

Although the need for intra-articular visualization often dictates portal placement, the hip joint is surrounded by several important neurovascular structures that can be damaged by portal incisions and manipulation. The femoral neurovascular bundle is present anteriorly, the lateral femoral cutaneous nerve (LFCN) anterolaterally, and the sciatic and gluteal vessels posteriorly.

The LFCN is the structure in closest proximity to the standard portal placement and at the highest risk for direct injury. Its course lies very close to the anterior portal, which traditionally is in line with anterior superior iliac spine.[25] Because of the risk of damaging the LFCN with the anterior portal, most practitioners use a modified anterior portal or midanterior portal, which can be placed a centimeter or more lateral to the anterior portal placement.[24,41] The LFCN can have an arborized branching pattern, so it is good practice whenever making a portal not to use stab incisions but instead cut only dermis and spread bluntly to create a window for the arthroscopic portal to minimize the risk of postoperative sensation changes.[41]

Although the LFCN is well known to be the most at-risk structure from a portal placement standpoint, many patients have some numbness to the anterolateral thigh following hip arthroscopy. Many of these reported cases are transient neurapraxia from traction or manipulation near the nerve, but direct laceration remains a possibility. The overall incidence of this complication has been hard to define. One series found the risk of injury to the LFCN or its branches using the traditional anterior portal to be 0.5%,[42] whereas other investigators have placed it somewhere between 1% and 10% and believe it is under-reported.[43] If lacerated, the nerve function often does not recover.[44,45] Even though the incidence and the morbidity associated with LFCN injury are small, patients should be counseled appropriately preoperatively.

Damage to the femoral and sciatic neurovascular bundles is a much rarer phenomenon, with only sparse case reports present in the literature. Applying traction may tension and lateralize these structures, placing them at higher risk for iatrogenic injury.[46,47] However, these structures should be well outside the working area for hip arthroscopy, even when performing acetabuloplasty and femoroplasty, and the overall safety of the traditional working portals for hip arthroscopy has been established.[41] There has been a single case report of a catastrophic result from an incorrectly placed posterolateral portal, which resulted in a severed inferior gluteal artery and permanent neurologic dysfunction caused by compressive hematoma on the sciatic nerve.[48] The femoral neurovascular structures can be avoided by making it a practice to not place a portal medial to the line connecting the anterior superior iliac spine (ASIS) down the femoral shaft.

Iatrogenic Chondral and Labral Damage

Because of the overall shape of the hip joint and difficulty with direct access, iatrogenic damage to the chondral surface or the acetabular labrum can occur (**Fig. 4**). It is thought that minor damage occurs with high frequency but is under-reported.[49]

When making the anterolateral portal, the superior labrum may be punctured. Even though this is performed using a modified Seldinger technique, it is not foolproof. The Byrd sign, or distal movement of the spinal needle with injection of saline, has been described to help ensure that the initial stick is not through the labrum, but it may have a high false-positive rate.[50,51] Although the rate of inadvertent labral punctures may be high, there is no evidence that these affect clinical results.[51]

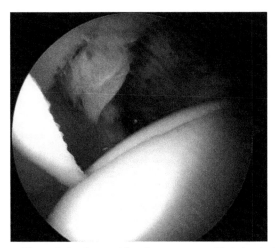

Fig. 4. Iatrogenic scuffing of the femoral head may occur with introduction of the spinal needle or cannulas.

Chondral scuffing generally affects the femoral head, and may be caused by the arthroscopist struggling for access in the setting of inadequate visualization from too little traction.[31,52] The rate of mild chondral scuffing has been described at 3%, primarily from instrument maneuvering.[52] These partial-thickness cartilage lesions are likely more common than reported and generally do not have any appreciable functional sequelae.[28,31] To avoid significant chondral undermining from portal placement, one trick is to ensure that the bevel of the spinal needle is facing the femoral head on insertion.

Overall, it seems that iatrogenic injury to the femoral chondral surface or acetabular labrum is common when placing portals or maneuvering instruments within the joint, but this may just be an incidental part of the procedure and has not been shown to negatively affect outcomes.

Iatrogenic Instability

Instability after hip arthroscopy can be related to damage to 1 or more of the hip stabilizers, and therefore loss of normal mechanics. Hip stability relies on a combination of osseous anatomy, acetabular labrum, and ligamentous hip capsule. When these structures are disrupted, instability, pain, or functional limitations can occur. When performing a surgical correction, intraoperative compromise of the acetabular-sided constraints can lead to instability. This compromise includes excessive resection or damage to any of the aforementioned stabilizers, including the anterior capsule and iliofemoral ligament, the acetabular labrum, or the bony acetabular rim during treatment of pincer impingement from a wide capsulotomy or aggressive labrectomy (**Fig. 5**).

The acetabular labrum is important for maintenance of hip stability, ensuring articular fluid seal, and helping modulate intra-articular lubrication and fluid pressure, which in turn protects the articular cartilage.[53–55]

As arthroscopic techniques improve and the biomechanical outcomes of hip arthroscopy are becoming more widely understood, labral resection and debridement have poorer functional outcomes with regard to those who underwent a labral

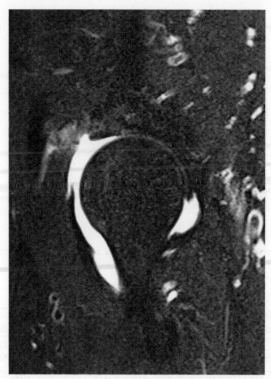

Fig. 5. Excessive capsular resection may lead to postoperative problems from capsular deficiency.

repair.[56–58] As labral repair becomes more standard of care, aggressive labrectomy as a cause for instability should become less common.

However, even during a labral repair, some labral debridement is necessary, and classically the labrum was detached to expose the acetabular rim.[59] This technique could theoretically lead to loss of normal hip stability, and constraint, and some clinicians have assessed the efficacy of preserving the chondrolabral junction when possible.[60] There are currently no good data in the literature to show that preserving the chondrolabral junction or fully detaching the labrum is superior or has differing clinical outcomes. Either way, the labrum has proved to serve a critical role in maintaining normal joint mechanics, so it is preferable to preserve it, if possible.

Matsuda[61] reported a patient with an anterior hip dislocation in the recovery room from anterior capsular excision and labral debridement, which was eventually converted to open capsular repair because of refractory instability. Other reports of instability exist in the literature, caused by some other underlying factor such as hip dysplasia or ligamentous laxity, but all suggest the utmost importance of preserving the labrum as a stabilizer and for longevity of the joint.[11,62,63]

Although frank instability is a rare complication, there are common features from these reports in the literature: female gender, narrow age range (late 30s to early 50s), occurrence either immediately or in the first few weeks, and anterior direction.[61–64] Much of the same literature recommends repair of the anterior capsule if there is any concern for predisposing factors for hip instability.

Inadequate Correction and Residual Femoroacetabular Impingement

Incomplete or inadequate surgical correction of FAI and persistent bony deformity have been identified as the primary reasons for revision hip arthroscopy[15,65,66] (**Fig. 6**). Philippon and colleagues[66] found that up to 97% of the patients in their series had radiographic evidence of residual FAI after arthroscopy. Others have found high rates of poor symptomatic improvement and residual FAI after initial arthroscopy, and that residual FAI is a common indication for revision surgery.[67,68] In a study including 3957 patients who underwent a hip arthroscopy, Kester and colleagues[69] found that the failure rate for all-comers was 9.7%, with 5.9% of patients being converted to total hip arthroplasty within 14.7 months. There is also evidence that lower-volume arthroscopists have higher rates of failure necessitating revision arthroscopy and higher conversion to total hip arthroplasty, suggesting incomplete or inadequate correction is associated with experience.

Preoperatively, thorough patient radiographic work-up, knowledge of the pathologic anatomy, and careful planning are necessary in order to fully understand and localize the areas of bony impingement that will be targeted during surgery. Practitioners often use cross-sectional imaging, including CT and magnetic resonance arthrography, in conjunction with several plain radiographic views in order to best understand the morphology of the proximal femur.[70,71]

Thorough intraoperative evaluation is necessary to confirm that bony resection is complete and to rule out any persistent bony impingement. Use of an image intensifier both preoperatively and intraoperatively is recommended for evaluating the adequacy of the bony decompression. The preoperative images can be compared with those taken intraoperatively to assess any residual FAI and evaluate completeness of the femoroplasty or acetabuloplasty.[72,73] When the surgeon believes the bony resection

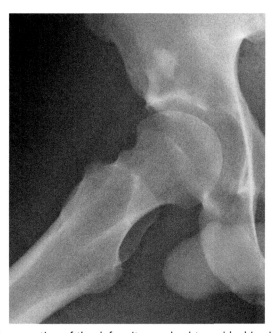

Fig. 6. Inadequate correction of the deformity may lead to residual impingement and is a common cause for revision hip arthroscopy. Intraoperative inspection with multiple fluoroscopic views is important to ensure complete correction.

has been completed, dynamic hip range of motion should be performed in extension, abduction, internal and external rotation, flexion abduction external rotation (FABER), and flexion adduction internal rotation (FADIR), as well as around-the-world views to fully evaluate the head-neck junction of the femur and residual cam deformity. The critical fluoroscopic images have been described by Ross and colleagues[73] in order to ensure thorough correction.

Obtaining these fluoroscopic views often requires fully mobilizing the foot and ankle and removing it from the secured traction apparatus. Although this may be tricky to perform while maintaining sterility of the surgical field, they are necessary to ensure that all points of preoperative bony impingement have been addressed. As with most technical aspects of surgery, there is a learning curve to this process, and adequacy of bony debridement and resultant functional hip scores have been correlated with surgeon experience.[74]

SURGICAL COMPLICATIONS
Fluid Extravasation

As with most arthroscopic procedures, visualization is improved from joint distension and bleeding tamponade effect by using irrigation fluid. This fluid may leak into the spaces around the joint, and significant extravasation into other anatomic spaces around the hip joint can be a dangerous complication. Fluid escapes from the capsulotomy incisions that are performed as a routine part of hip arthroscopy, but most reported cases of significant consequences from this extravasation involved some extracapsular procedure such as release of the iliopsoas tendon.[75–79] This fluid extravasation has been associated with prolonged surgical time, as well as with higher arthroscopic fluid pump pressures.[75,79,80] Although there is always some fluid extravasation during arthroscopic procedures using irrigation, one study measured a mean extravasation of 1132 mL into the periarticular tissues during a routine hip arthroscopy without negative sequelae.[81]

It is thought that exposure of the iliopsoas tendon sheath and iliac vessels provides a conduit for fluid to flow into the retroperitoneum. If this fluid tracks into the abdominal or retroperitoneal cavity, abdominal compartment syndrome can result, which has significant morbidity and mortality. If left untreated, intra-abdominal hypertension or abdominal compartment syndrome can progress to profound hemodynamic instability, end-organ failure, and even death. Thankfully, intra-abdominal fluid extravasation is rare; one survey found a 0.16% prevalence among 25,648 hip arthroscopies,[80] and there are only a few case reports of full abdominal compartment syndrome or serious sequelae in the literature.[77,79]

In general, an abdominal compartment syndrome diagnosis is made by serial physical examination, careful monitoring of hemodynamic status, intra-abdominal pressure measurement, and intra-abdominal imaging.[82] This diagnosis is not generally feasible when performing a hip arthroscopy, especially because this is done under general anesthesia and the surgical drapes may hide some of the telltale signs. If there is significant abdominal distension, subcutaneous edema, hypothermia, or change in vital signs noted by the physician or anesthesiologists, these may be clues. Signs of increased fluid extravasation during the procedure should also be a warning, such as difficulty keeping the joint distended, increased irrigation fluid requirements, or pump irrigation pressure warnings. If abdominal hypertension or compartment syndrome is suspected, urgent surgical consultation should be obtained, because treatment can consist of diuretics, change in body position, or even a need for an open abdominal decompression via laparotomy.[83]

Surgeons should be diligent in recognizing the clinical signs of fluid extravasation, especially into the abdominal compartment, as well as being aware of the pump pressures and amount of irrigant being used. Abdominal examinations have been recommended preoperatively and postoperatively to evaluate for gross signs of fluid extravasation.[84] Because of the pathway that fluid travels from the hip to the abdomen, if an arthroscopic psoas tendon release is to be performed, it is recommended that this be performed last to lessen the chance of abdominal extravasation.[70]

Femoral Neck Fracture and Avascular Necrosis

While performing bony resection around the femoral neck with an arthroscopic burr, there is the risk of overaggressive resection causing weakening of the femoral neck, and even femoral neck fracture. There have been reports in the literature of patients sustaining femoral neck fractures in the early postoperative period after arthroscopic or arthroscopically assisted correction of a cam deformity.[85,86] These fractures were associated with increased weight bearing or activity level in the early postoperative period.

Immediately after osteochondroplasty at the femoral head-neck junction, there is some theoretic weakness that is caused by resection of bone. This weakness takes time to heal, and osseous remodeling with complete recorticalization of the resected margins is thought to take on average 20 months.[87] One study showed that up to 30% of the diameter of the femoral neck could be resected safely, but this also decreases the energy required for a fracture.[88]

Although femoral neck fracture is very rare and there are only a few sporadic cases reported in the literature, this can be a devastating complication if the fracture displaces. However, a large administrative database study has shown that this complication is likely underreported and quotes the proximal femur fracture rate at 1% in 2581 hip arthroscopies.[89] Care should always be taken to avoid over-resection of the femoral neck, and it is recommended that patients be placed on modified or partial weight bearing for up to 6 weeks postoperatively to allow for adequate healing.

Another potentially devastating complication after hip surgery is avascular necrosis (AVN) of the femoral head caused by iatrogenic disruption of the blood supply. The medial femoral circumflex artery enters the hip joint at roughly the level of the superior gemellus, and gives rise to several intracapsular retinacular vessels (**Fig. 7**).

Although cam lesions causing FAI tend to be anterior along the femoral head and neck, there are some anatomic variations with posterolateral lesions causing symptomatic impingement. Femoroplasty along this posterolateral vascular region can theoretically disrupt the feeding vessels to the femoral head causing AVN. This possibility might be especially concerning in the pediatric or adolescent population, in which the femoral epiphyseal blood supply is more tenuous and subject to disruption.

Recent studies have found that, in the adult population, femoroplasty in the posterolateral region is not associated with AVN[90] and that there were no reported cases of AVN in 175 pediatric and adolescent hip arthroscopies.[91] There are only very rare and sporadic cases of AVN after hip arthroscopy present in the literature.[92] Although disruption of the femoral head blood supply is possible, careful dissection and technique should always be used, avoiding any vasculature, especially in the posterolateral region, and in particular when in the region posterior to the lateral synovial fold the peripheral compartment.[93] Overall, this seems to be more of a theoretical than actual complication of hip arthroscopy.

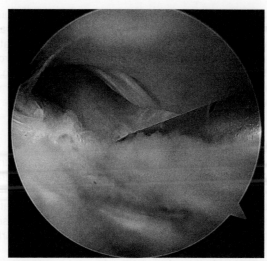

Fig. 7. The lateral retinacular vessels and medial synovial fold should be identified and protected during femoroplasty.

POSTOPERATIVE CONSIDERATIONS
Heterotopic Ossification

Heterotopic ossification (HO) is an osteogenic response that results in bone formation within the soft tissues, usually after a trauma or surgery to the area. In hip arthroscopy, the etiology for this ectopic bone formation within the gluteal musculature is the surgical trauma to the soft tissues and bony debris created during osteoplasty.[84]

HO is a very common complication after hip arthroscopy and can cause functional limitations by creating additional points of impingement, decreasing motion, and causing pain (**Fig. 8**). Rates of HO after hip arthroscopy vary from 0% to 44% in multiple studies.[94–98] Because of the prevalence of this complication and the significant restriction of movement, postoperative prevention is usually recommended in the form of chemoprophylaxis against the formation of HO.

The preferred method of HO prophylaxis is scheduled nonsteroidal antiinflammatory drug (NSAID) administration postoperatively for several weeks. In a randomized, placebo-controlled trial, Beckmann and colleagues[99] found that the prevalence of HO in the placebo group was 46% and only 4% in the group receiving naproxen 500 mg twice daily for 3 weeks. In addition to the administration of naproxen prophylaxis, mixed-type FAI was also a risk factor for developing HO compared with either isolated femoral or acetabular osteochondroplasty alone.[100] Indomethacin has also been used as an adjunct for HO chemoprophylaxis in addition to naproxen, with some suggestion of additional preventive effect.[101]

If the development of HO is severe enough to cause significant pain or functional limitations, surgical removal may be indicated. It is important, however, to ensure that these postoperative symptoms are being caused by the location of the HO, because radiologic ossification can often be clinically silent. There are many potential pain generators in the postoperative hip, so be wary of embarking on a surgical HO resection without confidence that it is the source of the patient's pain.

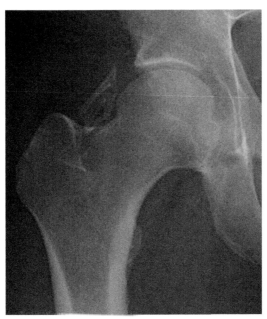

Fig. 8. Postoperative nonsteroidal antiinflammatory drug prophylaxis reduces the rate of potentially symptomatic HO.

Overall, it is recommended to thoroughly irrigate the joint to remove loose bony debris after osteochondroplasty to help prevent the formation of HO,[102] and there is good evidence that a scheduled NSAID chemoprophylaxis regimen postoperatively reduces the risk of HO.[99,100]

Rehabilitation

After surgery, the patients generally require several weeks of rehabilitation. This time period, although likely important for returning to function, has many differing opinions on weight-bearing status and physiotherapy without many strong data to support them.

A recent level I randomized controlled pilot study as well as a controlled trial evaluated the efficacy of adding physiotherapy after arthroscopic treatment of FAI, and found no differences in function or outcomes.[103,104] There is currently no strong literature that supports any physiotherapy regimen after hip arthroscopy. Also, in reviewing a large number of postoperative rehabilitation regimens, there are similar trends in the progression of activity after arthroscopy, but they vary in timing and are often not goal or benchmark dependent.[105,106] Patient adherence to the prescribed rehabilitation protocol may also be a concern, but there is no evidence to show that a lack of adherence leads to inferior outcomes.

Because of the lack of good evidence-based literature, most of what has been published on postoperative rehabilitation after hip arthroscopy is in the realm of expert opinion. Although this lacks hard data, some general trends have emerged. A survey of several high-volume arthroscopists found that most allow full immediate weight bearing as tolerated after acetabular chondroplasty or osteoplasty, psoas tenotomy, or labral resection. Most limit weight bearing for cartilage defects and have variable return-to-sport protocols.[107]

SUMMARY

Because of the recent increase in popularity of hip arthroscopy, as well as the technical expertise required, there are many complications that can be encountered. These complications can arise from any part of the surgery, from preoperative planning to positioning, and even postoperatively during the recovery and rehabilitation phase. By keeping all these potential complications in mind and paying attention to the recent body of clinical research, surgeons may be able to optimize outcomes for patients and improve clinical practice.

REFERENCES

1. Sing DC, Feeley BT, Tay B, et al. Age-related trends in hip arthroscopy: a large cross-sectional analysis. Arthroscopy 2015;31(12):2307–13.e2.
2. Frank JM, Harris JD, Erickson BJ, et al. Prevalence of femoroacetabular impingement imaging findings in asymptomatic volunteers: a systematic review. Arthroscopy 2015;31(6):1199–204.
3. Hack K, Di Primio G, Rakhra K, et al. Prevalence of cam-type femoroacetabular impingement morphology in asymptomatic volunteers. J Bone Joint Surg Am 2010;92(14):2436–44.
4. Jung KA, Restrepo C, Hellman M, et al. The prevalence of cam-type femoroacetabular deformity in asymptomatic adults. Bone Joint J 2011;93-B(10):1303–7.
5. Klaue K, Durnin CW, Ganz R. The acetabular rim syndrome. A clinical presentation of dysplasia of the hip. J Bone Joint Surg Br 1991;73(3):423–9. Available at: http://www.ncbi.nlm.nih.gov/pubmed/1670443. Accessed September 16, 2017.
6. McCarthy JC, Lee J-A. Acetabular dysplasia: a paradigm of arthroscopic examination of chondral injuries. Clin Orthop Relat Res 2002;(405):122–8. Available at: http://www.ncbi.nlm.nih.gov/pubmed/12461363. Accessed September 16, 2017.
7. Landa J, Benke M, Feldman DS. The limbus and the neolimbus in developmental dysplasia of the hip. Clin Orthop Relat Res 2008;466(4):776–81.
8. Ross JR, Clohisy JC, Baca G, et al, ANCHOR Investigators. Patient and disease characteristics associated with hip arthroscopy failure in acetabular dysplasia. J Arthroplasty 2014;29(9):160–3.
9. Ganz R, Klaue K, Vinh TS, et al. A new periacetabular osteotomy for the treatment of hip dysplasias: technique and preliminary results. 1988. Clin Orthop Relat Res 2004;(418):3–8. Available at: http://www.ncbi.nlm.nih.gov/pubmed/15052994. Accessed September 16, 2017.
10. Kirsch JM, Khan M, Bedi A. Does hip arthroscopy have a role in the treatment of developmental hip dysplasia? J Arthroplasty 2017;32(9S):S28–31.
11. Parvizi J, Bican O, Bender B, et al. Arthroscopy for labral tears in patients with developmental dysplasia of the hip: a cautionary note. J Arthroplasty 2009;24(6 Suppl):110–3.
12. Larson CM, Giveans MR, Taylor M. Does arthroscopic FAI correction improve function with radiographic arthritis? Clin Orthop Relat Res 2011;469(6):1667–76.
13. Ayeni OR, Alradwan H, de Sa D, et al. The hip labrum reconstruction: indications and outcomes—a systematic review. Knee Surg Sports Traumatol Arthrosc 2014;22(4):737–43.
14. Philippon MJ, Briggs KK, Carlisle JC, et al. Joint space predicts THA after hip arthroscopy in patients 50 years and older. Clin Orthop Relat Res 2013; 471(8):2492–6.

15. Bogunovic L, Gottlieb M, Pashos GB, et al. Why do hip arthroscopy procedures fail? Clin Orthop Relat Res 2013;471(8):2523–9. Available at: https://www.ncbi. nlm.nih.gov/pmc/articles/PMC3705062/pdf/11999_2013_Article_3015.pdf. Accessed August 18, 2017.
16. Horisberger M, Brunner A, Herzog RF. Arthroscopic treatment of femoral acetabular impingement in patients with preoperative generalized degenerative changes. Arthroscopy 2010;26(5):623–9.
17. McCarthy JC, Jarrett BT, Ojeifo O, et al. What factors influence long-term survivorship after hip arthroscopy? Clin Orthop Relat Res 2011;469(2):362–71.
18. Harris JD, McCormick FM, Abrams GD, et al. Complications and reoperations during and after hip arthroscopy: a systematic review of 92 studies and more than 6,000 patients. Arthroscopy 2013;29(3):589–95.
19. Cancienne JM, Mahon HS, Dempsey IJ, et al. Patient-related risk factors for infection following knee arthroscopy: an analysis of over 700,000 patients from two large databases. Knee 2017;24(3):594–600.
20. Werner BC, Higgins MD, Pehlivan HC, et al. Super obesity is an independent risk factor for complications after primary total hip arthroplasty. J Arthroplasty 2017;32(2):402–6.
21. Puvanesarajah V, Werner BC, Cancienne JM, et al. Morbid obesity and lumbar fusion in patients older than 65 years. Spine (Phila Pa 1976) 2017;42(2):122–7.
22. Collins JA, Beutel BG, Garofolo G, et al. Correlation of obesity with patient-reported outcomes and complications after hip arthroscopy. Arthroscopy 2015;31(1):57–62.
23. Gupta A, Redmond JM, Hammarstedt JE, et al. Does obesity affect outcomes in hip arthroscopy? Am J Sports Med 2015;43(4):965–71.
24. Simpson J, Sadri H, Villar R. Hip arthroscopy technique and complications. Orthop Traumatol Surg Res 2010;S68–76. https://doi.org/10.1016/j.otsr.2010. 09.010.
25. Smart LR, Oetgen M, Noonan B, et al. Beginning hip arthroscopy: indications, positioning, portals, basic techniques, and complications. Arthroscopy 2007; 23(12):1348–53.
26. Farjo LA, Glick JM, Sampson TG. Hip arthroscopy for acetabular labral tears. Arthroscopy 1999;15(2):132–7.
27. Griffin DR, Villar RN. Complications of arthroscopy of the hip. J Bone Joint Surg Br 1999;81(4):604–6. Available at: http://www.ncbi.nlm.nih.gov/pubmed/ 10463729. Accessed August 6, 2017.
28. Sampson TG. Complications of hip arthroscopy. Clin Sports Med 2001;20(4): 831–5. Available at: http://www.ncbi.nlm.nih.gov/pubmed/11675890. Accessed August 7, 2017.
29. Flierl MA, Stahel PF, Hak DJ, et al. Traction table-related complications in orthopaedic surgery. J Am Acad Orthop Surg 2010;18(11):668–75. Available at: http://www.ncbi.nlm.nih.gov/pubmed/21041801. Accessed August 6, 2017.
30. Funke EL, Munzinger U. Complications in hip arthroscopy. Arthroscopy 1996; 12(2):156–9. Available at: http://www.ncbi.nlm.nih.gov/pubmed/8776991. Accessed August 7, 2017.
31. Clarke MT, Arora A, Villar RN. Hip arthroscopy: complications in 1054 cases. Clin Orthop Relat Res 2003;(406):84–8.
32. Schröder e Souza BG, Dani WS, Honda EK, et al. Do complications in hip arthroscopy change with experience? Arthroscopy 2010;26(8):1053–7.

33. Gedouin J-E, May O, Bonin N, et al. Assessment of arthroscopic management of femoroacetabular impingement. A prospective multicenter study. Orthop Traumatol Surg Res 2010;S59–67. https://doi.org/10.1016/j.otsr.2010.08.002.

34. Coelho RF, Gomes CM, Sakaki MH, et al. Genitoperineal injuries associated with the use of an orthopedic table with a perineal posttraction. J Trauma 2008;65(4): 820–3.

35. Brumback RJ, Ellison TS, Molligan H, et al. Pudendal nerve palsy complicating intramedullary nailing of the femur. J Bone Joint Surg Am 1992;74(10):1450–5. Available at: http://www.ncbi.nlm.nih.gov/pubmed/1469004. Accessed August 6, 2017.

36. Byrd JWT. Hip arthroscopy: surgical indications. Arthroscopy 2006;22(12): 1260–2. Available at: http://www.ncbi.nlm.nih.gov/pubmed/17165215. Accessed August 12, 2017.

37. Merrell G, Medvecky M, Daigneault J, et al. Hip arthroscopy without a perineal post: a safer technique for hip distraction. Arthroscopy 2007;23(1):107.e1–3.

38. Pailhé R, Chiron P, Reina N, et al. Pudendal nerve neuralgia after hip arthroscopy: retrospective study and literature review. Orthop Traumatol Surg Res 2013;99(7):785–90.

39. Krueger A, Leunig M, Siebenrock KA, et al. Hip arthroscopy after previous surgical hip dislocation for femoroacetabular impingement. Arthroscopy 2007; 23(12):1285–9.e1.

40. Said HG, Steimer O, Kohn D, et al. Vascular obstruction at the level of the ankle joint as a complication of hip arthroscopy. Arthroscopy 2011;27:1594–6.

41. Robertson WJ, Kelly BT. The safe zone for hip arthroscopy: a cadaveric assessment of central, peripheral, and lateral compartment portal placement. Arthroscopy 2008;24(9):1019–26.

42. Byrd JWT. Hip arthroscopy. J Am Acad Orthop Surg 2006;14(7):433–44. Available at: http://www.ncbi.nlm.nih.gov/pubmed/16822891. Accessed August 12, 2017.

43. Dippmann C, Thorborg K, Kraemer O, et al. Symptoms of nerve dysfunction after hip arthroscopy: an under-reported complication? Arthroscopy 2014;30(2): 202–7.

44. Byrd JWT, Jones KS. Prospective analysis of hip arthroscopy with 10-year followup. Clin Orthop Relat Res 2010;468(3):741–6.

45. Goulding K, Beaulé PE, Kim PR, et al. Incidence of lateral femoral cutaneous nerve neuropraxia after anterior approach hip arthroplasty. Clin Orthop Relat Res 2010;468(9):2397–404.

46. Rodeo SA, Forster RA, Weiland AJ. Neurological complications due to arthroscopy. J Bone Joint Surg Am 1993;75(6):917–26. Available at: http://www.ncbi.nlm.nih.gov/pubmed/8314834. Accessed August 12, 2017.

47. Byrd JW, Pappas JN, Pedley MJ. Hip arthroscopy: an anatomic study of portal placement and relationship to the extra-articular structures. Arthroscopy 1995; 11(4):418–23. Available at: http://www.ncbi.nlm.nih.gov/pubmed/7575873. Accessed August 12, 2017.

48. Bruno M, Longhino V, Sansone V. A catastrophic complication of hip arthroscopy. Arthroscopy 2011;27(8):1150–2.

49. Ilizaliturri VM. Complications of arthroscopic femoroacetabular impingement treatment: a review. Clin Orthop Relat Res 2009;467(3):760–8.

50. Byrd JW. Avoiding the labrum in hip arthroscopy. Arthroscopy 2000;16(7): 770–3.

51. Badylak JS, Keene JS. Do iatrogenic punctures of the labrum affect the clinical results of hip arthroscopy? Arthroscopy 2011;27(6):761–7.
52. McCarthy JC, Lee J. Hip arthroscopy: indications, outcomes, and complications. Instr Course Lect 2006;55:301–8. Available at: http://www.ncbi.nlm.nih.gov/pubmed/16958465. Accessed August 12, 2017.
53. Cadet ER, Chan AK, Vorys GC, et al. Investigation of the preservation of the fluid seal effect in the repaired, partially resected, and reconstructed acetabular labrum in a cadaveric hip model. Am J Sports Med 2012;40(10):2218–23.
54. Crawford MJ, Dy CJ, Alexander JW, et al. The 2007 Frank Stinchfield Award. The biomechanics of the hip labrum and the stability of the hip. Clin Orthop Relat Res 2007;465:16–22.
55. Smith MV, Panchal HB, Ruberte Thiele RA, et al. Effect of acetabular labrum tears on hip stability and labral strain in a joint compression model. Am J Sports Med 2011;39(Suppl(1_suppl)):103S–10S.
56. Tibor LM, Leunig M. Labral resection or preservation during FAI treatment? A systematic review. HSS J 2012;8(3):225–9.
57. Larson CM, Giveans MR, Stone RM. Arthroscopic debridement versus refixation of the acetabular labrum associated with femoroacetabular impingement. Am J Sports Med 2012;40(5):1015–21.
58. Krych AJ, Thompson M, Knutson Z, et al. Arthroscopic labral repair versus selective labral debridement in female patients with femoroacetabular impingement: a prospective randomized study. Arthroscopy 2013;29(1):46–53.
59. Philippon MJ, Stubbs AJ, Schenker ML, et al. Arthroscopic management of femoroacetabular impingement. Am J Sports Med 2007;35(9):1571–80.
60. Redmond JM, El Bitar YF, Gupta A, et al. Arthroscopic acetabuloplasty and labral refixation without labral detachment. Am J Sports Med 2015;43(1):105–12.
61. Matsuda DK. Acute iatrogenic dislocation following hip impingement arthroscopic surgery. Arthroscopy 2009;25(4):400–4.
62. Benali Y, Katthagen BD. Hip subluxation as a complication of arthroscopic debridement. Arthroscopy 2009;25(4):405–7.
63. Ranawat AS, McClincy M, Sekiya JK. Anterior dislocation of the hip after arthroscopy in a patient with capsular laxity of the hip. A case report. J Bone Joint Surg Am 2009;91(1):192–7.
64. Mei-Dan O, McConkey MO, Brick M. Catastrophic failure of hip arthroscopy due to iatrogenic instability: can partial division of the ligamentum teres and iliofemoral ligament cause subluxation? Arthroscopy 2012;28(3):440–5.
65. Clohisy JC, Nepple JJ, Larson CM, et al, Academic Network of Conservation Hip Outcome Research (ANCHOR) Members. Persistent structural disease is the most common cause of repeat hip preservation surgery. Clin Orthop Relat Res 2013;471(12):3788–94.
66. Philippon MJ, Schenker ML, Briggs KK, et al. Revision hip arthroscopy. Am J Sports Med 2007;35(11):1918–21.
67. Heyworth BE, Shindle MK, Voos JE, et al. Radiologic and intraoperative findings in revision hip arthroscopy. Arthroscopy 2007;23(12):1295–302.
68. Cvetanovich GL, Harris JD, Erickson BJ, et al. Revision hip arthroscopy: a systematic review of diagnoses, operative findings, and outcomes. Arthroscopy 2015;31(7):1382–90.
69. Kester B, Mahure SA, Capogna B, et al. Independent risk factors for revision surgery or conversion to THA after hip arthroscopy: an analysis of 3,957 patients. Orthop J Sports Med 2017;5(7_suppl6). 2325967117S0041.

70. Papavasiliou AV, Bardakos NV. Complications of arthroscopic surgery of the hip. Bone Joint Res 2012;1(7):131–44.
71. Matsuda DK. Fluoroscopic templating technique for precision arthroscopic rim trimming. Arthroscopy 2009;25(10):1175–82.
72. Larson CM, Wulf CA. Intraoperative fluoroscopy for evaluation of bony resection during arthroscopic management of femoroacetabular impingement in the supine position. Arthroscopy 2009;25(10):1183–92.
73. Ross JR, Bedi A, Stone RM, et al. Intraoperative fluoroscopic imaging to treat cam deformities. Am J Sports Med 2014;42(6):1370–6.
74. Konan S, Rhee S-J, Haddad FS. Hip arthroscopy: analysis of a single surgeon's learning experience. J Bone Joint Surg Am 2011;93(Suppl 2):52–6.
75. Haupt U, Völkle D, Waldherr C, et al. Intra- and retroperitoneal irrigation liquid after arthroscopy of the hip joint. Arthroscopy 2008;24(8):966–8.
76. Ladner B, Nester K, Cascio B. Abdominal fluid extravasation during hip arthroscopy. Arthroscopy 2010;26(1):131–5.
77. Sharma A, Sachdev H, Gomillion M. Abdominal compartment syndrome during hip arthroscopy. Anaesthesia 2009;64(5):567–9.
78. Verma M, Sekiya JK. Intrathoracic fluid extravasation after hip arthroscopy. Arthroscopy 2010;26(9 Suppl):S90–4.
79. Fowler J, Owens BD. Abdominal compartment syndrome after hip arthroscopy. Arthroscopy 2010;26(1):128–30.
80. Kocher MS, Frank JS, Nasreddine AY, et al. Intra-abdominal fluid extravasation during hip arthroscopy: a survey of the MAHORN group. Arthroscopy 2012; 28(11):1654–60.e2.
81. Stafford GH, Malviya A, Villar RN. Fluid extravasation during hip arthroscopy. Hip Int 2011;21(6):740–3.
82. Cheatham ML, De Waele J, Kirkpatrick A, et al. Criteria for a diagnosis of abdominal compartment syndrome. Can J Surg 2009;52(4):315–6. Available at: http://www.ncbi.nlm.nih.gov/pubmed/19680517. Accessed August 18, 2017.
83. Kirkpatrick AW, Roberts DJ, Jaeschke R, et al. Methodological background and strategy for the 2012–2013 updated consensus definitions and clinical practice guidelines from the abdominal compartment society. Anestezjol Intens Ter 2015; 47(J):63–77.
84. Fabricant PD, Maak TG, Cross MB, et al. Avoiding complications in hip arthroscopy. Oper Tech Sports Med 2011;19(2):108–13.
85. Ayeni OR, Bedi A, Lorich DG, et al. Femoral neck fracture after arthroscopic management of femoroacetabular impingement: a case report. J Bone Joint Surg Am 2011;93(9):e47.
86. Laude F, Sariali E, Nogier A. Femoroacetabular impingement treatment using arthroscopy and anterior approach. Clin Orthop Relat Res 2009;467(3):747–52.
87. Nassif NA, Pekmezci M, Pashos G, et al. Osseous remodeling after femoral head-neck junction osteochondroplasty. Clin Orthop Relat Res 2010;468(2): 511–8.
88. Mardones RM, Gonzalez C, Chen Q, et al. Surgical treatment of femoroacetabular impingement: evaluation of the effect of the size of the resection. Surgical technique. J Bone Joint Surg Am 2006;88(Suppl 1 Pt 1):84–91.
89. Truntzer JN, Hoppe DJ, Shapiro LM, et al. Complication rates for hip arthroscopy are underestimated: a population-based study. Arthroscopy 2017;33(6): 1194–201.
90. Rupp RE, Rupp SN. Femoral head avascular necrosis is not caused by arthroscopic posterolateral femoroplasty. Orthopedics 2016;39(3):177–80.

91. Nwachukwu BU, McFeely ED, Nasreddine AY, et al. Complications of hip arthroscopy in children and adolescents. J Pediatr Orthop 2011;31(3):227–31.

92. Seijas R, Ares O, Sallent A, et al. Hip arthroscopy complications regarding surgery and early postoperative care: retrospective study and review of literature. Musculoskelet Surg 2017;101(2):119–31.

93. Nakano N, Khanduja V. Complications in hip arthroscopy. Muscles Ligaments Tendons J 2016;6(3):402–9.

94. Amar E, Sharfman ZT, Rath E. Heterotopic ossification after hip arthroscopy. J Hip Preserv Surg 2015;2(4):355–63.

95. Larson CM, Giveans MR. Arthroscopic management of femoroacetabular impingement: early outcomes measures. Arthroscopy 2008;24(5):540–6.

96. Clohisy JC, Zebala LP, Nepple JJ, et al. Combined hip arthroscopy and limited open osteochondroplasty for anterior femoroacetabular impingement. J Bone Joint Surg Am 2010;92(8):1697–706.

97. Randelli F, Pierannunzii L, Banci L, et al. Heterotopic ossifications after arthroscopic management of femoroacetabular impingement: the role of NSAID prophylaxis. J Orthop Traumatol 2010;11(4):245–50.

98. Rath E, Sherman H, Sampson TG, et al. The incidence of heterotopic ossification in hip arthroscopy. Arthroscopy 2013;29(3):427–33.

99. Beckmann JT, Wylie JD, Potter MQ, et al. Effect of naproxen prophylaxis on heterotopic ossification following hip arthroscopy. J Bone Joint Surg Am 2015; 97(24):2032–7.

100. Beckmann JT, Wylie JD, Kapron AL, et al. The effect of NSAID prophylaxis and operative variables on heterotopic ossification after hip arthroscopy. Am J Sports Med 2014;42(6):1359–64.

101. Bedi A, Zbeda RM, Bueno VF, et al. The incidence of heterotopic ossification after hip arthroscopy. Am J Sports Med 2012;40(4):854–63.

102. Matsuda DK, Calipusan CP. Adolescent femoroacetabular impingement from malunion of the anteroinferior iliac spine apophysis treated with arthroscopic spinoplasty. Orthopedics 2012;35(3):e460–3.

103. Bennell KL, Spiers L, Takla A, et al. Efficacy of adding a physiotherapy rehabilitation programme to arthroscopic management of femoroacetabular impingement syndrome: a randomised controlled trial (FAIR). BMJ Open 2017;7(6): e014658.

104. Kemp J, Moore K, Fransen M, et al. A pilot randomised clinical trial of physiotherapy (manual therapy, exercise, and education) for early-onset hip osteoarthritis post-hip arthroscopy. Pilot Feasibility Stud 2018;4(1):16.

105. Kraeutler MJ, Anderson J, Chahla J, et al. Return to running after arthroscopic hip surgery: literature review and proposal of a physical therapy protocol. J Hip Preserv Surg 2017;4(2):121–30.

106. Adler KL, Cook PC, Geisler PR, et al. Current concepts in hip preservation surgery: part II–rehabilitation. Sports Health 2016;8(1):57–64.

107. Rath E, Sharfman ZT, Paret M, et al. Hip arthroscopy protocol: expert opinions on post-operative weight bearing and return to sports guidelines. J Hip Preserv Surg 2017;4(1):60–6.

Knee Anterior Cruciate Ligament Injuries
Common Problems and Solutions

James E. Christensen, MD, Mark D. Miller, MD*

KEYWORDS

- Anterior cruciate ligament reconstruction • Complications • Knee arthroscopy
- Knee surgery • Autograft

KEY POINTS

- Anterior cruciate ligament (ACL) complications are rare entities, but the complications can represent significant morbidities for patients.
- More common complications for ACL reconstruction include tunnel malposition, infection, tunnel osteolysis, fixation failure, fracture, arthrofibrosis, graft site morbidity, and deep vein thrombosis or pulmonary embolism.
- When complications can be anticipated, proper planning, such as computed tomography and proper bone graft options in osteolysis, can help decrease the morbidity associated with them.

 Video content accompanies this article at http://www.sportsmed.theclinics.com.

INTRODUCTION

Anterior cruciate ligament (ACL) reconstruction is one of the most commonly performed orthopedic procedures in the United States, with more than 127,000 performed in 2006.[1] Complications are rare in ACL surgery, but given the amount of ACL surgeries performed each year, it does represent a significant amount of patient complications, with the potential for short- and long-term morbidity. ACL complications can include technical failures as well as patient-related factors.

COMPLICATIONS

One of the most common technical errors that can occur in ACL reconstruction is aberrant tunnel placement, which can lead to ACL failure because it places excessive

Disclosure Statement: No disclosures.
Department of Orthopaedic Surgery, University of Virginia, 400 Ray C Hunt Drive, Charlottesville, VA 22903, USA
* Corresponding author.
E-mail address: MDM3P@hscmail.mcc.virginia.edu

Clin Sports Med 37 (2018) 265–280
https://doi.org/10.1016/j.csm.2017.12.006
0278-5919/18/© 2017 Elsevier Inc. All rights reserved.

stress on the graft. Aberrant tunnel placement can lead to poorer outcomes based on their location and whether the aberrant tunnel is in the tibia or femur, with the femoral side accounting for 80% of aberrant tunnels. When transtibial ACL reconstruction was more common, tunnel placement would often be more vertical and anterior. Transtibial reconstruction can lead to stable-appearing knees, especially in the anteroposterior plane as evidenced with a negative Lachman, but they tend to leave residual rotational instability with a positive pivot shift.

Aberrant tunnel placement in the tibia can cause dysfunction depending on the location of the tunnel. If placed too anteriorly, patients can experience loss of extension as the graft impinges on the roof. Conversely, when the tunnel is placed too posteriorly, posterior cruciate ligament (PCL) impingement can occur, which places greater tension on the graft and can lead to decreased flexion as well as anterior laxity. A tunnel placed too medially can lead to iatrogenic medial plateau fracture. A tunnel placed too laterally can lead to impingement on the lateral wall and lead to attenuation of the graft as well.

As with the tibia, aberrant femoral tunnel placement can lead to ACL failure. For a tunnel placed too far anteriorly, the patient can experience difficulty with achieving full flexion because the graft will impinge on the roof. On the other hand, for a tunnel placed too far posteriorly, the patient can struggle to achieve full extension while having laxity in flexion. If placed too far posteriorly, there is also the risk of posterior wall blowout, which will affect the fixation technique used. Fluoroscopy can be a good intraoperative tool to visualize proper tunnel placement.

One of the common issues encountered with ACL reconstruction, especially as it pertains to revision ACL cases, is tunnel osteolysis or widening. Although the full cause is not fully understood, it may be explained by several factors, including mechanical factors and biologic factors. Mechanical factors can include improper graft tunnel placement and fixation methods. Graft suspension methods can lead to a windshield-wiper effect or bungee cord motion within the tunnels. Biologic factors that may lead to osteolysis include graft type and donor type (allograft or autograft) as well as synovial fluid propagation. Synovial fluid propagation and gravity may also be responsible for the fact that tibial tunnel osteolysis tends to be greater than femoral tunnel osteolysis.

For ACL reconstruction, there are multiple methods of fixation from cortical buttons and suspensory fixation to biodegradable or metal interference screws to tying over a post. As discussed in the section on tunnel widening, suspensory fixation can lead to abnormal motion within the tunnel during the process of incorporation, but it is also important at the time of implantation to ensure that the cortical button properly deploys or that the cortex is competent to avoid early failure. When using interference fixation, it is important that the screws properly "interfere." When screws diverge more than 15° to 30°, there is an increased risk of bone plug pullout.[2–4]

Postoperative infection is always a concern no matter which surgery is being performed, and ACL reconstruction is no different. Infection is a rare complication in ACL reconstruction (<1%) but can lead to significant morbidity if unrealized and untreated because articular destruction can occur in 11 days. There are some factors that increase the risk of infection after ACL reconstruction. Tobacco use, which has been established through multiple studies to be a preventable cause of morbidity and mortality, has also been associated with an increased risk of infection after ACL reconstruction.[5] Recently, there have been multiple studies that have shown ACL reconstruction performed with hamstring autograft has a higher infection rate than those with bone-patellar tendon-bone (BTB) autograft.[6,7] Studies have not shown an increased risk of infection with BTB autograft compared with allograft reconstruction.[6,8,9] Although rare, infections should be handled expediently.

Fracture can occur as a complication of harvest after BTB autograft and usually occurs as a later complication, usually 8 to 12 weeks postoperatively. There are different techniques to decrease the risk of fracture, including using a smaller saw blade and cutting the undersurface of the patella.

The 2 most commonly used grafts, hamstring autograft and BTB autograft, do differ in their incisions with the hamstring incision usually being a smaller incision and centered more inferiorly. However, they are both more slightly medially based incisions, and because of this, they both risk injury to the infrapatellar branch of the saphenous nerve, which can cause paresthesias over the lateral aspect of the anterior proximal leg or a painful neuroma in rare cases. Most patients eventually have minimal residual paresthesias over a small area of the proximal leg. An additional potential complication associated with hamstring harvest is premature graft amputation, necessitating graft augmentation with a contralateral hamstring harvest, an allograft, or another graft option entirely.

Arthrofibrosis can complicate ACL reconstruction and lead to poorer outcomes. Loss of motion can be due to many factors, including preoperative factors, intraoperative factors, and postoperative factors. Preoperative factors leading to arthrofibrosis may include poor range of motion (ROM), effusion, quadriceps tone, and poor gait. Intraoperative factors that can affect postoperative ROM include tunnel positioning and graft tensioning. Postoperatively, hemarthrosis and poor patient-directed motion can lead to poor ROM after ACL reconstruction.

As is a concern with any surgery and especially lower-extremity surgeries, venous thromboembolism (VTE) is a possible complication with ACL reconstruction. Studies of symptomatic deep vein thrombosis (DVT) and pulmonary embolism (PE) incidence in ACL reconstruction range from 0% to 2% and 0% to 0.2%, respectively.[10–12] Asymptomatic DVT incidence is up to 14%, although their treatment would be controversial. Not many studies have been performed, though, to analyze the use of prophylactic agents after surgery. Kaye and colleagues[13] looked at aspirin as VTE prophylaxis but found no difference in rates of VTE. The level and type of VTE prophylaxis are not well studied at this point, and it is not completely clear what should be used after ACL reconstruction.

The most common cause of graft failure, which accounts for 32% of failures, is due to trauma.[14] In that same study by Wright and colleagues,[14] the second most common mode of failure, and the most correctable issue, was technical failure, which was thought to contribute to failure in 24% of cases. Of the technical errors, 80% of them were attributed to femoral tunnel placement, and the next most common technical error was tibial tunnel placement. These 2 technical causes were considerably more likely to lead to ACL failure than any other technical failure with the next most common accounting for 7% (allograft source). Similarly, Diamantopoulos and colleagues[15] showed that tunnel malposition accounted for a significant amount of failures, though, in their study tunnel malposition accounted for 63% of failures. Sommer and colleagues[16] showed in their study that, in their cohort, the most common error in femoral placement was a tunnel placed too anteriorly, and they also showed a correlation between femoral placement and functional scores.

As described earlier, there are multiple factors posited as the cause of tunnel enlargement with biologic and mechanical factors playing a role, although the process of tunnel widening is not fully understood. Although tunnel widening has not been shown to affect outcomes in a functioning ACL, it can present issues when it comes to ACL revision surgery. In a recent study by Ayala-Mejias and colleagues,[17] they found that at 10-year follow-up, most patients who underwent ACL reconstruction had some level of tunnel widening. Tibial tunnel widening was more common, with 85% undergoing widening, compared with 57% of femoral tunnels undergoing widening. Tibial tunnels also widened more than femoral tunnels did, and further dilatation was seen at later follow up at intermediate follow-up and at 10 years. Tibial tunnel widening was also observed more commonly in vertically oriented tunnels. Tunnel expansion tends to happen at the aperture, and in Weber and colleagues,[18] they discussed that it tends to happen early but tends to decrease over a 2-year period, contrary to the Ayala-Meijas 10-year study. In their study, they also found that younger patients (<30 years), men, and those with delayed ACL reconstruction from injury (<1 year) had a greater probability of having tunnel expansion.

Wilson and colleagues[19] and Maak and colleagues[20] also give a comprehensive overview of tunnel widening and its causes. In both articles, they discuss the mechanical and biologic factors that have been postulated to cause tunnel osteolysis. In addition to tunnel malposition leading to graft failure, poorly placed tunnels can also lead to tunnel widening because the impingement force may be transmitted to the graft-tunnel interface, especially before graft incorporation. Graft fixation technique also is thought to play a role because suspensory fixation can lead to a "bungee cord effect" with elongation and retraction of the graft leading to widening coupled with a "windshield-wiper effect" of the graft within the tunnel can cause abrasion at the tunnel entrance.

Biologic factors in tunnel widening also vary. Cytokine levels have been postulated as a potential factor in tunnel widening because the proinflammatory state can lead to increased osteoclast activity, although the contribution of cytokines to widening is unknown. Furthermore, although some investigators have questioned its contribution as well,[21] synovial fluid propagation into the tunnels is also thought to be a contributing factor especially when coupled with the windshield-wiper effect. Hamstring tendon grafts have shown greater widening than BTB grafts with widening up to 25%.

Infections in ACL reconstruction are rare complications, estimated at 0.1% to 1.7% of patients,[22] with the potential to cause long-term morbidity with delayed diagnosis as well as incurring a significant cost with estimates as much as 6 times as much as the index procedure.[23] The most common isolates are Staphylococcus aureus and coagulase-negative staph[22]; this would suggest skin flora as a potential source. Inoculation is likely at the time of surgery or shortly after surgery. Hantes and colleagues[24] showed that intraoperative autograft contamination rates of BTB and hamstring were similar (~10%) but showed no correlation with postoperative inflammatory marker levels. Hamstring grafts may have an increased risk of infection compared with BTB grafts as Maletis and colleagues[7] found an incidence of 0.61% in hamstring graft ACL compared with 0.07% rate in BTB and has been shown in other studies.[6] The overall infection rate was 0.48%. They also found no difference in the allograft and BTB autograft infection rates as has been shown in multiple studies.[6,8,9] Because dropping a graft is a feared complication intraoperatively, chlorhexidine wash has been shown to decrease the amount of bacterial growth after a simulated drop onto the floor. Molina and colleagues[25] showed that chlorhexidine was superior to povidone-iodine and antibiotic washes. When septic arthritis is diagnosed, typically arthroscopic debridement is undertaken, and repeat irrigation and debridement (I&D) may be needed in 35% of cases.[26] Graft retention is attempted when possible if the graft does not appear grossly infected or unstable. Cadet and colleagues[22] showed in multiple studies that graft retention could be accomplished with early intervention with an average number of procedures of 1 to 2.8. Some of these studies did show normal to near-normal functional outcomes, but other studies have shown more than half of their patients with postoperative infections had only fair or poor results.[27,28] Prompt diagnosis is an important aspect of postoperative infections.

Patella fracture is another rare complication of ACL reconstruction when using BTB but can lead to good outcomes nonetheless. Patella fractures tend to occur 2 to

4 months postoperatively with an incidence of 0.2% to 1.3%.[29–32] Some of these fractures were treated nonoperatively if they were non-displaced, but displaced fractures
were treated with internal fixation. Most were transverse patella fractures with patients
undergoing indirect and direct trauma. Viola and Vianello[32] and Papageorgiou and colleagues[33] showed no difference in outcomes compared with normal ACL reconstruction, and 75% of patients had good to excellent results in Stein and colleagues.[29]

Any time immobilization is needed after ACL reconstruction or even in the absence
of immobilization, arthrofibrosis is a concern. Early studies reported a high incidence
of arthrofibrosis (35%),[34] but after improvements in surgical techniques and rehabilitation protocols incidence decreased with estimates only up to 5% when one ex-
cludes concurrent collateral reconstructions.[35–37] In their study, Csintalan and
colleagues[38] observed that female sex and previous knee surgery were risk factors
for arthrofibrosis and reoperation. The key to preventing arthrofibrosis is early postoperative motion. Noyes and colleagues[39] reported 93% return of full motion with early
active and passive knee motion, and 98% regained motion without needing arthroscopic lysis of adhesions. For those who do require manipulation and/or lysis of adhesions, positive results can occur because Noyes and colleagues in that same paper
had 9 patients who had flexion to 90° at 6 weeks and after manipulation or lysis, all
achieved flexion to at least 135°. Manipulation is recommended within 4 to 12 weeks.

CASE EXAMPLES

Tunnel osteolysis does require preoperative planning in order to help decide whether
ACL revision reconstruction can be accomplished in one stage or whether it requires
2 stages. Computed tomography (CT), in addition to an MRI, which can show any
intra-articular abnormality, can be helpful in determining the size of the tunnels as
well as tunnel location. Generally, if the previous tunnel locations do not compromise
the planned tunnels and tunnel enlargement is less than 14 mm, a single-stage revision
can be undertaken with allograft bone dowels. The remnant graft is debrided (**Fig. 1**),
and after adequate debridement, a center guide pin can be placed in the previous tunnel (**Fig. 2**). The previous tunnel is serially drilled to debride the remaining tissue within
the tunnel and the surrounding sclerotic bone. After this is accomplished, a bone

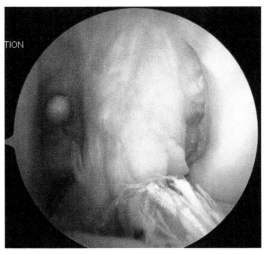

Fig. 1. Prior graft debridement.

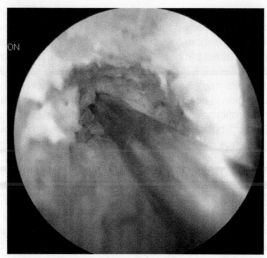

Fig. 2. Center guide pin in previous tunnel.

dowel of the size of the tunnel can be impacted into the previous tunnel with the bone dowel sized to the last reamer used (**Figs. 3**A and **4**). Once this is impacted into the previous tunnel, the new tunnel can be drilled (**Figs. 3**B and C). Video 1 shows a bone dowel being impacted into the tibial tunnel. **Fig. 5** shows a one-stage revision using a bone dowel at 4 months post-operatively.

For those tunnels that have massive osteolysis with widening greater than 14 mm, poor biologic milieu, or convergent tunnels, a 2-stage revision may be indicated. These revisions would require the first stage consisting of bone grafting followed by graft reconstruction after incorporation of the graft. For bone grafting, one can use allograft bone dowels, like in one-stage revisions, autogenous iliac crest, local autogenous graft, or femoral head allograft. In a case example in **Figs. 5** and **6**, the patient had massive osteolysis on CT. Again, the steps are similar to those involved in a one-stage revision. The graft and tunnels are debrided after placing a centering pin in the previous tunnels. A dowel is placed in the femoral tunnel, and after serial debridements of the tibial tunnel (**Fig. 6**), 2 dowels are used to fill the tibial defect in this case (**Fig. 7**). After grafting, it is prudent to wait at least 4 months for graft incorporation. In **Fig. 8**, incorporation on CT as well as on histology can be seen.

Dowels can be very useful in revision cases with tunnels that require grafting, but they can have their drawbacks. They can be brittle and fracture during insertion of

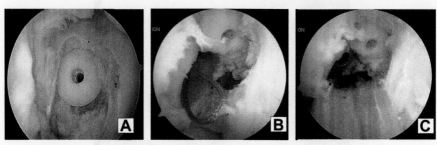

Fig. 3. (*A*) Bone dowel impacted into previous tunnel; (*B*) new tunnel drilled; (*C*) new tunnel beside dowel.

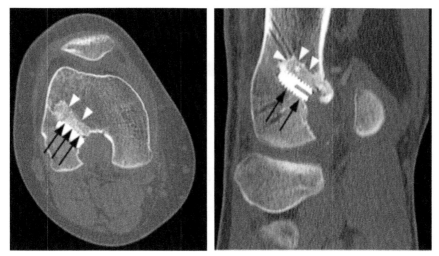

Fig. 4. Incorporation of dowel bone graft, 4 months postoperatively. *Black arrows* indicate screw-graft interface without osteolysis, *White arrowheads* indicate healing at femur-allograft bone dowel interface, Asterisk indicates bone dowel.

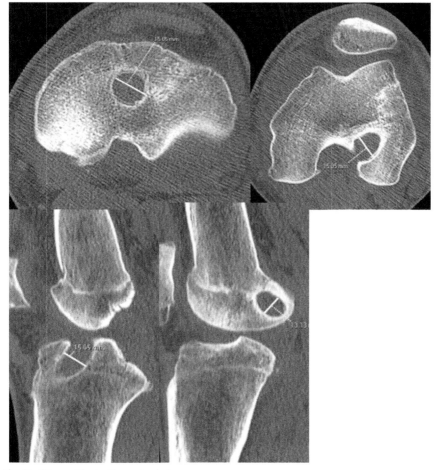

Fig. 5. CT scan illustrating osteolysis.

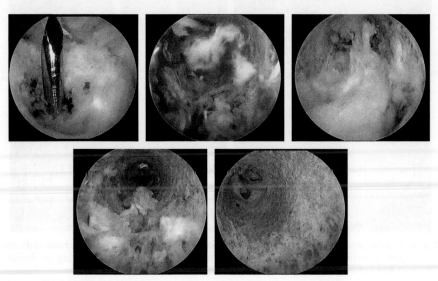

Fig. 6. Tibial serial reamings.

the dowel (**Fig. 9**). Dowels can also fail to incorporate into the tunnel, which may then require revision bone grafting (**Figs. 10** and **11**).

In the rare event of a presumed infection, the joint should be aspirated to confirm the diagnosis and should be followed by prompt and aggressive I&D because articular destruction can occur in 11 days. Aggressive I&D should be followed by 4 to 6 weeks of intravenous antibiotics. As mentioned, if the graft does not show instability and does not appear grossly infected, it can be retained if the infection is acute. It may require

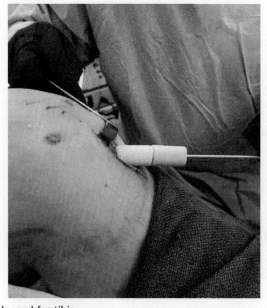

Fig. 7. Two dowels used for tibia.

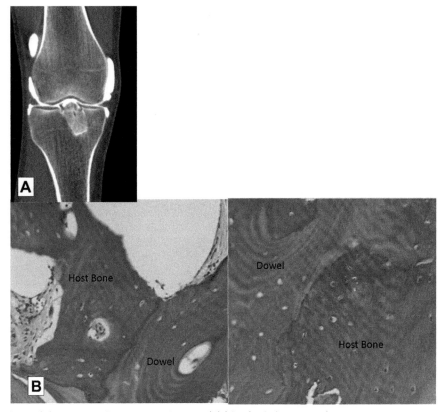

Fig. 8. (*A*) Incorporation seen on CT scan; (*B*) histologic incorporation.

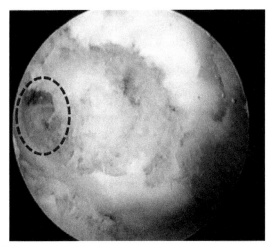

Fig. 9. Fracture of dowel (*dotted line*).

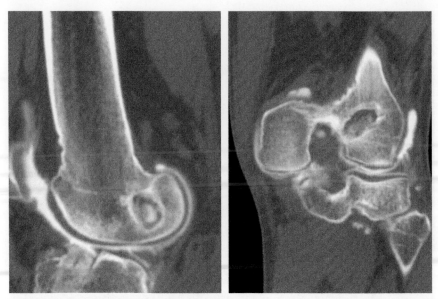

Fig. 10. Failure of dowel incorporation on CT scan.

graft removal. In the case of a graft being dropped on the floor, although the graft is contaminated quickly, the graft can be saved. After cleaning the graft off with saline, the sutures should be removed. The graft can be washed with a chlorhexidine pulsed lavage followed by serial antibiotic soaks.

Patella fracture after BTB harvest can be a complication that can set a patient back but ultimately leads to good results. They are a rare complication, but steps can be taken in order to decrease their incidence: use of a smaller saw blade, cutting the undersurface of the bone interface, drilling holes at the corners of the graft harvest site, cutting a less rectangular graft, and bone grafting defects with one from the tunnels or extra bone from the bone blocks that was trimmed in order to fit the graft. **Fig. 12** shows a patella fracture after BTB harvest in a PCL reconstruction. It was treated with wire and screw fixation.

The tibial tunnel reamings can be saved as a slurry and can be placed in the patellar defect. The paratenon can then be closed over the defect to contain the graft (**Fig. 13**). **Fig. 14** shows a patella at 4 months and 8 years after bone grafting from the tibial slurry.

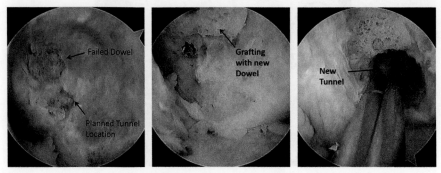

Fig. 11. Failure of dowel incorporation with revision grafting and tunnel placement.

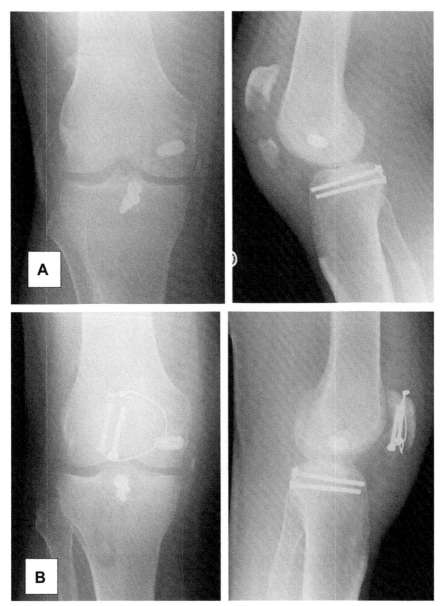

Fig. 12. (A) Patella fracture after PCL reconstruction with BTB; (B) ORIF of patella fracture. ORIF, open reduction internal fixation.

A rare fracture complication can also occur in the femur. In a case example, a 31-year-old petite woman with an ACL tear had an ipsilateral hamstring harvest. After her hamstrings were quadrupled, they only sized to a 7-mm graft. Magnussen and colleagues[40] showed that grafts 8 mm or less has a 2.2 higher odd ratio of failure compared with larger grafts. Because of this, the decision was made to make a larger graft with contralateral semitendinosus harvest, which brought the graft to 9 mm. The tunnel was reamed up to 10 mm, and after the femoral tunnel was dilated for the soft tissue interference screw sheath, a coronal split or Hoffa fracture of the lateral femoral

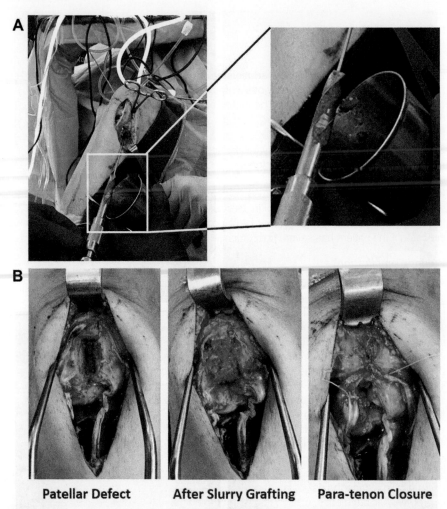

Patellar Defect   **After Slurry Grafting**   **Para-tenon Closure**

Fig. 13. (*A*) Reamings for patella grafting from tibial tunnel drilling. (*B*) Reamings placed in patella void with paratenon closure over top.

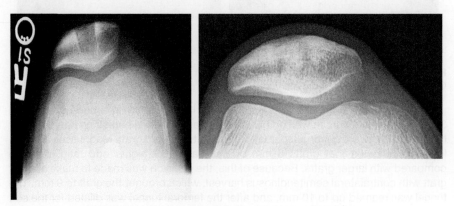

Fig. 14. Four months (*left*) and 8 years (*right*) after harvest and grafting.

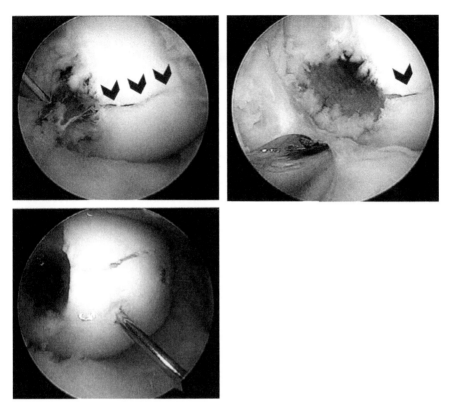

Fig. 15. (*Top*) Coronal split seen during arthroscopy; (*bottom*) Guide wire for screw fixation. *Arrowheads* indicate fracture line of lateral condyle.

condyle was noted on arthroscopy. Fluoroscopy did not show the split. **Fig. 15** shows the coronal split on arthroscopy. The femoral fixation was changed to a cortical suspensory device. The split was internally fixed with 2 headless screws as seen in **Fig. 16**. Her weight-bearing was limited for 6 weeks with close monitoring of the

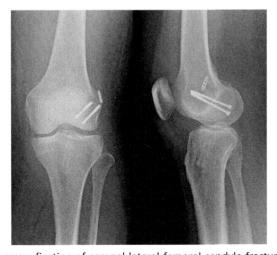

Fig. 16. Headless screw fixation of coronal lateral femoral condyle fracture.

radiographs. At 3 months, the patient was doing well, although she did have slow union. CT at 4 months showed bridging callus. This case illustrates the fixation methods for this rare complication as well as rethinking graft size depending on the patient size.

SUMMARY

Complications in ACL reconstruction are rare, but given that many of ACL reconstructions are performed in young, active individuals, complications can create significant short- and long-term morbidities for this population. More common complications include tunnel malposition, tunnel osteolysis or widening, infection, arthrofibrosis, venothromboembolism, graft site morbidity, fixation problems, and fracture. Tunnel malposition is the most common technical error in ACL reconstruction and can lead to early failure as well as tunnel osteolysis and arthrofibrosis, 2 other more commonly encountered complications. The risk of poor tunnel placement can be reduced with adequate preoperative and intraoperative planning. Tunnel osteolysis can present a dilemma if revision ACL reconstruction is needed. Depending on the size and placement of the tunnels, bone grafting with possible staging may be needed for successful revision. Infection, although rare, if not identified promptly, can lead to significant long-term morbidity for patients and may require loss of the graft in recalcitrant or severe cases. Arthrofibrosis can be due to technical causes or patient factors but can often be remedied with proper therapy. Venothromboembolic disease should be addressed, especially with higher-risk individuals. Fracture can be a complication encountered early or late, but most patients still have satisfactory outcomes. When complications are encountered with ACL reconstruction, adequate awareness and planning can help mitigate the morbidity that can be associated with them.

SUPPLEMENTARY DATA

Supplementary data related to this article can be found online at https://doi.org/10.1016/j.csm.2017.12.006.

REFERENCES

1. Buller LT, Best MJ, Baraga MG, et al. Trends in anterior cruciate ligament reconstruction in the United States. Orthop J Sports Med 2015;3(1). 2325967114563664.
2. Ninomiya T, Tachibana Y, Miyajima T, et al. Fixation strength of the interference screw in the femoral tunnel: the effect of screw divergence on the coronal plane. Knee 2011;18(2):83–7.
3. Dworsky BD, Jewell BF, Bach BR. Interference screw divergence in endoscopic anterior cruciate ligament reconstruction. Arthroscopy 1996;12(1):45–9.
4. Lemos MJ, Jackson DW, Lee TQ, et al. Assessment of initial fixation of endoscopic interference femoral screws with divergent and parallel placement. Arthroscopy 1995;11(1):37–41.
5. Cancienne JM, Gwathmey FW, Miller MD, et al. Tobacco use is associated with increased complications after anterior cruciate ligament reconstruction. Am J Sports Med 2016;44(1):99–104.
6. Barker JU, Drakos MC, Maak TG, et al. Effect of graft selection on the incidence of postoperative infection in anterior cruciate ligament reconstruction. Am J Sports Med 2010;38(2):281–6.

7. Maletis GB, Inacio MCS, Reynolds S, et al. Incidence of postoperative anterior cruciate ligament reconstruction infections: graft choice makes a difference. Am J Sports Med 2013;41(8):1780–5.

8. Greenberg DD, Robertson M, Vallurupalli S, et al. Allograft compared with autograft infection rates in primary anterior cruciate ligament reconstruction. J Bone Joint Surg Am 2010;92(14):2402–8.

9. Katz LM, Battaglia TC, Patino P, et al. A retrospective comparison of the incidence of bacterial infection following anterior cruciate ligament reconstruction with autograft versus allograft. Arthroscopy 2008;24(12):1330–5.

10. Erickson BJ, Saltzman BM, Campbell KA, et al. Rates of deep venous thrombosis and pulmonary embolus after anterior cruciate ligament reconstruction. Sports Health 2015;7(3):261–6.

11. Gaskill T, Pullen M, Bryant B, et al. The prevalence of symptomatic deep venous thrombosis and pulmonary embolism after anterior cruciate ligament reconstruction. Am J Sports Med 2015;43(11):2714–9.

12. Janssen RPA, Reijman M, Janssen DM, et al. Arterial complications, venous thromboembolism and deep venous thrombosis prophylaxis after anterior cruciate ligament reconstruction: a systematic review. World J Orthop 2016;7(9):604.

13. Kaye ID, Patel DN, Strauss EJ, et al. Prevention of venous thromboembolism after arthroscopic knee surgery in a low-risk population with the use of aspirin. A randomized trial. Bull Hosp Jt Dis (2013) 2015;73(4):243–8.

14. Wright RW, Huston LJ, Spindler KP, et al. Descriptive epidemiology of the multicenter ACL revision study (MARS) cohort. Am J Sports Med 2010;38(10):1979–86.

15. Diamantopoulos AP, Lorbach O, Paessler HH. Anterior cruciate ligament revision reconstruction: results in 107 patients. Am J Sports Med 2008;36(5):851–60.

16. Sommer C, Friederich NF, Müller W. Improperly placed anterior cruciate ligament grafts: correlation between radiological parameters and clinical results. Knee Surg Sports Traumatol Arthrosc 2000;8(4):207–13.

17. Ayala-Mejias JD, Garcia-Gonzalez B, Alcocer-Perez-España L, et al. Relationship between widening and position of the tunnels and clinical results of anterior cruciate ligament reconstruction to knee osteoarthritis: 30 patients at a minimum follow-up of 10 years. J Knee Surg 2017;30(6):501–8.

18. Weber AE, Delos D, Oltean HN, et al. Tibial and femoral tunnel changes after ACL reconstruction: a prospective 2-year longitudinal MRI study. Am J Sports Med 2015;43(5):1147–56.

19. Wilson TC, Kantaras A, Atay A, et al. Tunnel enlargement after anterior cruciate ligament surgery. Am J Sports Med 2004;32(2):543–9.

20. Maak TG, Voos JE, Wickiewicz TL, et al. Tunnel widening in revision anterior cruciate ligament reconstruction. J Am Acad Orthop Surg 2010;18(11):695–706.

21. L'Insalata JC, Klatt B, Fu FH, et al. Tunnel expansion following anterior cruciate ligament reconstruction: a comparison of hamstring and patellar tendon autografts. Knee Surg Sports Traumatol Arthrosc 1997;5(4):234–8.

22. Cadet ER, Makhni EC, Mehran N, et al. Management of septic arthritis following anterior cruciate ligament reconstruction: a review of current practices and recommendations. J Am Acad Orthop Surg 2013;21(11):647–56.

23. McAllister DR, Parker RD, Cooper AE, et al. Outcomes of postoperative septic arthritis after anterior cruciate ligament reconstruction. Am J Sports Med 1999;27(5):562–70.

24. Hantes ME, Basdekis GK, Varitimidis SE, et al. Autograft contamination during preparation for anterior cruciate ligament reconstruction. J Bone Joint Surg Am 2008;90(4):760–4.

25. Molina ME, Nonweiller DE, Evans JA, et al. Contaminated anterior cruciate ligament grafts: the efficacy of 3 sterilization agents. Arthroscopy 2000;16(4):373–8.

26. Saper M, Stephenson K, Heisey M. Arthroscopic irrigation and debridement in the treatment of septic arthritis after anterior cruciate ligament reconstruction. Arthroscopy 2014;30(6):747–54.

27. Schulz AP, Götze S, Schmidt HGK, et al. Septic arthritis of the knee after anterior cruciate ligament surgery: a stage-adapted treatment regimen. Am J Sports Med 2007;35(7):1064–9.

28. Judd D, Bottoni C, Kim D, et al. Infections following arthroscopic anterior cruciate ligament reconstruction. Arthroscopy 2006;22(4):375–84.

29. Stein DA, Hunt SA, Rosen JE, et al. The incidence and outcome of patella fractures after anterior cruciate ligament reconstruction. Arthroscopy 2002;18(6):578–83.

30. Lee GH, McCulloch P, Cole BJ, et al. The incidence of acute patellar tendon harvest complications for anterior cruciate ligament reconstruction. Arthroscopy 2008;24(2):162–6.

31. Milankov M, Rasović P, Kovacev N, et al. Fracture of the patella after the anterior cruciate ligament reconstruction. Med Pregl 2012;65(11–12):476–82.

32. Viola R, Vianello R. Three cases of patella fracture in 1,320 anterior cruciate ligament reconstructions with bone–patellar tendon–bone autograft. Arthroscopy 1999;15(1):93–7.

33. Papageorgiou CD, Kostopoulos VK, Moebius UG, et al. Patellar fractures associated with medial-third bone-patellar tendon-bone autograft ACL reconstruction. Knee Surg Sports Traumatol Arthrosc 2001;9(3):151–4.

34. Strum GM, Friedman MJ, Fox JM, et al. Acute anterior cruciate ligament reconstruction. Analysis of complications. Clin Orthop Relat Res 1990;(253):184–9.

35. Werner BC, Cancienne JM, Miller MD, et al. Incidence of manipulation under anesthesia or lysis of adhesions after arthroscopic knee surgery. Am J Sports Med 2015;43(7):1656–61.

36. Hettrich CM, Dunn WR, Reinke EK, et al. The rate of subsequent surgery and predictors after anterior cruciate ligament reconstruction: two- and 6-year follow-up results from a multicenter cohort. Am J Sports Med 2013;41(7):1534–40.

37. Magit D, Wolff A, Sutton K, et al. Arthrofibrosis of the knee. J Am Acad Orthop Surg 2007;15(11):682–94.

38. Csintalan RP, Inacio MCS, Funahashi TT, et al. Risk factors of subsequent operations after primary anterior cruciate ligament reconstruction. Am J Sports Med 2014;42(3):619–25.

39. Noyes FR, Berrios-Torres S, Barber-Westin SD, et al. Prevention of permanent arthrofibrosis after anterior cruciate ligament reconstruction alone or combined with associated procedures: a prospective study in 443 knees. Knee Surg Sports Traumatol Arthrosc 2000;8(4):196–206.

40. Magnussen RA, Lawrence JTR, West RL, et al. Graft size and patient age are predictors of early revision after anterior cruciate ligament reconstruction with hamstring autograft. Arthroscopy 2012;28(4):526–31.

Knee MLI Injuries
Common Problems and Solutions

Niv Marom, MD, Joseph J. Ruzbarsky, MD, Naomi Roselaar, BS, Robert G. Marx, MD*

KEYWORDS

- Multiple ligament injury • Knee dislocation • Complications • Surgical reconstruction
- Surgical repair • Cruciate ligaments • Collateral ligaments

KEY POINTS

- Multiligament injuries are complex injuries with the potential for an array of significant complications.
- Prevention of these complications is based on comprehensive understanding of knee anatomy and biomechanics, detailed surgical planning, careful execution in the operation room, close postoperative monitoring, and a proper rehabilitation program.
- Early recognition of complications with appropriate management is critical for satisfactory outcomes.

INTRODUCTION

The multiple ligament injured knee presents a challenge with regard to management and treatment. Recent evidence suggests that the incidence of knee dislocations and multiple ligament injured knees is 0.072 events per 100 patient-years. This rate is considered by many as an underestimation based on the unique characteristics of this injury and possible spontaneous reduction of the dislocation, which can lead to a missed diagnosis.[1–3]

The immediate management of the acute injury requires special attention and thorough examination because knee dislocations have been associated with vascular complications such as popliteal artery injury in 5% to 40% of cases, neurologic complications including peroneal nerve injury in 16% to 40% of cases, tibial nerve injuries, associated fractures in 10% to 20% of cases, open wounds and soft tissue injuries, and visceral injuries.[1,4–6] Additional associated knee injuries include meniscal tears in up to 37% of cases, knee articular cartilage damage in up to 20% of cases in the acute setting, patellar dislocations in 5% of cases, and patellar tendon rupture in nearly 2% of cases.[6]

Disclosure Statement: All authors have no commercial or financial conflicts of interest and deny any funding sources relevant to this article.
Sports Medicine, Hospital for Special Surgery, 535 East 70th Street, New York, NY 10021, USA
* Corresponding author.
E-mail address: MarxR@hss.edu

Treatment options range from closed reduction and immobilization to surgical repair and/or reconstruction of the injured ligaments using allograft, autograft, synthetic ligaments, or combinations thereof.[7] The optimal timing of these procedures is still debatable, with more and more evidence supporting superior clinical outcomes with early intervention.[7–9]

This article focuses on complications that may result from surgical treatments of the multiple ligament injured knee.

SURGICAL COMPLICATIONS
Vascular Injury

Missed popliteal artery injury at presentation
A missed or subclinical popliteal artery injury that was not diagnosed at presentation can manifest itself during or after surgery on a multiligament injured knee (**Fig. 1**). The risk is thought to increase with use of a thigh tourniquet. Reports of large intimal tears and pseudoaneurysms of the popliteal artery requiring urgent revascularization procedures postoperatively owing to a pulseless limb are described in the literature.[10–12]

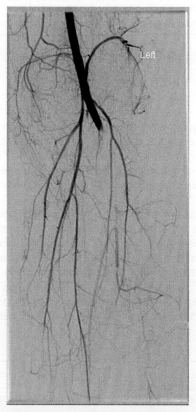

Fig. 1. Conventional arteriogram demonstrating collateral flow to the distal part of the lower extremity despite complete popliteal artery occlusion. In the dislocated knee, a palpable pulse may be present distal to a complete popliteal arterial occlusion. (*From* Fanelli GC, Stannard JP, Stuart MJ, et al. Management of complex knee ligament injuries. J Bone Joint Surg Am 2010;92(12):2236; with permission.)

The surgeon performing multiligament surgeries must be aware of these potential risks and conduct repeated and meticulous neurovascular examinations to the involved limb before and after surgery. Any abnormality requires urgent attention and a thorough evaluation.

In the surgery itself, special consideration should be given to tourniquet use. The tourniquet should be placed very proximal on the patient's thigh, as far as possible from the zone of injury, adequate padding should be used if using a pneumatic tourniquet, all-in-one exsanguination devices should be avoided, and the tourniquet should be inflated to an appropriate pressure for as brief a duration as possible. If an extensive tourniquet time is planned, it is recommended to periodically deflate the tourniquet for approximately 10 to 15 minutes to allow reperfusion before reinflation.

Iatrogenic vascular injury

In addressing a multiligamentous injured knee, the reconstruction of the posterior cruciate ligament (PCL) presents a risk for an iatrogenic intraoperative injury to the popliteal artery. Drilling the tibial tunnel in a transtibial fashion, vigorous retraction, or improper dissection in the tibial inlay technique all put the popliteal artery at risk for injury.[13] The distance of the popliteal artery from the tibial attachment of the PCL in the sagittal plane has been shown to be 9.3 mm in average with knee flexion of 100°, but only as little as 5.4 mm in average in full extension.[14]

Preventing iatrogenic injuries can potentially be facilitated with the use of commercially available PCL tibial guides and retractors designed for protecting guide pin penetration into the posterior capsule. Additional strategies include fluoroscopic imaging, direct visualization of the guide pin exiting the PCL tibial footprint by using the 70° arthroscope through an accessory portal, and the use of commercially available pin blocker (or curette) for protection during tunnel reaming. Regardless of the method used, careful and deliberate surgical technique, especially while reaming the tibial tunnel, should be carried out to allow for slow penetration of the PCL footprint.

Nerve Injury

Iatrogenic peroneal nerve injury

Repair and reconstruction of the posterolateral corner of the knee presents a risk for iatrogenic injuries to the peroneal nerve that crosses in close proximity to the posterolateral structures.[15,16] The nerve is at greatest risk during fibular tunnel drilling during reconstructions or when performing a biceps femoris repair.[10] Another potential nerve injury risk is the use of tourniquets during the surgeries.

Prevention of peroneal nerve injury is based on identifying and protecting the peroneal nerve early in the surgical dissection. The nerve is best identified in the distal thigh posterior to the biceps femoris tendon.[17] During closure, the fascial plane posterior to the biceps femoris should be left open to prevent potential nerve compression owing to postoperative edema.

Iatrogenic saphenous nerve injury

Repair and reconstruction of the medial corner of the knee present a risk for iatrogenic injuries to the saphenous nerve and its branches. The saphenous nerve courses deep to the sartorius muscle and the gracilis tendon. The main branch of this nerve, the sartorial branch, travels distally to supply sensation to the medial aspect of the leg. Injury to the sartorial branch may result in numbness or sensory disturbances in this distribution or a painful neuroma at the site of injury.[10] The risk of such injury is increased when using a posteromedial arthroscopic portal, harvesting the pes anserine tendons, or performing medial collateral ligament reconstruction or repair. The infrapatellar branch of the saphenous nerve is potentially at risk for injury when performing anteromedial incisions around the knee or when establishing a medial arthroscopic portal. Injury to this branch would lead to sensory disturbance over the anterolateral aspect of the knee and may also lead to a painful neuroma.[18,19] It is thought that flexing of the knee during pes tendon harvesting may put the nerve at a lesser risk for injury.

Venous Thromboembolic Events

Although there is no reported specific data regarding the specific incidence of deep venous thrombosis and pulmonary embolism in patients after multiligament surgery, it is well-accepted that these patients are at a higher risk for such complications given the risk factors of a complex injury, lengthy operation, the intraoperative use of a tourniquet, venous stasis, a possible endothelial injury, and postoperative immobilization. Rates of 3.5% have been reported for knee dislocations[20] and a recently published case report presented an asymptomatic 43-year-old woman who was diagnosed with deep venous thrombosis and bilateral massive pulmonary embolism 10 days postoperatively after revision multiligament reconstruction.[21]

Despite these risks, there is no consensus on the use of drug prophylaxis for thromboembolic disease or the indications for an inferior vena cava filter. A surgeon should use his or her best judgment for appropriate pharmacologic or mechanical thromboembolic prophylaxis, especially in the setting of restricted weightbearing or knee range of motion. In addition to prophylaxis, evaluation for deep venous thromboses before the planned surgery is of paramount importance before any intervention so that appropriate treatment can ensue.

Arthrofibrosis

Functional range of motion is a key factor in return to daily life activities and especially in athletes who wish to return to sports. Many factors influence the risk of arthrofibrosis, including the severity of trauma, preoperative range of motion, tunnel position, heterotopic ossification, infection, rehabilitation, compliance, and genetic predisposition. Previously, arthrofibrosis was a more commonly encountered complication when multiple ligament injured knees were treated definitively with long term cast immobilization. Even in those knees treated surgically, however, the mean incidence of this complication has been high with reports up to 29%.[22] A high rate of these patients, up to 21%, goes on to require subsequent manipulation procedures.[23] Some authors have suggested that early surgical intervention in the first 3 weeks after injury might promote arthrofibrosis, whereas others found improved outcomes with early surgical intervention.[24–30] Recent systematic reviews reported superior clinical outcomes with early intervention.[8,24]

Prevention strategies for arthrofibrosis include careful handling of soft tissue, arthroscopic techniques where possible, minimization of autografts from the injured knee, postoperative protocols that address swelling and inflammation (rest, ice, compression, elevation, early range of motion exercises), and adherence to a proven rehabilitation protocol. If arthrofibrosis develops, there is a spectrum of treatment modalities available. These include rigorous physiotherapy accompanied with proper pain and inflammation management; manipulation under anesthesia with therapy after manipulation; surgical intervention with arthroscopic synovectomy, lysis of adhesions, and fat pad debridement; or open procedures for the debridement of excessive scar tissue.

Compartment Syndrome and Fluid Extravasation

Knee dislocation injuries can involve a significant capsular disruption and/or fascial damage. These anatomic defects can predispose to fluid extravasation during arthroscopy, if performed in the first 1 to 2 weeks after injury. Extravasation of arthroscopic fluid has the potential to cause a compartment syndrome.[31–33]

Strategies for avoiding the extravasation of fluid and potential compartment syndrome are postponing the surgery to allow for capsular and fascial healing when an extensive injury is diagnosed. When reconstruction is performed early, using a low-flow pump, gravity flow, dry arthroscopy, or doing the arthroscopy after the open surgery for the medial or lateral side to allow for an external fluid leak may all be beneficial for prevention.

Regardless of the specific preventive technique, when the arthroscopy is performed, it is essential that compartments of the involved limb be assessed both preoperatively and postoperatively with inpatient evaluation as warranted.

Wound Problems and Infection

Wound complications and infection are of particular concern because many patients with knee dislocations have severely traumatized soft tissues around the knee, both superficial and deep. Special consideration should be taken when managing an open knee dislocation, as it may require emergent debridement, irrigation, intravenous antibiotics, and external fixation. Generally, surgical intervention should be delayed until swelling and/or ecchymosis have resolved, wounds around the knee have healed, and there are no signs of infection.

Intraoperative methods to prevent potential wound healing problems include avoiding new incisions that cross previous scars or wounds, maintaining sufficient skin bridges (>10 cm) between incisions, practicing meticulous skin and soft tissue management with full tissue skin flaps, performing appropriate hemostasis before wound closure, closing the wound without tension, and using drains when deemed necessary for prevention of hematoma formation.[10] Postoperatively, surgical wounds should be monitored closely during the first few weeks for infection or wound complications.

Heterotopic Ossification

Heterotopic ossification is a less reported complication in the multiple ligament injured knee; however, it is common, with a published incidence of 26% to 43%.[34–36] The timing of surgery or number of ligaments reconstructed does not seem to affect the development of heterotopic ossification. Symptoms described in the literature include pain and limited range of motion, with minority of cases presenting as ankylosis.[34–36]

Prevention modalities such as prophylactic antiinflammatory drugs or low-dose radiation have not been investigated in the dislocated knee. Manipulation under anesthesia and intensive physiotherapy remain the mainstay of treatments in the mild to moderate cases, whereas surgical lysis of adhesions and release of soft tissue is recommended in more severe and complicated cases.

Fractures and Avascular Necrosis

Multiligament reconstruction surgeries require drilling of multiple tunnels in the proximal tibia and distal femur. Weakening of the femoral condyles secondary to multiple tunnels drilled and hardware installed in the bone presents the risk of fracture or avascular necrosis (**Fig. 2**). Sporadic cases have been reported in the literature.[37]

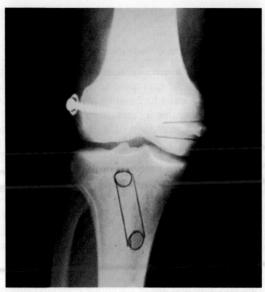

Fig. 2. Medial femoral condyle osteonecrosis after multiligament reconstruction surgery with low posterior cruciate ligament tunnel leading to avascular necrosis. (*Courtesy of Dr Greg Fanelli, Danville, PA; with permission.*)

Tunnels Placement

Tunnel placement in cruciate ligament reconstruction is crucial for anatomically placed grafts, which allow for adequate stability and full range of motion. Tunnel malposition and graft impingement are among the more common complications seen in cruciate ligament reconstructions. The orientation of the tunnels and the exact position of the intraarticular tunnel aperture are important factors that must be considered before and during the surgery. It is well-accepted, for instance, that vertical femoral tunnels in isolated anterior cruciate ligament (ACL) reconstruction provide suboptimal rotational stability and that anterior tibial tunnels may cause notch impingement and loss of extension.[38,39] As for reconstructions of the PCL, a high tunnel aperture on the posterior tibia will lead to suboptimal lever arm and potential graft failure (**Fig. 3**). The multiligament injured knee is much less tolerant to tunnel placement errors, especially when both cruciate ligaments are reconstructed. Intraoperative fluoroscopy can be helpful for correct placement of tunnels.

Tunnel Convergence

Drilling multiple tunnels, especially in the distal femur, raises the potential risk of convergence of tunnels or hardware. Convergence of tunnels may result in graft damage and fixation impairment that can result in reconstruction failure. In the distal femur, the ACL tunnel is at risk of convergence with the lateral and posterolateral reconstruction tunnels and the PCL tunnel is at risk for convergence with the medial and posteromedial reconstruction tunnels. In the tibia, the PCL tunnel is at risk for convergence, with both the posterior oblique ligament tunnel and the superficial medial collateral ligament tunnel. Surgeons must preplan tunnel placement and make sure they are prepared for intraoperative complications such as convergence, because these complications often require backup fixation methods. Recent published data provide

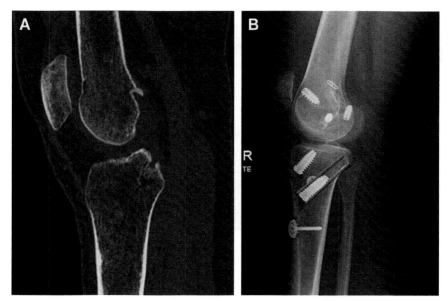

Fig. 3. (*A*) Computed tomography scan (sagittal view) of the right knee after failed multi-ligament reconstruction and removal of hardware. The posterior cruciate ligament (PCL) tunnel aperture is shown high on the posterior proximal tibia. (*B*) Lateral radiographic view of the same knee after revision multiligament reconstruction showing a proper placement of the PCL tunnel and tunnel aperture lower on the posterior proximal tibia, proving a better lever arm.

recommendations for reducing the risk of convergence in the multiple ligament reconstructed knee.[40,41]

Graft Tensioning

The position of the knee and sequence in which each graft is tensioned and fixed, as well as the tensioning techniques, are all important factors that play a significant role in achieving good stability and full range of motion for the multiple ligament injured knee. For instance, tensioning and fixation of the ACL graft in flexion and before tensioning and fixation of the PCL may result extension lag and an anteriorly subluxed knee. Typically, the PCL is the first graft that should be tensioned and fixed, followed by the ACL, posterolateral complex ligaments, and finally the medial ligament complex.[42] Modifications can be made if knee stability and range of motion are not compromised.

Malalignment

Osseous malalignment can be a contributing factor to knee ligament surgery failure and realignment surgery can improve function and stability in those instances.[43] Unrecognized malalignment of the lower limb will place additional forces on repaired or reconstructed ligaments and increase the risk of failure.[44,45] Malalignment can be either preexisting or the result of malunited intraarticular or extraarticular fractures (**Fig. 4**). The most common deformity contributing to graft failure is varus malalignment leading to premature failure of posterolateral corner reconstructions. Tibial slope should also be taken to consideration, especially in revision cases.[43,46] When suspicion exists, preoperative full-length standing lower extremity radiographs or EOS should be obtained to identify potential cases of malalignment. Corrective

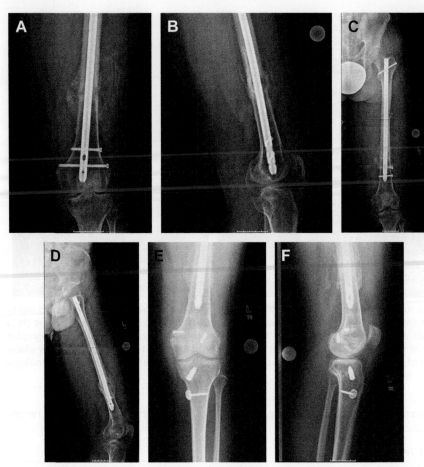

Fig. 4. A 38-year-old man presented with malunited left open femoral shaft fracture (external rotation deformity) that was internally fixed with intramedullary nail and failed isolated medial collateral ligament (MCL) reconstruction in an anterior cruciate ligament (ACL)-deficient knee. (*A, B*) Anteroposterior (AP) and lateral views of the left femur, demonstrating a healed fracture with long intramedullary nail. On the medial side of the knee, suboptimal reconstructed MCL attachments can be seen: slightly distal on the femur and slightly proximal on the tibia in relation to the anatomic insertion sites. (*C, D*) AP and lateral views of the left femur after removal of the long nail, corrective femoral, osteotomy and shorter intramedullary nail fixation. (*E, F*) Standing AP and lateral views of the left knee after ACL and MCL anatomic reconstruction using Achilles tendon allograft for both ligaments.

osteotomies or other procedures can then be performed at the time of surgery or at in a staged fashion.

SUMMARY

Multiligament injuries are complex injuries with the potential for an array of significant complications. Prevention of these complications is based on a comprehensive understanding of knee anatomy and biomechanics, detailed surgical planning, careful execution in the operation room, close postoperative monitoring, and a proper rehabilitation program. Early recognition of complications with appropriate management is critical for satisfactory outcomes.

REFERENCES

1. Arom GA, Yeranosian MG, Petrigliano FA, et al. The changing demographics of knee dislocation: a retrospective database review. Clin Orthop Relat Res 2014; 472(9):2609–14.
2. Wilson SM, Mehta N, Do HT, et al. Epidemiology of multiligament knee reconstruction. Clin Orthop Relat Res 2014;472(9):2603–8.
3. Brautigan B, Johnson DL. The epidemiology of knee dislocations. Clin Sports Med 2000;19:387–97.
4. Rihn JA, Groff YJ, Harner CD, et al. The acutely dislocated knee: evaluation and management. J Am Acad Orthop Surg 2004;2(5):334–46.
5. Henrichs A. A review of knee dislocations. J Athl Train 2004;39:365–9.
6. Cole BJ, Harner CD. The multiple ligament injured knee. Clin Sports Med 1999;8: 241–62.
7. Moatshe G, Dornan GJ, Løken S, et al. Demographics and injuries associated with knee dislocation: a prospective review of 303 patients. Orthop J Sports Med 2017;5(5):232.
8. Dwyer T, Marx RG, Whelan D. Outcomes of treatment of multiple ligament knee injuries. J Knee Surg 2012;25(4):317–26.
9. Hohmann E, Glatt V, Tetsworth K. Early or delayed reconstruction in multiligament knee injuries: a systematic review and meta-analysis. Knee 2017. https://doi.org/10.1016/j.knee.2017.06.011.
10. Tay AK, MacDonald PB. Complications associated with treatment of multiple ligament injured (dislocated) knee. Sports Med Arthrosc 2011;19(2):153–61.
11. Natividad TT, Wascher CD. Complications associated with the treatment of the multiple ligament injured knee. In: Fanelli GC, editor. The multiple ligament injured knee: a practical guide to management. New York: Springer; 2013. p. 443–50.
12. McDonough EB Jr, Wojtys EM. Multi-ligamentous injuries of the knee and associated vascular injuries. Am J Sports Med 2009;37:156–9.
13. Kaufman SL, Martin LG. Arterial injuries associated with complete dislocation of the knee. Radiology 1992;184:153–5.
14. Jackson DW, Proctor CS, Simon TM. Arthroscopic assisted PCL reconstruction: a technical note on potential neurovascular injury related to drill bit configuration. Arthroscopy 1993;9:224–7.
15. Matava MJ, Sethi NS, Totty WG. Proximity of the posterior cruciate ligament insertion to the popliteal artery as a function of the knee flexion angle: implications for posterior cruciate ligament reconstruction. Arthroscopy 2000;16:796–804.
16. Shapiro MS, Freedman EL. Allograft reconstruction of the anterior and posterior cruciate ligaments after traumatic knee dislocation. Am J Sports Med 1995;23:580–7.
17. Luo H, Yu JK, Ao YF, et al. Relationship between different skin incisions and the injury of the infrapatellar branch of the saphenous nerve during anterior cruciate ligament reconstruction. Chin Med J (Engl) 2007;120:1127–30.
18. Yates SK, Hurst LN, Brown WF. The pathogenesis of pneumatic tourniquet paralysis in man. J Neurol Neurosurg Psychiatry 1981;44:759–67.
19. Figueroa D, Calvo R, Vaisman A, et al. Injury to the infrapatellar branch of the saphenous nerve in ACL reconstruction with the hamstrings technique: clinical and electrophysiological study. Knee 2008;15:360–3.

20. Terry GC, LaPrade RF. The posterolateral aspect of the knee. Anatomy and surgical approach. Am J Sports Med 1996;24:732–9.
21. Engebretsen L, Risberg MA, Robertson B, et al. Outcome after knee dislocations: a 2-9 years follow-up of 85 consecutive patients. Knee Surg Sports Traumatol Arthrosc 2009;17:1013–26.
22. Takigami J, Hashimoto Y, Yamasaki S, et al. A case of asymptomatic bilateral massive pulmonary embolism after arthroscopic multiple knee ligament reconstruction. Knee Surg Sports Traumatol Arthrosc 2017;25(1):260–2.
23. Stannard JP, Schenck RC Jr, Fanelli GC. Knee dislocations and fracture-dislocation. In: Bucholz RW, Court-Brown C, Heckman JD, editors. Rockwood and Green's fractures in adults. Philadelphia: Lippincott, Williams, and Wilkins; 2009. p. 1832–66.
24. Harner CD, Waltrip RL, Bennett CH, et al. Surgical management of knee dislocations. J Bone Joint Surg Am 2004;86-A:262–73.
25. Harner CD, Irrgang JJ, Paul J, et al. Loss of motion after anterior cruciate ligament reconstruction. Am J Sports Med 1992;20:499–506.
26. Shelbourne KD, Nitz P. Accelerated rehabilitation after anterior cruciate ligament reconstruction. Am J Sports Med 1990;18:292–9.
27. Shelbourne KD, Wilckens JH, Mollabashy A, et al. Arthrofibrosis in acute anterior cruciate ligament reconstruction. The effect of timing of reconstruction and rehabilitation. Am J Sports Med 1991;19:332–6.
28. Mohtadi NG, Webster-Bogaert S, Fowler PJ. Limitation of motion following anterior cruciate ligament reconstruction. A case-control study. Am J Sports Med 1991;19:620–5.
29. Fanelli GC, Giannotti BF, Edson CJ. Arthroscopically assisted combined posterior cruciate ligament/posterior lateral complex reconstruction. Arthroscopy 1996;12:521–30.
30. Liow RY, McNicholas MJ, Keating JF, et al. Ligament repair and reconstruction in traumatic dislocation of the knee. J Bone Joint Surg Br 2003;85:845–51.
31. Levy BA, Dajani KA, Whelan DB, et al. Decision making in the multiligament-injured knee: an evidence-based systematic review. Arthroscopy 2009;25:430–8.
32. Bomberg BC, Hurley PE, Clark CA, et al. Complications associated with the use of an infusion pump during knee arthroscopy. Arthroscopy 1992;8:224–8.
33. Ekman EF, Poehling GG. An experimental assessment of the risk of compartment syndrome during knee arthroscopy. Arthroscopy 1996;12:193–9.
34. Amendola A, Faber K, Willits K, et al. Compartment pressure monitoring during anterior cruciate ligament reconstruction. Arthroscopy 1999;15:607–12.
35. Levy BA, Krych AJ, Shah JP, et al. Staged protocol for initial management of the dislocated knee. Knee Surg Sports Traumatol Arthrosc 2010;18:1630–7.
36. Stannard JP, Wilson TC, Sheils TM, et al. Heterotopic ossification associated with knee dislocation. Arthroscopy 2002;18:835–9.
37. Patton WC, Tew WM. Periarticular heterotopic ossification after multiple knee ligament reconstructions. A report of three cases. Am J Sports Med 2000;28(3):398–401.
38. Konan S, Haddad FS. Femoral fracture following knee ligament reconstruction surgery due to an unpredictable complication of bioabsorbable screw fixation: a case report and review of literature. J Orthop Traumatol 2010;11:51–5.
39. Trojani C, Sbihi A, Djian P, et al. Causes for failure of ACL reconstruction and influence of meniscectomies after revision. Knee Surg Sports Traumatol Arthrosc 2011;19(2):196–201.
40. Petsche TS, Hutchinson MR. Loss of extension after reconstruction of the anterior cruciate ligament. J Am Acad Orthop Surg 1999;7:119–27.

41. Moatshe G, Brady AW, Slette EL, et al. Multiple ligament reconstruction femoral tunnels: intertunnel relationships and guidelines to avoid convergence. Am J Sports Med 2017;45(3):563–9.
42. Moatshe G, Slette EL, Engebretsen L, et al. Intertunnel relationships in the tibia during reconstruction of multiple knee ligaments: how to avoid tunnel convergence. Am J Sports Med 2016;44(11):2864–9.
43. LaPrade RF, Resig S, Wentorf F, et al. The effects of grade III posterolateral knee complex injuries on anterior cruciate ligament graft force. A biomechanical analysis. Am J Sports Med 1999;27:469–75.
44. Tischer T, Paul J, Pape D, et al. The impact of osseous malalignment and realignment procedures in knee ligament surgery: a systematic review of the clinical evidence. Orthop J Sports Med 2017;5(3). 2325967117697287.
45. Bretin P, O'Loughlin PF, Suero PM, et al. Influence of femoral malrotation on knee joint alignment and intraarticular contact pressures. Arch Orthop Trauma Surg 2011;131:1115–20.
46. Fanelli GC, Orcutt DR, Edson CJ. The multiple-ligament injured knee: evaluation, treatment, and results. Arthroscopy 2005;21(4):471–86.

Knee Meniscus Injuries
Common Problems and Solutions

Matthew H. Blake, MD[a],*, Darren L. Johnson, MD[b]

KEYWORDS

- Meniscus • Complication • Infection • Tear • Repair • Chondrolysis • Implant
- Nerve injury

KEY POINTS

- The rates of arthroscopic meniscus repair continue to increase with excellent reported outcomes.
- Complications, sometimes catastrophic, following meniscus repair may occur.
- The rate of postoperative complications may be reduced by adequate diagnosis, appropriate patient selection, meniscus repair selection, surgical techniques, and postoperative management.
- When complications occur, the provider must identify and take steps to rectify as well as prevent further complications from occurring.
- The purpose of this article is to detail the common diagnostic, technical, and postoperative pitfalls that may result in poor patient outcomes.

INTRODUCTION

The menisci were once thought to be functionless remnants of intra-articular leg muscles; however, now they are recognized as important structures that provide lubrication, stability, joint congruity, load transmission, and functionally act as "shock absorbers" for joint preservation.[1,2] Injuries to the menisci alter normal knee kinematics, increase peak contact stress, and can result in early degenerative changes of the knee.[3–8] A structure once excised with impunity, the menisci are now preserved and repaired to protect articular cartilage from accelerated degeneration as well as provide important stabilization to the cruciate injured knee.

Partial meniscectomy has been reported to be the most common orthopedic surgical procedure in America.[9] Improved arthroscopic instrumentation and surgical techniques combined with increased knowledge of the form and function of the meniscus have led to a doubling of arthroscopic meniscal repairs from 2005 to

[a] Department of Orthopaedic Surgery and Sports Medicine, Avera McKennan Hospital and University Health Center, 911 East 20th Street, Suite 300, Sioux Falls, SD 57105, USA; [b] Department of Orthopaedic Surgery, University of Kentucky School of Medicine, 740 South Limestone, K403, Lexington, KY 40536-0284, USA
* Corresponding author.
E-mail address: Matthew.Blake@Avera.org

Clin Sports Med 37 (2018) 293–306
https://doi.org/10.1016/j.csm.2017.12.007
0278-5919/18/© 2017 Elsevier Inc. All rights reserved.

sportsmed.theclinics.com

2011.[10] The success rate of meniscal repairs has been reported to be between 87% and 91%.[11-14] Despite excellent success rates, failures, sometimes catastrophic, may occur.[15-18] The purpose of this article is to detail the common diagnostic, technical, and postoperative pitfalls that may result in poor patient outcomes.

PATIENT SELECTION

Appropriate patient and meniscus selection is paramount to successful meniscus repair. The ideal candidate is a patient who has had a recent traumatic episode causing mechanical symptoms that can be localized and re-created by physical examination. During evaluation, it is important that the patient's symptoms correlate with both their physical examination and their diagnostic studies. Surgery for problems that do not correlate with their examination and diagnostic findings will not be beneficial, and one must look for other potential sources of their knee pain.

The physician must assess important risk factors, such as smoking and obesity, as well as patient-specific postoperative expectations that may lead to repair failure.[19] The physician must discuss with the patient and determine if the patient will be compliant with the postoperative protocol.[18] A partial meniscectomy may be appropriate if the patient is unable or unwilling to follow a conservative postoperative protocol or if the patient has had a prior failed meniscal repair.

There is not a patient chronologic age limit when meniscal repairs should not be performed. The physiologic age of the knee and activity level of the patient often dictates treatment. Isolated meniscal repair in patients older than 40 years old may have a higher failure rate[18,20-22]; however, this has recently come under debate.[23-25] Dr Steadman and colleagues[25] recently reported 136 meniscal repairs in patients younger than 40 years old to those older than 40 years old and found no difference in meniscal repair failure rates.

Meniscal tears that are more degenerative in nature or chronic may not be amenable to repair. These meniscal tears are often found in patients with a long-standing history of knee pain, usually without a traumatic event, that are identified by MRI ordered for generalize knee pain. Likewise, radiographic findings of knee arthritis (Outerbridge grades 3 and 4) with an MRI finding of a meniscal tear have a low likelihood of success following repair.[26,27] Greater than 2 mm of joint space narrowing on weight-bearing radiographs is strongly correlated with Outerbridge grade 3 and 4 cartilage degeneration.[28] Joint space narrowing is not influenced by meniscectomy and thus is pathognomonic for osteoarthritis (**Fig. 1**).[29]

Patients with a body mass index >30 have been shown to have a higher incidence of repair failure.[21,30] Smoking has also been shown to have a 3.8 times higher rate of meniscal repair failure compared with patients who do not smoke.[19] Joint stability after cruciate ligament injury and reconstruction is very dependent upon intact medial and lateral menisci. The force experienced by the medial meniscus in the anterior cruciate ligament (ACL) -deficient knee is increased by 52% in full extension and by 197% at 60° of flexion under a 134-N load.[31] In patients with an unstable knee, the meniscal repair failure rate is as high as 18%.[32,33] If meniscal repair is to be performed, concomitant ligament reconstruction should always be performed. Any meniscal lesion in the ACL injured knee must be given strong consideration for repair versus reconstruction. The medial meniscus acts as a strong restraint against anterior translation, and the lateral meniscus assists greatly in rotatory stability. Absence of either of these structures will drastically decrease the ACL reconstruction success rate. One could argue, based on recent available literature, that the importance of the menisci to knee stability is greater than that of chondroprotection.

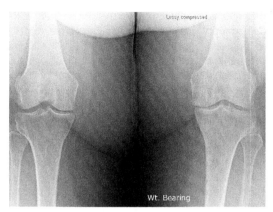

Fig. 1. Rosenberg view depicting left knee medial joint space narrowing greater than 2 mm in comparison to contralateral knee. This is equivalent to grade III or IV chondromalacia. Wt., weight.

DIAGNOSIS

Many meniscal tear patterns are easily diagnosed on MRI as well as during arthroscopy. Three tear patterns that may be easily missed on poor-quality MRI scans or one who is not "looking" for them are meniscal root tears, ramp lesions, and popliteomeniscal fasciculi tears.[34,35]

Meniscal root tears are avulsions from the bone or radial tears of the meniscus that occur at the meniscal attachment to the tibial plateau. Lateral meniscal root tears are present in up to 20% of the acutely injured ACL knee. Meniscal root tears change the biomechanics and kinematics of the knee to equal the biomechanics and kinematics of a total meniscectomy.[36] Coronal MRI sequences reveal high T2 signal between the meniscus and posterior cruciate ligament (PCL) (**Fig. 2**A). Meniscal extrusion greater than 3 mm as well as the "ghost sign" near the root on sagittal images highly correlates with a meniscal root tear (**Fig. 2**B).[36] Failure to diagnosis and repair these lesions may lead to increased incidence of osteoarthritis as well as an increased failure rate of ACL reconstruction.

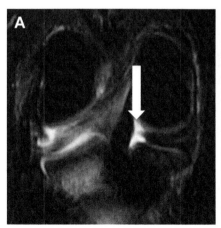
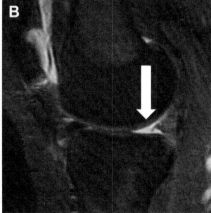

Fig. 2. (*A*) Arrow pointing to increase signal between medial meniscus root and PCL. (*B*) Arrow pointing to the ghost sign of the medial meniscus.

A ramp lesion is a longitudinal tear of the peripheral attachment of the posterior horn of the medial meniscus commonly seen in the ACL injured knee.[37] MRI sensitivity in diagnosing a ramp lesion has been reported to be 0% to 77%.[38–40] MRI findings of a thin fluid signal interposed between the posterior horn of the medial meniscus and the posteromedial capsule, high signal irregularity of the capsular margin of the medial meniscus posterior horn, and a posteromedial tibial bone bruise are 3 subtle findings that should alert the surgeon to have a higher index of suspicion of a ramp lesion (**Fig. 3**).[41–43]

The anteroinferior, posterosuperior, and posteroinferior fasciculi comprise the popliteomeniscal fasciculi and secure the lateral meniscus at the popliteal hiatus (**Fig. 4**A).[44] Disruption of the popliteomeniscal fasciculi results in lateral joint line pain with increased lateral meniscus mobility that may cause mechanical symptoms of locking or catching, particularly in the figure-4 position or if the patient sits "Indian style."[45–47] Isolated popliteomeniscal fascicle tears can best be evaluated on sagittal T2-weighted MRI with disruption of the posterosuperior popliteomeniscal fascicle having a high positive-predictive value for arthroscopically confirmed tears of the posterior horn of the lateral meniscus (**Fig. 4**B).[48,49] Most patients seen in the office that have this problem have an MRI reading that says "the lateral meniscus appears normal." A high index of suspicion must be made by the clinician with confirmation done at the time of arthroscopy. At the time of arthroscopy, if more than half of the lateral meniscus shows abnormal mobility, a popliteomeniscal fascicle tear should be suspected (**Fig. 4**C).[50] Inside-out repair of the lateral meniscus back to the popliteomeniscal fascicles and popliteus tendon has yielded good results (**Fig. 4**D).[45,51,52]

The size of tear, location of tear, and the complexity of tear are readily evaluated at the time of arthroscopy. Evaluation of the substance of the tear and adjacent tissue helps determine the meniscus' capacity to heal. The size and location of the tear can be assessed using calibrated probes. Tears that are less than 1 cm and partial thickness tears generally heal without intervention.[7,53] Peripheral tears that do not displace with probing may be treated with abrasion and trephination without repair.[7,18]

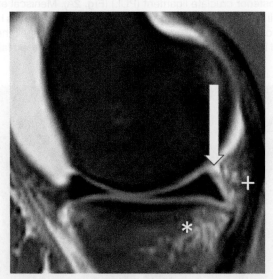

Fig. 3. Subtle findings consistent with a posteromedial meniscus ramp lesion. Arrow pointing to fluid interposed between the posterior horn of the medial meniscus and the posteromedial capsule. Asterisk on the posteromedial tibial bone bruise. Plus sign depicting high signal of the posterior capsular margin.

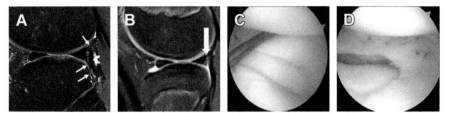

Fig. 4. (*A*) Normal popliteomeniscal fasciculi. Single arrow pointing to the posterosuperior fasciculi. Double arrow pointing to the posteroinferior fasciculi. Greater than sign pointing to the popliteal tendon. (*B*) Arrow pointing to a tear of the popliteomeniscal fasciculi. (*C*) Increased anterior translation of the lateral meniscus to probing. (*D*) Repair of the lateral meniscus.

Tears within 3 mm of the meniscosynovial junction, in the red-red zone, have adequate blood supply, and repair should be performed (**Fig. 5**).[53] Likewise, tears in the red-white zone should also be considered for repair with biologic augmentation, particularly in the cruciate injured knee. Tears that occur in the white zone of the meniscus do not heal and should be excised.[54,55] Persistent pain, recurrent effusion, or return of symptoms after surgery may indicate failure of repair and MRI with arthrogram performed.

Tears occurring in more than one plane are described as complex tears and should be excised because of the high incidence of repair failure (**Fig. 6**).[18,56] These types of tears are usually degenerative and are often associated with chondral damage. Complex meniscal tears associated with chondral damage and joint space narrowing on weight-bearing radiographs without malalignment are best treated with nonsteroidal anti-inflammatory drugs, periodic steroid injections, weight loss, and physical therapy but eventually may require total knee replacement. Complex tears causing mechanical symptoms may require partial meniscectomy if the "mechanical symptoms" and not pain are the primary symptom of the patient. If a complex tear has been repaired and the patient continues to be symptomatic, then a postoperative MRI and arthroscopic evaluation may need to be performed.[27,57]

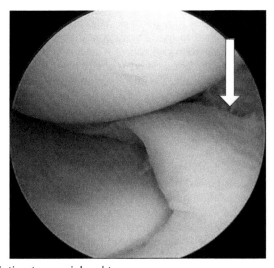

Fig. 5. Arrow pointing to a peripheral tear.

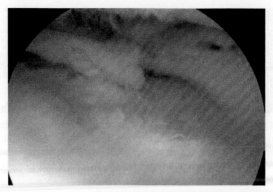

Fig. 6. A complex tear with radial, horizontal, and oblique tears.

TECHNIQUE

Without appropriate surgical techniques, including visualization, instrumentation, suture choice and configuration, and augmentation, repair failure can occur.

An anterolateral portal is established 1 cm lateral to the inferior pole of the patella. The anteromedial portal is established under direct arthroscopic observation directly proximal to the anterior horn of the medial meniscus allowing for adequate instrumentation and visualization of the posterior horns of the menisci. Using a 70° arthroscope may also improve visualization. Portal placement may change based on body habitus as well as the exact location of the tear. If one needs to make additional portals that enable superior visualization and suture placement, then there is no limit on portal placement. The morbidity of an additional portal is zero compared with damaged articular cartilage or a poorly performed meniscal repair.

Visualization is necessary for any surgery and is of paramount importance for arthroscopic meniscal repair, particularly to avoid iatrogenic injury to the articular cartilage. Inadequate visualization increases the risk for poor portal placement, poor meniscal repair, missed identification of meniscal tears, and chondral damage. Visualization of the lateral meniscus can be easily obtained by the "**Fig. 4**" position, whereas a varus load is placed on the knee. Varying amounts of knee flexion can further open the joint. Visualizing the medial joint space may be more difficult. A leg holder or a lateral post placed a handbreadth proximal to the femoral condyles will provide an appropriate fulcrum to aid in opening the medial joint space. A valgus force with the knee flexed at ~20° increases the visualization and working space of the medial joint. In order to see posteriorly medially, one must extend the knee fully while maintaining a valgus load. In the ACL-deficient knee that wants to "pivot" and close down the working space, the assistant must externally rotate the foot to keep the medial space open in the nonpivoted position. Changing the amount of flexion and/or increasing the valgus load may increase the working space. If adequate visualization cannot be achieved by knee manipulation, the medial collateral ligament (MCL) can be pie-crusted underneath the medial meniscus with an 18-gauge needle (**Fig. 7**) thus opening the medial joint space. Post-operatively the patient may have to be placed into a hinged brace until the MCL tightens.

With visualization obtained and appropriate portals made, the surgeon is able to adequately assess the meniscus. If repair is chosen, the surgeon must adequately prepare the tear for repair. Meniscal tears in the red-red and red-white zone must be prepared by rasping the meniscus tissue and periphery to increase vascularity at the repair site (**Fig. 8**). Trephination of the peripheral meniscal rim with an 18-gauge needle from inside out or outside in may also be performed. The repair can be

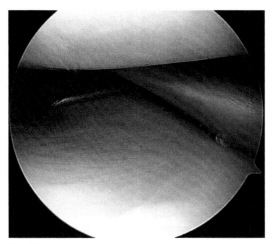

Fig. 7. Puncturing the MCL underneath the medial meniscus open the medial joint space.

augmented with a fibrin clot, or a microfracture of the lateral wall of the intercondylar notch above the femoral attachment of the ACL may also promote an inflow of pluripotent stem cells (**Fig. 9**).

The gold standard of meniscal repair is an inside-out technique for the body and posterior horns of the mensci; however, all inside techniques have also been described.[58–61] An outside-in technique should be used for tears of the anterior horn of the meniscus.[62] Intraoperatively, if a tear cannot be addressed by one repair technique, alternative techniques should be tried or hybrid repairs can be used. It is of paramount importance that an ACL surgeon be comfortable with multiple meniscal repair techniques because clearly "one size does not fit all."

Permanent suture is recommended because it allows for longer, more stable fixation, allowing the meniscal repair more time to complete maturation and remodeling. The meniscus heals with scar tissue and therefore never regains the absolute normal

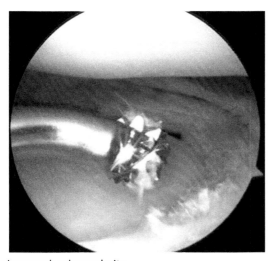

Fig. 8. Rasping to increase local vascularity.

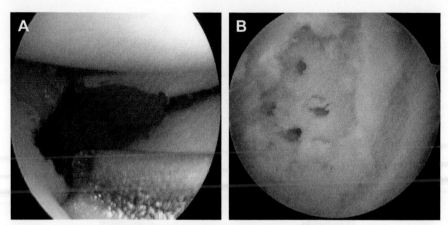

Fig. 9. (*A*) Fibrin clot. (*B*) Anterolateral notchplasty with microfracture.

collagen tensile strength it did before the tear happened. A braided suture has less risk of cut through than a monofilament and should be used. A 2-0 braided suture provides adequate strength and stability.[54,63] If using a meniscal repair kit or device, it is imperative that it is appropriately used as directed by manufacturer specifications.

Suture that is placed using improper suture pattern can lead to a biomechanically inferior repair with persistent pain and a nonhealing meniscus. Zone-specific cannulas aid in placing proper sutures in the specified zones of the meniscus. Sutures should be placed 3 to 5 mm apart throughout the length of the repair. Vertical mattress repairs are biomechanically superior to horizontal repairs with lower rates of pullout (**Fig. 10**).[64,65] One should alternate sutures on the superior and inferior meniscus surface so that the meniscus will lay flat on the tibial plateau.

Inappropriate tensioning of the suture can lead to nonhealing or iatrogenic meniscal injury.[66] Once the sutures are passed, the surgeon should tie the sutures while arthroscopically visualizing the repair allowing the surgeon, in real time, to assess the reduction of the meniscus without pulling the suture through the meniscal tissue. If too little tension is placed, then the meniscus will not be adequately reduced, leading to impaired healing

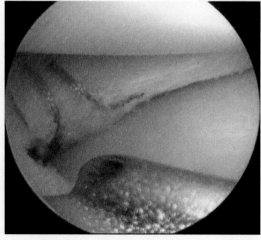

Fig. 10. Vertical mattress sutures spaced 3 to 5 mm apart.

and/or persistent instability. Medial meniscal repairs should be tied with the knee in full extension and lateral repairs with the knee in 90° of flexion so that tethering to the capsule leading to decreased range of motion does not occur.[22,55] Tying of the sutures medially in flexion will "capture" the knee and make it very difficult for the patient to regain normal extension postoperatively.

NERVE INJURY

A thorough knowledge of knee anatomy is a necessity so as not to injure any neurovascular structure. Injury to the saphenous nerve and vein, peroneal nerve, popliteal vessels, posterior tibial nerve, and geniculate arteries has been described.[67,68]

Injury to the saphenous nerve and vein are associated with medial meniscus repairs.[69] Clinically, the patient will have decreased sensation on the medial foot and possibly a painful neuroma at the injury site. The nerve travels on the undersurface of the sartorius anterior to the gracilis and superficial to the semimembranosus. Identification of the vein by transillumination of the vein through the inferolateral portal helps to identify the location of the nerve and vein.[69] During surgery, one may flex or extend the knee to move the nerve into a safer position during the repair. If injury to the saphenous nerve occurs and the patient has neuropathic pain or a positive tinel's sign, the nerve may require surgical exploration and/or excision.[70]

Injury to the peroneal nerve may cause deficits in dorsal and lateral leg and foot sensation. Injury can also cause weak or absent ankle and toe dorsiflexion. The common peroneal nerve lies on the medial side of the biceps muscle and on the lateral side of the lateral head of the gastrocnemius. It also lies posterior and deep to the biceps at the level of the joint line. Suture passing should be performed between the posterior edge of the iliotibial (IT) band and the biceps.[71] The nerve is at higher risk with most posterior repairs and divergent sutures. If one flexes the knee to 90°, the nerve will move away from the posterior horn of the lateral meniscus. Nonoperative treatment of purely sensory deficits is adequate. If one has neuropraxia or motor loss that does not resolve, this may need exploration, neurolysis, primary nerve repair, or nerve grafting.[72]

Injury to the popliteal vessels is a surgical emergency that, if missed, can lead to amputation. The popliteal neurovascular bundle resides posterior to the posterior root of the lateral meniscus. The vessels are usually posterior the popliteal muscle; however, in 2% of cases, the vessels pass anterior to the muscle belly.[73] The vessels must be protected with retractors or a spoon before passing sutures. Arthroscopic visualization in this area is a must and the use of a 70° arthroscope may aid in observation of the posterior knee. After repair of the posterior horn of the lateral meniscus, the tourniquet should be deflated, excess intraoperative bleeding assessed, pulsatile bleeding assessed, and pulses assessed. If there are asymmetric distal pulses, expanding hematoma, or brisk pulsatile bleeding from the posterior lateral knee, urgent vascular consultation is required with possible fasciotomy and vessel repair.[74]

POSTOPERATIVE

Complications such as implant migration and fragmentation, arthrofibrosis, hemarthrosis, and recurrence of the tear may all occur.[69]

Early all-inside ridged devices had a higher incidence of device fracture and migration leading to chondral wear and early arthritis.[75–77] Newer suture-based all-inside devices have decreased incidence of loosening and migration; however, this may still occur. It is important to avoid overpenetration by using calibrated devices so that capture of the IT band and other structures do not occur (**Fig. 11**). Intraoperatively one must probe the meniscus and tear after each device has been deployed to ensure

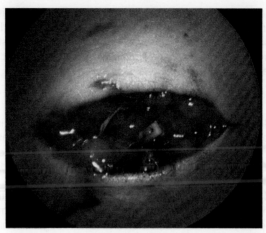

Fig. 11. Prominent suture anchor that has pierced the MCL lying in subcutaneous fat.

appropriate deployment. If a patient has recurrent effusions, pain, or mechanical symptoms, one should obtain an MR arthrography to assess for meniscal or chondral injury that would be associated with implant failure or migration. If there is failure or migration, the implant must be removed and repeat repair or meniscectomy with possible chondral surgery performed. Recently, foreign body reaction has been reported with placement of an all inside meniscal device. Ultrasound (US), after a negative MRI, identified bursal tissue surrounding the anchor and suture material. Diagnostic injection under US resulted in temporary resolution of pain and resolution of symptoms following surgical excision of the anchor and reactive tissue.[78]

Adequate pain control after meniscal surgery combined with an appropriate physical therapy protocol will reduce the risk of arthrofibrosis.[79] A manipulation under anesthesia with or without an arthroscopic lysis of adhesions and posterior medial capsulotomy may be needed to improve range of motion in refractory cases if motion has not been obtained by 3 to 4 months.[80] To prevent arthrofibrosis, avoidance of excessive immobilization, not plicating the posterior capsule in the repair, as well as possibly staging procedures if concomitant ligament reconstruction needs to be performed.[70]

As stated before, a surgeon should not repair menisci in unstable knees. Postoperatively, the patient should be partial weight-bearing and should not perform deep knee bends. Return to high-level sports in a high school, collegiate, and professional athlete should be delayed a minimum of 4 to 6 months after meniscal repair.

If patients return with continued swelling, effusion, and motion loss, an aspiration with analysis of the aspirated fluid for infection or inflammatory cause should be performed. Repeat arthroscopy may be necessary. Typically, drains are not routinely recommended.

Patients who initially do well postoperatively and then symptoms such as locking, buckling, and giving way occur may have a recurrence of the meniscal tear. MR arthrography is superior to conventional MR for evaluation of retear, and second look arthroscopy is the gold standard.[18] If the tear is present, one must consider partial meniscectomy versus repeat repair. Isolated revision repair should rarely be performed unless a technical factor played a significant role in the early failure of primary repair.

SUMMARY

Increased knowledge of the form and function of the meniscus as well as newer arthroscopic meniscal repair techniques and instrumentation has led to an overall increase in meniscal repairs in the last 20 years. Despite excellent repair rates, complications still arise. A proactive approach must be established to prevent and correct these complications. Satisfactory patient outcomes are predicated on correct patient selection, diagnosis, meniscal tear characteristics, surgical technique and instrumentation, and postoperative management. Most complications may be easily prevented with superior visualization and technical skill. When complications transpire, the provider must identify and take steps to rectify as well as prevent further complications from occurring.

REFERENCES

1. Sutton JB. The nature of certain ligaments. J Anat Physiol 1884;18(Pt 3):i2–238.
2. Fox AJ, Wanivenhaus F, Burge AJ, et al. The human meniscus: a review of anatomy, function, injury, and advances in treatment. Clin Anat 2015;28(2):269–87.
3. Koenig JH, Ranawat AS, Umans HR, et al. Meniscal root tears: diagnosis and treatment. Arthroscopy 2009;25(9):1025–32.
4. Kopf S, Colvin AC, Muriuki M, et al. Meniscal root suturing techniques: implications for root fixation. Am J Sports Med 2011;39(10):2141–6.
5. Kim JG, Lee YS, Bae TS, et al. Tibiofemoral contact mechanics following posterior root of medial meniscus tear, repair, meniscectomy, and allograft transplantation. Knee Surg Sports Traumatol Arthrosc 2013;21(9):2121–5.
6. Papalia R, Vasta S, Franceschi F, et al. Meniscal root tears: from basic science to ultimate surgery. Br Med Bull 2013;106:91–115.
7. Shelbourne KD, Roberson TA, Gray T. Long-term evaluation of posterior lateral meniscus root tears left in situ at the time of anterior cruciate ligament reconstruction. Am J Sports Med 2011;39(7):1439–43.
8. Sung JH, Ha JK, Lee DW, et al. Meniscal extrusion and spontaneous osteonecrosis with root tear of medial meniscus: comparison with horizontal tear. Arthroscopy 2013;29(4):726–32.
9. Garrett WE Jr, Swiontkowski MF, Weinstein JN, et al. American Board of Orthopaedic Surgery practice of the orthopaedic surgeon: part-II, certification examination case mix. J Bone Joint Surg Am 2006;88(3):660–7.
10. Abrams GD, Frank RM, Gupta AK, et al. Trends in meniscus repair and meniscectomy in the United States, 2005-2011. Am J Sports Med 2013;41(10):2333–9.
11. Quinby JS, Golish SR, Hart JA, et al. All-inside meniscal repair using a new flexible, tensionable device. Am J Sports Med 2006;34(8):1281–6.
12. Kotsovolos ES, Hantes ME, Mastrokalos DS, et al. Results of all-inside meniscal repair with the FasT-Fix meniscal repair system. Arthroscopy 2006;22(1):3–9.
13. Noyes FR, Heckmann TP, Barber-Westin SD. Meniscus repair and transplantation: a comprehensive update. J Orthop Sports Phys Ther 2012;42(3):274–90.
14. Shieh AK, Edmonds EW, Pennock AT. Revision meniscal surgery in children and adolescents: risk factors and mechanisms for failure and subsequent management. Am J Sports Med 2016;44(4):838–43.
15. Sonnery-Cottet B, Archbold P, Thaunat M, et al. Rapid chondrolysis of the knee after partial lateral meniscectomy in professional athletes. Knee 2014;21(2):504–8.
16. Sonnery-Cottet B, Mortati R, Gadea F, et al. Osteolysis of the tibial plateau after meniscal repair with hybrid suture anchor. Knee Surg Sports Traumatol Arthrosc 2013;21(9):2137–40.
17. Wendt MC, Spinner RJ, Shin AY. Iatrogenic transection of the peroneal and partial transection of the tibial nerve during arthroscopic lateral meniscal debridement and removal of osteochondral fragment. Am J Orthop (Belle Mead NJ) 2014;43(4):182–5.

18. Gwathmey FW Jr, Golish SR, Diduch DR. Complications in brief: meniscus repair. Clin Orthop Relat Res 2012;470(7):2059–66.
19. Blackwell R, Schmitt LC, Flanigan DC, et al. Smoking increases the risk of early meniscus repair failure. Knee Surg Sports Traumatol Arthrosc 2016;24(5):1540–3.
20. Lyman S, Hidaka C, Valdez AS, et al. Risk factors for meniscectomy after meniscal repair. Am J Sports Med 2013;41(12):2772–8.
21. Hwang BY, Kim SJ, Lee SW, et al. Risk factors for medial meniscus posterior root tear. Am J Sports Med 2012;40(7):1606–10.
22. Barber FA, McGarry JE. Meniscal repair techniques. Sports Med Arthrosc 2007; 15(4):199–207.
23. Ahn JH, Lee YS, Yoo JC, et al. Results of arthroscopic all-inside repair for lateral meniscus root tear In patients undergoing concomitant anterior cruciate ligament reconstruction. Arthroscopy 2010;26(1):67–75.
24. Kenji T, Kumangai G, Nohmi S, et al. Arthroscopic repair of meniscus tear in patients 40 years age and over. Asia Pac J Sports Med Arthrosc Rehabil Technol 2016;6:55–8.
25. Steadman JR, Matheny LM, Singleton SB, et al. Meniscus suture repair: minimum 10-year outcomes in patients younger than 40 years compared with patients 40 and older. Am J Sports Med 2015;43(9):2222–7.
26. Harris B, Miller MD. Biomedical devices in meniscal repair. Sports Med Arthrosc 2006;14(3):120–8.
27. Belzer JP, Cannon WD Jr. Meniscus tears: treatment in the stable and unstable knee. J Am Acad Orthop Surg 1993;1(1):41–7.
28. Rosenberg TD, Paulos LE, Parker RD, et al. The forty-five-degree posteroanterior flexion weight-bearing radiograph of the knee. J Bone Joint Surg Am 1988; 70(10):1479–83.
29. Prove S, Charrois O, Dekeuwer P, et al. Comparison of the medial femorotibial joint space before and immediately after meniscectomy. Rev Chir Orthop Reparatrice Appar Mot 2004;90(7):636–42 [in French].
30. Laurendon L, Neri T, Farizon F, et al. Prognostic factors for all-inside meniscal repair. A 87-case series. Orthop Traumatol Surg Res 2017;103(7):1017–20.
31. Allen CR, Wong EK, Livesay GA, et al. Importance of the medial meniscus in the anterior cruciate ligament-deficient knee. J Orthop Res 2000;18(1):109–15.
32. Hanks GA, Gause TM, Handal JA, et al. Meniscus repair in the anterior cruciate deficient knee. Am J Sports Med 1990;18(6):606–11 [discussion: 612–3].
33. Steenbrugge F, Van Nieuwenhuyse W, Verdonk R, et al. Arthroscopic meniscus repair in the ACL-deficient knee. Int Orthop 2005;29(2):109–12.
34. Lee SY, Jee WH, Kim JM. Radial tear of the medial meniscal root: reliability and accuracy of MRI for diagnosis. AJR Am J Roentgenol 2008;191(1):81–5.
35. Jones AO, Houang MT, Low RS, et al. Medial meniscus posterior root attachment injury and degeneration: MRI findings. Australas Radiol 2006;50(4):306–13.
36. Bhatia S, LaPrade CM, Ellman MB, et al. Meniscal root tears: significance, diagnosis, and treatment. Am J Sports Med 2014;42(12):3016–30.
37. Strobel M. Manual of arthroscopic surgery. New York: Springer; 1988.
38. Bollen SR. Posteromedial meniscocapsular injury associated with rupture of the anterior cruciate ligament: a previously unrecognised association. J Bone Joint Surg Br 2010;92(2):222–3.
39. Liu X, Feng H, Zhang H, et al. Arthroscopic prevalence of ramp lesion in 868 patients with anterior cruciate ligament injury. Am J Sports Med 2011;39(4):832–7.
40. Edgar C, Ware JK, Obopilwe E, et al. Posteromedial meniscocapsular tear: prevalence, detection sensitivity, biomechanics, and repair technique. Paper presented at: AAOS Annual Meeting; March 24-28, 2015; Las Vegas, NV.

Available at: http://aaos2015.conferencespot.org/58906-aaos-1.1965581/t004-1.1971711/f004-1.1971712/a096-1.1971713/se81-1.1971728.

41. Kaplan PA, Gehl RH, Dussault RG, et al. Bone contusions of the posterior lip of the medial tibial plateau (contrecoup injury) and associated internal derangements of the knee at MR imaging. Radiology 1999;211(3):747–53.

42. Hash TW 2nd. Magnetic resonance imaging of the knee. Sports Health 2013;5(1): 78–107.

43. Hatayama K, Kimura M, Ogoshi A, et al. Ramp lesion associated with anterior cruciate ligament rupture. ePoster ISAKOS 2013 meeting. Available at: https://www.isakos.com/meetings/2013congress/onsite/AbstractView?EventID=7751.

44. Cohn AK, Mains DB. Popliteal hiatus of the lateral meniscus. Anatomy and measurement at dissection of 10 specimens. Am J Sports Med 1979;7(4):221–6.

45. Simonian PT, Sussmann PS, Wickiewicz TL, et al. Popliteomeniscal fasciculi and the unstable lateral meniscus: clinical correlation and magnetic resonance diagnosis. Arthroscopy 1997;13(5):590–6.

46. Kimura M, Shirakura K, Hasegawa A, et al. Anatomy and pathophysiology of the popliteal tendon area in the lateral meniscus: 2. Clinical investigation. Arthroscopy 1992;8(4):424–7.

47. Kimura M, Shirakura K, Hasegawa A, et al. Anatomy and pathophysiology of the popliteal tendon area in the lateral meniscus: 1. Arthroscopic and anatomical investigation. Arthroscopy 1992;8(4):419–23.

48. Johnson RL, De Smet AA. MR visualization of the popliteomeniscal fascicles. Skeletal Radiol 1999;28(10):561–6.

49. Peduto AJ, Nguyen A, Trudell DJ, et al. Popliteomeniscal fascicles: anatomic considerations using MR arthrography in cadavers. AJR Am J Roentgenol 2008; 190(2):442–8.

50. Shin HK, Lee HS, Lee YK, et al. Popliteomeniscal fascicle tear: diagnosis and operative technique. Arthrosc Tech 2012;1(1):e101–6.

51. Camarillo M, Johnson DL. Popliteomeniscal fascicle tears. Orthopedics 2014; 37(3):187–90.

52. LaPrade RF, Konowalchuk BK. Popliteomeniscal fascicle tears causing symptomatic lateral compartment knee pain: diagnosis by the figure-4 test and treatment by open repair. Am J Sports Med 2005;33(8):1231–6.

53. DeHaven KE. Decision-making factors in the treatment of meniscus lesions. Clin Orthop Relat Res 1990;(252):49–54.

54. Morgan CD, Wojtys EM, Casscells CD, et al. Arthroscopic meniscal repair evaluated by second-look arthroscopy. Am J Sports Med 1991;19(6):632–7 [discussion: 637–8].

55. Watson FA, Arciero RA. Inside out meniscus repair. Oper Tech Sports Med 2003;(11):104–26.

56. Fox MG. MR imaging of the meniscus: review, current trends, and clinical implications. Radiol Clin North Am 2007;45(6):1033–53, vii.

57. Boyd KT, Myers PT. Meniscus preservation; rationale, repair techniques and results. Knee 2003;10(1):1–11.

58. Rosso C, Kovtun K, Dow W, et al. Comparison of all-inside meniscal repair devices with matched inside-out suture repair. Am J Sports Med 2011;39(12):2634–9.

59. Barber FA, Herbert MA, Bava ED, et al. Biomechanical testing of suture-based meniscal repair devices containing ultrahigh-molecular-weight polyethylene suture: update 2011. Arthroscopy 2012;28(6):827–34.

60. Rosso C, Muller S, Buckland DM, et al. All-inside meniscal repair devices compared with their matched inside-out vertical mattress suture repair: introducing 10,000 and 100,000 loading cycles. Am J Sports Med 2014;42(9):2226–33.

61. Elkousy H, Higgins LD. Zone-specific inside-out meniscal repair: technical limitations of repair of posterior horns of medial and lateral menisci. Am J Orthop (Belle Mead NJ) 2005;34(1):29–34.
62. Rodeo SA. Arthroscopic meniscal repair with use of the outside-in technique. Instr Course Lect 2000;49:195–206.
63. Barrett GR, Richardson K, Ruff CG, et al. The effect of suture type on meniscus repair. A clinical analysis. Am J Knee Surg 1997;10(1):2–9.
64. Rimmer MG, Nawana NS, Keene GC, et al. Failure strengths of different meniscal suturing techniques. Arthroscopy 1995;11(2):146–50.
65. Kocabey Y, Taser O, Nyland J, et al. Pullout strength of meniscal repair after cyclic loading: comparison of vertical, horizontal, and oblique suture techniques. Knee Surg Sports Traumatol Arthrosc 2006;14(10):998–1003.
66. Allum R. Complications of arthroscopy of the knee. J Bone Joint Surg Br 2002; 84(7):937–45.
67. In den Kleef NJ, Konings PC, Smeets L. Sural artery injury with arteriovenous fistula: case report about a rare complication following arthroscopic medial meniscectomy. J Surg Case Rep 2015;2015(2) [pii:rju156].
68. Bernard M, Grothues-Spork M, Georgoulis A, et al. Neural and vascular complications of arthroscopic meniscal surgery. Knee Surg Sports Traumatol Arthrosc 1994;2(1):14–8.
69. Jan N, Sonnery-Cottet B, Fayard JM, et al. Complications in posteromedial arthroscopic suture of the medial meniscus. Orthop Traumatol Surg Res 2016;102(8S): S287–93.
70. Austin KS, Sherman OH. Complications of arthroscopic meniscal repair. Am J Sports Med 1993;21(6):864–8 [discussion: 868–9].
71. Deutsch A, Wyzykowski RJ, Victoroff BN. Evaluation of the anatomy of the common peroneal nerve. Defining nerve-at-risk in arthroscopically assisted lateral meniscus repair. Am J Sports Med 1999;27(1):10–5.
72. Kim TK, Savino RM, McFarland EG, et al. Neurovascular complications of knee arthroscopy. Am J Sports Med 2002;30(4):619–29.
73. Kil SW, Jung GS. Anatomical variations of the popliteal artery and its tibial branches: analysis in 1242 extremities. Cardiovasc Intervent Radiol 2009;32(2):233–40.
74. Mullen DJ, Jabaji GJ. Popliteal pseudoaneurysm and arteriovenous fistula after arthroscopic meniscectomy. Arthroscopy 2001;17(1):E1.
75. Ganko A, Engebretsen L. Subcutaneous migration of meniscal arrows after failed meniscus repair. A report of two cases. Am J Sports Med 2000;28(2):252–3.
76. Gliatis J, Kouzelis A, Panagopoulos A, et al. Chondral injury due to migration of a Mitek RapidLoc meniscal repair implant after successful meniscal repair: a case report. Knee Surg Sports Traumatol Arthrosc 2005;13(4):280–2.
77. Ross G, Grabill J, McDevitt E. Chondral injury after meniscal repair with bioabsorbable arrows. Arthroscopy 2000;16(7):754–6.
78. Warth LC, Bollier MJ, Hoffman DF, et al. New complication associated with all-inside meniscal repair device: ultrasound-aided diagnosis and operative localization of foreign body reaction. Orthop J Sports Med 2016;4(9). 2325967116664882.
79. Barber FA, Click SD. Meniscus repair rehabilitation with concurrent anterior cruciate reconstruction. Arthroscopy 1997;13(4):433–7.
80. Dean CS, Chahla J, Mikula JD, et al. Arthroscopic posteromedial capsular release. Arthrosc Tech 2016;5(3):e495–500.

Knee Cartilage Repair and Restoration: Common Problems and Solutions

Kristina Linnea Welton, MD[a], Stephanie Logterman, MD[b,c],*,
Justin H. Bartley, MD[a], Armando F. Vidal, MD[d,e],
Eric C. McCarty, MD[a]

KEYWORDS

- Cartilage defects • Osteochondral defects • Knee • Complications
- Osteochondral autograft • Osteochondral allograft • Microfracture
- Autologous chondrocyte implantation

KEY POINTS

- There are a wide variety of surgical techniques to repair or restore symptomatic focal cartilage defects of the knee and each is associated with its own profile of potential complications.
- Complications associated with microfracture commonly include poor defect filling, osseous overgrowth, and deterioration over time.
- Autologous chondrocyte implantation (ACI) can be impeded by graft hypertrophy, insufficient regenerative cartilage, and disturbed fusion while osteochondral autograft transfer (OAT) can be complicated by donor site morbidity, donor-to-recipient site incongruity, and hemarthrosis.
- Complications encountered with particulated juvenile allograft cartilage (PJAC) are graft hypertrophy and displacement while loosening, fragmentation, subchondral collapse, and nonunion are potential complications encountered with osteochondral allografts (OCA).

Disclosure Statement: K.L. Welton, S. Logterman, and J.H. Bartley have no disclosures to report. A.F. Vidal acts as a Stryker consultant. E.C. McCarty receives institutional support from Stryker, Smith and Nephew, Depuy, and Arthrex. He acts as a consultant for Zimmer Biomet and receives book royalties for Elsevier.

[a] Department of Orthopedic Surgery – Sports Medicine, University of Colorado, CU Sports Medicine and Performance Center, 2150 Stadium Drive, Boulder, CO 80309, USA; [b] Department of Orthopedic Surgery, University of Colorado, 12631 E. 17th Avenue, Mailstop B202, Aurora, CO 80045, USA; [c] Department of Orthopedic Surgery, University of Colorado, Anschutz Medical Campus, 13001 East 17th Place, AO1 Building – 4th Floor, Aurora, CO 80045, USA; [d] Department of Orthopedic Surgery – Sports Medicine, University of Colorado, 2150 Stadium Drive, Boulder, CO 80309, USA; [e] Department of Orthopedic Surgery, CU Sports Medicine Center, 2000 South Colorado Boulevard, The Colorado Center Tower One, Suite 4500, Denver, CO 80222, USA
* Corresponding author. Department of Orthopedic Surgery, University of Colorado, Anschutz Medical Campus, 13001 East 17th Place, AO1 Building – 4th Floor, Aurora, CO 80045.
E-mail address: Stephanie.Logterman@ucdenver.edu

INTRODUCTION AND BACKGROUND

Articular cartilage injuries of the knee are common with a reported incidence of up to 66% in diagnostic knee arthroscopies performed to investigate knee pain.[1–3] Cartilage injuries can result from multiple causes including trauma and osteochondritis dissecans; typical symptoms include swelling, mechanical symptoms, and pain that is equivalent to that of end-stage arthritis.[4,5] In addition, cartilage lesions (9 mm or greater) have been reported to be biomechanically unstable with a high propensity of progression to degenerative joint disease.[6,7] History and physical examination vary and MRI is helpful to evaluate cartilage lesions; factors to consider include lesion size, depth, location, leg alignment, and concomitant meniscal and/or ligamentous injury. Patient factors, such as age and activity level, should also be considered. There is limited self-healing potential because of the poor regenerative capacity and avascular nature of cartilage, therefore surgery is often necessary in the symptomatic setting.[8,9] Surgical treatment consisting of microfracture or chondroplasty can temporarily relieve symptoms but heals with fibrocartilage and likely does not address the potential for long-term joint degeneration.[10,11] Unfortunately, fibrocartilage has been found to exhibit diminished resiliency, less stiffness, and poor wear characteristics in comparison with native articular cartilage.[12,13] Because of this, the ideal treatment of focal articular cartilage defects is an approach that restores organized hyaline cartilage with minimal morbidity and pain-free survivability over a long period of time.[14] Current advanced surgical treatment options that continue to be investigated and potentially offer these advantages include autologous chondrocyte implantation (ACI), osteochondral autograft transfer (OAT), and osteochondral allograft transplantation (OCA). In addition, new techniques that use implantation of particulate juvenile allograft cartilage (PJAC; DeNovo Natural Tissue, Zimmer, Warsaw, IN) have promise but clinical outcome data remain limited.[8,15] Multiple treatment algorithms have been proposed; however, they continue to evolve as additional information and long-term follow-up are acquired.[8] The focus of this case-based review is to highlight common complications associated with common surgical techniques that restore focal articular cartilage defects of the knee, emphasizing how these complications were recognized, how they were addressed, and techniques on how they are avoided.

MICROFRACTURE

Microfracture was developed by Steadman and colleagues[16] to treat full-thickness chondral defects of the knee because articular cartilage has severely limited regenerative capacity. It is the most commonly used technique for treating small articular cartilage lesions in the knee. Microfracture is a bone marrow stimulation technique that aims to surgically induce the formation of a marrow-rich clot to cover the lesion. Mesenchymal stem cells and growth factors induce the remodeling of the fibrin clot into fibrocartilage composed primarily of type I collagen, with only minimal type II collagen.[8] Indications for microfracture include grade III or IV articular cartilage defects in a weight-bearing area of the knee (femoral condyle, tibia, patella, or trochlear groove), unstable cartilage overlying subchondral bone, and focal degenerative changes in a knee with proper coronal alignment.[17]

Although meta-analysis of microfracture demonstrates positive short-term functional improvement, there is a paucity of data exploring long-term results of this procedure. Factors positively affecting outcome following microfracture include age less than 40 year old, symptoms less than 12 months, defect less than 4 cm^2, body mass index less than 30 kg/m^2, and repair cartilage volume (defect fill) of greater than 66%.[18] This technique is limited by its ability to consistently provide adequate hyaline repair tissue, variable repair volume, or lack of defect filling, and deterioration of healing cartilage over time.[19] Early revision rates demonstrated in randomized control trials was 2.5% at 2 years and increased to 23% to 31% at the 2- to 5-year mark postoperatively.[18] Complications following microfracture are rare. A large study with 1275 patients reported no perioperative complications following the procedure,[16,20] whereas three randomized control trials also failed to report any postoperative adverse effects.[21–23] The most commonly reported complication is arthralgia (57%) followed by knee effusion (5%) and crepitation (1.6%).[24] These reported complications, as they relate to the surgery itself, can be caused by poor defect filling, osseous hypertrophy, or deterioration of the fibrocartilage over time.

Microfracture Case

A 44-year-old woman presented to clinic with left knee pain after being involved in an airplane crash. Her initial left knee MRI was significant only for a bone contusion to her tibial plateau. She was treated conservatively with physical therapy but her symptoms failed to resolve. A repeat MRI was obtained that demonstrated a 1.9-cm^2 full-thickness chondral lesion in the lateral aspect of the medial femoral condyle (**Fig. 1**). The patient underwent arthroscopic microfracture of her left medial femoral condyle with no other pathology noted during her surgical intervention (**Fig. 2**). The procedure involved debriding the exposed bone of all remaining unstable cartilage in addition to removing all minimally attached cartilage from the surrounding rim of the lesion. Once the lesion was prepared, any remaining calcified cartilage within the lesion was removed with a curette. An awl was then used to make multiple holes, or microfactures, to a depth of 2 to 4 mm and no closer than 3 to 4 mm apart within the subchondral bone plate, protecting the subchondral plate between the holes from fracturing. Once complete, the water was turned off to visualize marrow droplets and blood emanating from each microfracture hole. Postoperatively the patient was kept non–weight bearing for 6 weeks, with use of a continuous passive motion

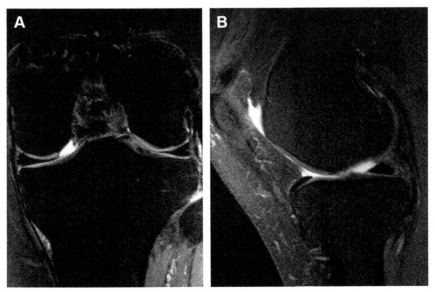

Fig. 1. MRI image of the patient's focal cartilage defect in the weight-bearing surface of the medial femoral condyle. (*A*) Coronal image. (*B*) Sagittal image.

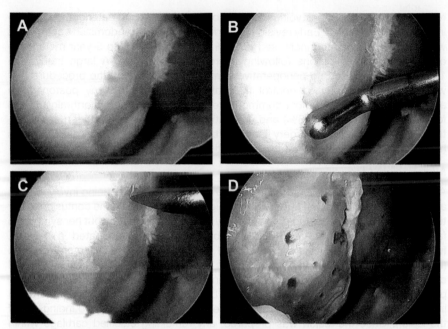

Fig. 2. Intraoperative arthroscopic images of microfracture procedure. (*A*) Cartilage defect after debridement to stable cartilage borders and curettage of calcified base. (*B*) Measurement of cartilage defect. (*C*) Placement of microfracture tip before impaction. (*D*) Evidence of bleeding, marrow extravasation after microfracture; ensuring proper depth.

machine, early physical therapy, and a medial unloader brace starting at 6 weeks through 6 months. At her 6-month postoperative visit she continued to have anteriomedial knee pain and a pinching sensation with extension. MRI was obtained at that time, which revealed the area of microfracture had failed to reconstitute with fibrocartilage (**Fig. 3**). Given her continued symptoms, a discussion was had about further interventions including viscosupplementation, ACI, or getting a second opinion. The patient decided to undergo revision surgery with ACI.

Discussion of Complications

Poor defect filling
Poor defect filling is a potential complication encountered with microfracture. The technique relies on formation of a stable blood clot to maximally fill the chondral defect. Suboptimal results occur when the blood clots only fill a portion of the lesion or are only partially adherent to the base of the defect.[19] To improve clot stability following microfracture, several adjuncts exist, such as chitosan, platelet-derived growth factor, and insulin-like growth factor. Although promising, these adjuncts have unproven clinical efficacy at this point because they have not been tested in clinic trials.[19] Mithoefer and colleagues[18] found that the grade of fill on MRI correlated with better clinic outcomes. In this study, 54% of patients had good fill with reparative fibrocartilage, 29% had moderate fill, and 17% had poor fill on MRI.

Osseous overgrowth
Osseous overgrowth is another complication following microfracture. Bone overgrowth is also referred to as intralesional osteophyte or elevation of subchondral

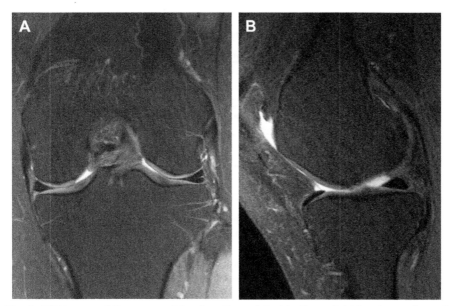

Fig. 3. MRI image of the recurrent focal cartilage defect in the weight-bearing surface of the medial femoral condyle. (A) Coronal image. (B) Sagittal image.

bone plate and occurs after errant removal of subchondral bone during the microfracture. It is hypothesized that osseous overgrowth causes thinning of the overlying repair cartilage with associated alterations in normal cartilage biomechanics. The incidence ranges from 10% to 99% in different studies.[25–27] Mithoefer and colleagues[25] observed that most bone overgrowth (64%) was low grade and usually developed in the first year after surgery. Furthermore, they also found that there was no statistically significant difference in Knee Injury and Osteoarthritis Outcome scores in those patients with and without overgrowth. Osseous overgrowth is associated with increased rate of postoperative failure (25%) after microfracture and 93% of patients who failed microfracture had evidence of bone overgrowth. Risk factors for bone overgrowth include increased body mass index; lesion location on the lateral femoral condyle; and aggressive, deep removal of the calcified cartilage layer.

Deterioration over time

Deterioration over time has been documented by several studies. One study found that 47% of patients who underwent microfracture had reduction in clinical outcomes after initially showing clinical improvement.[18] This is especially true in larger lesions. Gobbi and colleagues[28] found that 80% of patients had a decline in activity at approximately 72 months follow-up. In addition to functional decline, deterioration of healing cartilage is seen on MRI 18 months postoperatively.[19]

Microfracture is a common procedure for chondral injuries; however, as with all surgical interventions, it is associated with its own unique profile of potential complications. Poor filling defects, osseous overgrowth, and deterioration of function over time are all well documented in the literature. Patient selection has an impact on the success of the procedure because younger patients with smaller defects benefit most. **Table 1** summarizes technical pearls reducing the risk of these potential complications.

Table 1
Technical pearls of microfracture technique to reduce potentially encountered complications

Common Complications	Methods of Prevention
Poor defect filling	Ensure proper spacing and depth of microfracture holes
	Consider use of adjuvants to help form and maintain a stable clot
Subchondral fracture	Place microfracture holes no closer than 3–4 mm apart
Osseous overgrowth	Avoid errant subchondral bone removal
	Consider increased risk in younger patient
Deterioration over time	Consider patient selection: procedure works best for patients <40 years old and in smaller lesions

AUTOLOGOUS CHONDROCYTE IMPLANTATION

ACI is a technique used to treat full-thickness cartilage defects that involves restoration of cartilage cells into the lesions. Unlike microfracture, ACI results in the development of hyaline cartilage that more closely resembles the native knee articular surface. ACI involves two separate procedures. First, cells are arthroscopically harvested from the intercondylar notch and the size of the lesion is estimated to help approximate cell density at the time of culture. The chondrocytes are isolated and allowed to reproduce in vitro for 4 to 6 weeks. The chondrocytes are then implanted in the lesion in combination with a membrane (periosteal or biomembrane covered) or incorporated into a scaffold matrix (matrix-associated). Outcomes following ACI have been largely positive. One prospective clinical trial found that 76% of patients had pain relief and improved quality of life following ACI.[29] Furthermore, Minas and colleagues[30] found the 10-year survivorship of ACI to be 71% with functional improvement in 75% of patients.

Limitations to this surgical technique exist. One obvious limitation to ACI is that it involves two surgeries. Wood and colleagues[31] reported that graft failure accounted for 24.8% of all adverse events following ACI. The most common complication of ACI is graft hypertrophy, which is most often associated with the periosteal patch-covered ACI procedure with an incidence of 36%.[32] Niemeyer and colleagues[33] found the revision rate for ACI to be 17%, with the periosteum-covered ACI technique most commonly requiring revision. These data are supported by a study that found a 16% revision rate among patients undergoing ACI.[34] Niemeyer and colleagues[33] observed four pathologic changes arthroscopically following ACI including graft hypertrophy, insufficient integration of regenerated cartilage at the borders with native cartilage, deficient regenerative cartilage, and delamination of intact cartilage.

Autologous Chondrocyte Implantation Case

A 45-year-old woman with left knee pain after being involved in an airplane crash was found to have a chondral defect of her medial femoral condyle and underwent microfracture surgery. At 6 months out from her procedure, she continued to have anteromedial knee pain and a pinching sensation. MRI of her left knee revealed a residual 2.5-cm^2 chondral defect in the area of microfracture because it had failed to reconstitute with fibrocartilage (see **Fig. 3**). She was counseled on the options of viscosupplementation, ACI, or referral for a second opinion. At 18 months from out from her microfracture surgery she decided to undergo ACI (**Fig. 4**). She had an uncomplicated postoperative course. At her 1-year follow-up appointment, she was able to perform her normal activities of daily living, but her recreational activities remained somewhat limited. On examination, she had full range of motion with minimal quad atrophy and

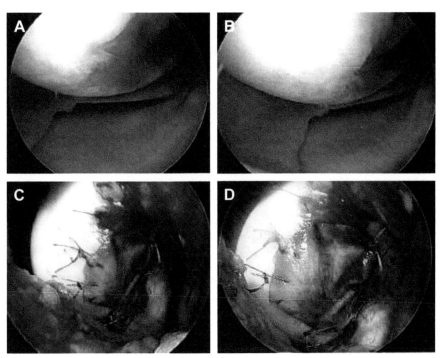

Fig. 4. Arthroscopic intraoperative images of ACI. (*A, B*) Chondral defect 18 months after microfracture. (*C, D*) Defect after ACI with periosteal patch.

mild tenderness to palpation along the medial femoral condyle, similar to her preoperative pain. Postoperative MRI (**Fig. 5**) showed decent infill but was not full thickness in the most medial aspect. The patient was counseled on continued nonoperative and operative measures; she chose to proceed without further intervention.

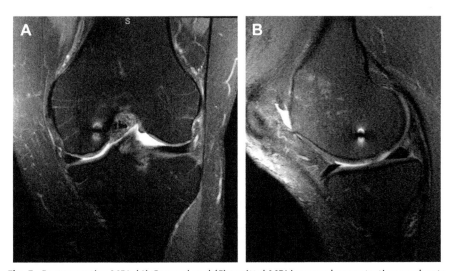

Fig. 5. Postoperative MRI. (*A*) Coronal and (*B*) sagittal MRI images demonstrating moderate but incomplete infill of the defect.

Discussion of Complications

Insufficient regenerative cartilage

Insufficient regenerative cartilage is a complication following ACI and refers to failure of the graft to regenerate as expected. Insufficient regenerative cartilage was found to occur in 17.3% and was diagnosed on MRI in patients with persistent pain and other symptoms after initial surgery.[33] This complication occurred more often in the periosteum-covered and matrix-associated groups at rates of 3.8% and 3.7%, respectively, whereas occurring only 1.9% in the biomembrane covered ACI group. Revision surgery for insufficient cartilage regeneration depends on the size of the defect. Smaller defects (<2 cm^2) can be managed with microfracture or transplantation of OAT, whereas larger defects can be treated with repeat ACI or consideration of OCA.

Graft hypertrophy

Graft hypertrophy is the most common complication of ACI, with an incidence of 28% to 36%.[32,33,35] It occurs most often in those treated with a periosteal flap-covered ACI. Hypertrophy frequently causes clinical symptoms, such as persistent pain or loss of knee function. The most common site of graft hypertrophy was found in defects of the patella with an incidence of 8.1% to 50% followed by the medial and lateral femoral condyles (both 3.5%).[33] Graft hypertrophy typically occurs within the first 12 months following surgery and Pietschmann and colleagues[32] observed no new cases of graft hypertrophy in patients after 24 months. Decision to undergo revision surgery, usually arthroscopic shaving or partial resection of the excess graft, is based on clinical symptoms and amount of hypertrophy seen on MRI.

Disturbed or inadequate fusion

Disturbed or inadequate fusion refers to failure of the regenerative cartilage to incorporate with the healthy surrounding cartilage. Niemeyer and colleagues[33] found an incidence of insufficient fusion of 23.1%. Disturbed fusion occurred most commonly in the matrix-associated ACI group (4.8%) followed by the biomembrane covered ACI group (3.7%) with no cases of disturbed fusion in the periosteal patch–covered group. Marrow stimulation techniques, such as anterograde drilling or microfracture, are frequently used in cases of disturbed fusion.

Delamination

Delamination is another complication following ACI and refers to the separation of cartilage from the underlying bone. This is caused by shearing forces that result in the cartilage layer sliding over the subchondral bone before fusion of the two layers occurs, as can transpire with noncompliance or returning to weight bearing prematurely. Intraoperatively it occurs more frequently in larger or uncontained defects.[36] Delamination was documented in 22.1% of cases in one study reporting adverse outcomes to the US Food and Drug Administration.[31] Delamination is managed by complete removal of the delaminated cartilage with further treatment dependent on the size of the remaining defect, similar to the treatment of insufficient regeneration.

In summary, unsatisfactory results requiring further intervention after ACI occurs in up to 16.8%. Graft hypertrophy, delamination, disturbed fusion, and insufficient regenerative cartilage account for approximately 88% of complications following ACI. Hypertrophy usually occurs in younger patients, whereas insufficient regenerative tissue formation is more commonly seen in older patients.[33] MRI and clinical findings are not highly specific and sometimes do not result in a preoperative diagnosis, thus treating surgeons should have a low threshold for diagnostic arthroscopy in patients with persistent symptoms following initial ACI. **Table 2** provides a summary of technical pearls to reduce complications and poor outcomes that may occur with ACI.

PARTICULATED JUVENILE ALLOGRAFT CARTILAGE

Particulated articular cartilage grafting procedures are also used to treat focal articular cartilage defects. It can be harvested as an autograft but often off-the-shelf allogenic juvenile grafts are used because juvenile tissue has theoretic increased proliferative and restorative potential. This technique involves the mechanical mincing of cartilage into 1- to 2-mm pieces, which allows chondrocytes to escape from their encasing extracellular matrix and diffuse into the surrounding tissues where they form new hyaline-like cartilage.[37] Use of PJAC is advantageous in that it is performed as a single-stage procedure. The procedure first requires debridement of the defect to a bleeding base. Fibrin glue is then applied to the base of the lesion and the PJAC fragments (DeNovo Natural Tissue, Zimmer) are inserted, spaced every 1 to 2 mm. A final layer of fibrin glue is then used to secure the graft in place. Two recent studies found improved International Knee Documentation Committee and Knee Injury and Osteoarthritis Outcome scores at 2 years with MRI evidence of chondral defect resolution at greater than 18 months postoperatively.[38,39] Potential limitations of PJAC are cost, requires an open approach (ie, cannot be done arthroscopically), and a low risk of disease transmission.

Discussion of Complications

Graft hypertrophy
Graft hypertrophy is also a complication for PJAC. Patients typically present with knee effusion and stiffness. Tompkins and colleagues[39] reported that 5 of 15 patients developed graft hypertrophy following PJAC with only two of those patients requiring arthroscopic debridement.

Graft displacement
Graft displacement can occur intraoperatively while the fibrin glue is setting. This is caused by improper patient positioning, overfilling the defect (graft should sit recessed 1 mm), or inadequate defect preparation (eg, not debriding the border of the defect to stable cartilaginous vertical walls or incompletely clearing the base of calcified

Table 2	
Technical pearls of ACI to reduce potentially encountered complications	
Common Complications	**Methods of Prevention**
Insufficient regenerative cartilage	Consider patient age (older patients at higher risk) Consider membrane used with fixation (periosteal patch carries higher risk)
Graft hypertrophy	Consider patient age (younger patients have higher risk) Consider membrane used with fixation (periosteal patch carries higher risk) Consider location of defect (patellar defects associated with increased chance)
Disturbed/inadequate fusion	Consider fixation technique of cells (matrix carries highest risk) Use of microfracture concomitantly
Delamination	Use biodegradable bone anchors or limited suture fixation if lesion is uncontained Limit weight bearing for at least 8–12 wk

cartilage).[37] This complication is prevented through the use of proper surgical technique and by avoiding the previously mentioned pitfalls.

In summary, PJAC is a newer therapy for chondral defects. Limited data exist and further studies are needed to compare its clinical efficacy with ACI. Complications of PJAC are similar to ACI.

OSTEOCHONDRAL AUTOGRAFT TRANSPLANTATION/MOSAICPLASTY

OAT is a surgical technique developed to treat small- to medium-sized focal grade III and IV chondral defects in the knee. The procedure entails harvesting one or more osteochondral grafts from a donor site in the ipsilateral knee (usually from limited weight bearing areas, such as the far medial or lateral aspects of the trochlea or the lateral aspect of the intercondylar notch) and transplanting into the area of cartilage damage in press-fit fashion. The main benefits of this technique are that it is a single-stage procedure and there is rapid subchondral bone healing with restoration of native type II hyaline cartilage at the articular surface. Limitations and common complications associated with this technique include donor site availability and morbidity, especially of larger defects, and the technically demanding precision required to prevent donor-to-recipient-site mismatch, overreduction or underreduction of the graft, and chondrocyte injury or graft fracture at the time of impaction. Overall clinical studies have shown good to excellent outcomes at short- and long-term follow-up with higher return to athletic activity when compared with microfracture.[40–43] Patients in whom rate of failure is elevated seem to be those older than 40 years of age, women, and those in whom the defect size is greater than 3 cm^2.[40]

Osteochondral Autograft Transplantation/Mosaicplasty Case

A 24-year-old woman presented to the sports medicine clinic with 1 year of superolateral right knee pain. She was previously a Division I collegiate gymnast who sustained an anterior horn lateral meniscus tear and small, focal lateral femoral cartilage defect from a dismounting injury at the age of 19. At that time she underwent an arthroscopic surgery by her team surgeon who did a partial lateral meniscectomy and microfracture of her 1.5-cm^2 cartilage defect. Unfortunately, her cartilage defect did not fill in over the proceeding months and she continued to have persisting lateral knee pain with weight bearing. A second treating surgeon performed an OAT procedure 14 months later, taking two 10-mm diameter donor plugs from her lateral trochlea. She recovered from this surgery and was able to continue as a competitive collegiate gymnast. On graduation from college she became a gymnastics coach. However, because of continued crepitance and pain in the superior-lateral aspect of her knee with walking downhill, squatting, and prolonged periods of sitting she returned to her treating surgeon.

Examination revealed crepitus with range of motion and tenderness to palpation over the superior lateral aspect of her trochlea, near her previous donor sites. No joint line pain was present nor tenderness along the distal, posterior portion of her lateral femur, the location of her previous cartilage defect. An MRI was performed and showed incongruity and hypertrophy of the cartilage surface from her donor sites with a small amount of cystic change in the subchondral bone (**Fig. 6**). Her OAT grafts in the lateral femoral condyle appeared to have incorporated well into the surrounding bone with congruent cartilage surfaces (**Fig. 7**). It was believed that her presenting symptoms were caused by donor site morbidity and she was offered an arthroscopic debridement of this area versus a trial of physical therapy; she opted for the former.

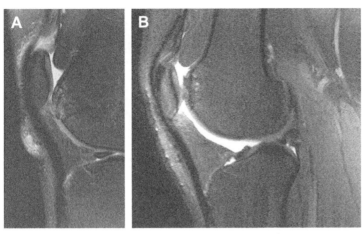

Fig. 6. Sequential MRI of patient's lateral femoral condyle. (*A, B*) Demonstrating cartilage hypertrophy and subchondral cystic changes at her donor sites.

At the time of her arthroscopic surgery careful assessment of her prior OAT grafts was performed. They were found to be stable and congruous. On evaluation of her donor sites, these were found to be filled with fibrocartilage. The surface of this area was noted to be hypertrophied, fibrillated, and irregular on the surface (**Fig. 8**). This area was gently debrided down to a smooth base using an arthroscopic shaver. Postoperatively the patient's symptoms improved and she was able to return to running, hiking, and skiing.

Discussion of Complications

Donor site morbidity

Donor site morbidity is the most unique complication of OAT surgery. A recent systematic review by Andrade and colleagues[44] found a 0% to 92% reporting of donor site morbidity, with a pooled rate of 5.9%. When this was broken down into specific donor-site issues the most common complaints were patellofemoral disturbances (23%), crepitation (31%), and stairs/kneeling pain (2.3%). Gudas and colleagues[11] noted that larger grafts yielded greater chance of donor site morbidity and prefer 8-mm grafts. The taking of multiple plugs, minimal spacing (<2 mm) between donor sites, and poor harvesting technique also can lead to increased donor site

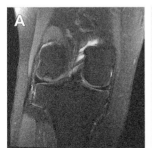
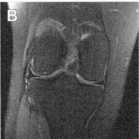
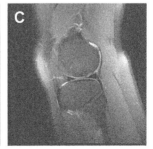

Fig. 7. MRI of OAT recipient site. (*A, B*) Sequential coronal images showing congruity of articular surface of recipient site. (*C*) Sagittal view of healed OATs recipient site.

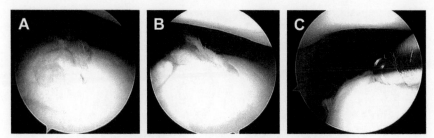

Fig. 8. Arthroscopic images of OAT donor site. (*A, B*) Hypertrophy and fibrillation of fibro-cartilage fill in former lateral trochlea donor site. (*C*) Gentle debridement was performed with an arthroscopic shaver to establish a smooth base.

morbidity.[43,45] Although less common, hypertrophy of fibrocartilage at the donor sites of mosaicplasty procedures has also been reported in several studies, often requiring a second surgery to trim the excess growth.[41,46]

Donor-to-recipient site incongruity

Donor-to-recipient site incongruity is another potential complication. Ideally the harvest site would come from areas of low-weight-bearing stress and provide a donor with similar contour of the defect and chondral depth. In a finite element model of the knee, D'Lima and colleagues[47] demonstrated that donor grafts lacking uniform curvature to that of the defect leads to higher stresses and strains to the cartilage surface. This study along with a sheep-based study also depicted the importance of not leaving the grafts proud nor countersinking them more than 1 mm.[48] Incongruity of the graft to the native chondral surface leads to higher rates of resorption, necrosis, and worse clinical outcomes.[49,50] The potential for an incongruous surface and gapping increases with the more grafts used during a mosaicplasty. Not only is congruity lost, but the fill between plugs is fibrocartilaginous in nature.[45,51] As such, some recommend the use of OATs with no more than two or three plugs.[52] It is also paramount to make sure that the depth of the recipient hole matches and is filled completely by the recipient graft. Having an unbottomed graft reduces stability, relying solely on circumferential frictional forces, and can lead to graft subsidence over time.[53,54] Multiple plugs in mosaicplasty further compromises stability because gaps between round plugs reduces frictional forces.

Graft fracture and chondral injury

Graft fracture and chondral injury are complications that can occur intraoperatively and can lead to surgical failure. Graft fracture can occur during its harvest from the donor site if the harvester is toggled instead of turned to release and cut the graft from the site. Use of a mallet instead of a tamp has also been reported to yield graft fracture.[52] Increased and/or uneven forces to impact the graft into the recipient site has been well shown to reduce cartilage cell viability (**Fig. 9**).[47,55–57] Specifically, the magnitude of the impact loads seems to affect chondrocyte viability in a dose–response relationship, whereas the number of impacts plays less of a role, favoring multiple, lower load impacts to properly seat an OAT graft.[58,59]

Hemarthrosis and arthrofibrosis

Hemarthrosis and arthrofibrosis postoperatively have been encountered and in higher percentages compared with other cartilage-based procedures because of the bleeding that occurs from the donor-sites. Although the donor tunnels have been

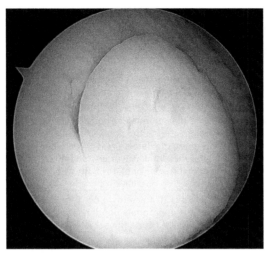

Fig. 9. Arthroscopic image of OAT graft after impaction into the defect. Note the rutted cartilages surface of the donor graft depicting a suboptimal, uneven impaction technique.

shown to fill in with cancellous bone in 4 weeks and with a fibrocartilagenous cap developing by 8 to 12 weeks,[60,61] in an 8-year follow-up study of 652 patients treated with mosaicplasty, 38 (5.8%) developed postoperative bleeding complications with four of these going onto developing a septic joint.[62] Other studies have corroborated this as a potential complication.[41,45] For this reason some resurfacing techniques with biodegradable materials, such as hydroxyapatite, carbon fiber, polyglyconate, compressed collagen, and polycaprolactones, have been tested.[63] In Feczkó and colleagues[63] canine study all of the previously mentioned materials reduced postoperative hemarthrosis, although compressed collagen provided the best substrate for healing of the defects with bone and fibrocartilage.

In summary, complications can arise with OAT or mosaicplasty procedures for restoring small- to medium-sized high-grade chondral and osteochondral defects. However, the surgeon has a direct impact on the success of these surgical procedures not only because of patient and cartilage defect selection parameters, but also because outcome is directly linked to the care and precision used during the employment of this surgical technique. **Table 3** provides a summary of technical pearls to reduce complications and poor outcomes that can arise from OAT/mosaicplasty.

OSTEOCHONDRAL ALLOGRAFT

OCA transplant is a common cartilage resurfacing procedure that entails transplantation of a viable, articular cartilage, cadaver graft along with underlying subchondral bone into an existing cartilage defect. Chondrocyte viability directly correlates with OCA transplant success and fresh OCAs have been found to have the highest level of chondrocyte viability; typical procedural timeline includes transplant of these grafts within 1 week of harvest.[19,64,65]

Primary advantages of this technique include no donor site morbidity, the ability to achieve precise articular surface congruity, it is a single-stage procedure, and maintains the ability to treat larger defects throughout the knee. Limitations include limited graft availability, cost, risk of immunologic rejection, and the potential for disease transmission. Outcomes of OCA transplant for cartilage defects are reportedly good to

Table 3
Technical pearls of OAT technique to reduce potentially encountered complications

Common Complications	Methods of Prevention
Donor site morbidity	Minimize size of graft taken as able Take as few grafts as possible Take graft from far lateral, far medial aspects of trochlea vs lateral aspect of intercondylar notch
Donor-to-recipient mismatch	Ensure the harvester is perpendicular to the donor site to achieve congruency at the donor-plug interface Make sure the defect site is prepared to the appropriate depth to prevent subsidence or an "unbottomed" graft Impact the graft until it is flush with the surrounding cartilage surface; do not leave it proud
Graft injury	To avoid graft fracture do not toggle the harvester Once the appropriate depth has been reached during graft acquisition rotate the harvester 180° to cut and disengage the graft During seating of the graft into the defect, use a great number of impacts with a tamp and mallet with low force to reduce chondrocyte damage and cell death
Hemarthrosis	Take the smallest size and number of grafts as possible Consider placing the recipient bone plug into the donor site defect or fill with cancellous allograft chips or other biocompatible material

excellent. Levy and colleagues[66] published results on a cohort of 122 patients demonstrating 82% survivorship at 10 years, 74% at 15 years, and 66% at 20 years. Failure rate was 24% at a mean of 7.2 years and was found to be associated with patients older than 30 and those with two or more previous surgeries at the time of the surgery. In addition, a recent study with 2.5-year follow-up demonstrated 80% of athletes were able to return to sport at their preinjury level following osteochondral allograft procedures; risk factors for not returning to sport included patients older than 25 years of age and preoperative symptoms for longer than 12 months.[67] A study by Bugbee and Convery[65] reported an 86% success rate following OCA in the treatment of large unipolar defects; however, the survival drops quickly in the setting of bipolar defects (54%). In a systematic review performed by Chahal and colleagues,[68] short-term complication rates of fresh, prolonged-fresh, and fresh-frozen allograft is reportedly low (2.3%); however, failure rates were 18% at an average follow-up of 58 months.

Osteochondral Allografts Case 1

A 17-year-old male baseball player presented to clinic with lateral joint line pain in his right knee 5 months after an injury sustained while sliding into third base. On examination, he had full range of motion but had a positive McMurray test and lateral joint line tenderness with palpation. An MRI revealed a displaced bucket-handle tear of the lateral meniscus and a small cartilage lesion of the lateral femoral condyle (**Fig. 10**). His initial surgery required a partial lateral meniscectomy because of the chronicity of his injury and thus irreparable nature of his meniscus tear, and chondroplasty following initial evaluation of the large grade 3 area of cartilage wear on the lateral femoral condyle (**Fig. 11**). A lateral unloader brace was used during his recovery, although he continued to experience lateral joint line pain 6 months after surgery and further work-up including long-alignment films revealed neutral lower extremity

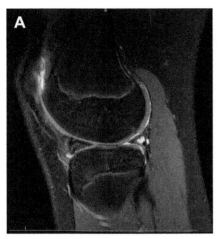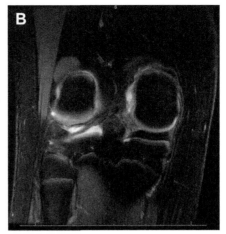

Fig. 10. MRI of cartilage lesion of the lateral femoral condyle. (*A*) Sagittal. (*B*) Coronal.

alignment. On physical examination, he maintained full range of motion and quadriceps tone, but did have a large effusion and significant lateral joint line pain. Surgical treatment options were discussed and OCA to the lateral femoral condyle (**Fig. 12**).

Initially the patient did well postoperatively; he had no swelling 3 months after surgery, great quad development, full range of motion, and no joint line tenderness. However, 6 months after surgery, the patient was riding his bike around campus, swerved to miss another cyclist, and collided with a concrete wall resulting in a traumatic impact to his operative knee with immediate swelling and pain of the knee. MRI was conducted that noted shearing of the cartilage off the allograft with free-floating cartilage in the joint (**Fig. 13**). On repeat arthroscopic examination, the loose body was removed and the area of cartilage delamination at the previous allograft site was evaluated (**Fig. 14**). The patient's cartilage defect was then revised using an open approach with PJAC cartilage transplant to the defect. The patient was followed for to 2 years after the procedure, returning to all desired activities without restriction.

Osteochondral Allografts Case 2

A 29-year-old male rugby player presented to clinic with a history of three right knee surgeries including microfracture, partial medial meniscectomy, and OAT procedure

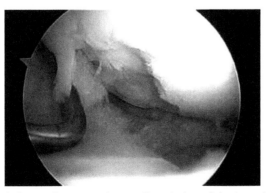

Fig. 11. Arthroscopic image demonstrating cartilage lesion of the lateral femoral condyle.

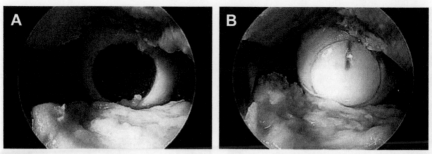

Fig. 12. Arthroscopic images of initial osteochondral allograft transplant. (*A*) Site of lesion following reaming. (*B*) Final osteochondral graft implanted.

to the medial femoral condyle over a 6-year time period. Approximately 10 months after his OAT surgery he developed an abrupt deterioration of his symptoms with significant knee pain and recurrent effusions. On examination, he had significant medial joint line tenderness and effusion. Long alignment films demonstrated that his knee was in a large amount of varus with the weight-bearing axis passing through the medial compartment (**Fig. 15**). MRI demonstrated that the entire osteochondral autograft had deteriorated and a recurrent osteochondral defect in the medial femoral condyle measuring 3.6 cm² was present (**Fig. 16**). This failed osteochondral defect (OCD) lesion of the medial femoral condyle was believed to be secondary to varus malalignment of the lower extremity. An opening wedge, varus-producing high tibial osteotomy was conducted with revision of the medial femoral condyle cartilage defect using OCA (**Fig. 17**). He progressed well in the postoperative period and at most recent follow-up had returned to running and rugby without pain.

Discussion of Complications

Early loosening
Early loosening of an osteochondral allograft can occur secondary to mismatch of the graft to the prepared recipient socket or inadequate fixation. Typically, it is suggested that the graft is press-fit into the recipient socket in a fashion to achieve congruency of

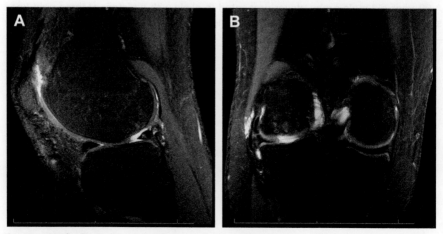

Fig. 13. MRI findings demonstrating recurrent cartilage lesion. (*A*) Sagittal. (*B*) Coronal.

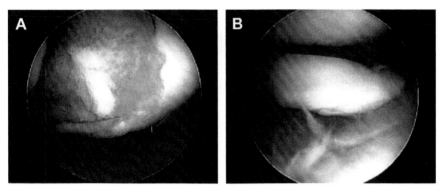

Fig. 14. Arthroscopic images of failed osteochondral allograft site. (*A*) Site of osteochondral graft with intact bone but cartilage sheared off. (*B*) Loose cartilaginous body associated with failed graft.

the graft to the surrounding native cartilage and a tight circumferential fit of the graft. If an adequate press-fit is obtained, fixation should naturally exist without supplemental fixation. A common reason for compromised stability of the graft is interruption of the circumferential structure of the recipient site secondary to blow-out, resulting in interruption of hoop stresses and compromise of the structural integrity of the recipient site. The key to avoid this is adequate exposure, using the cannulated cylindrical sizing guide to ensure 1 to 2 mm of native cartilage and bone remains circumferentially following reaming, and lastly maintaining a perpendicular orientation to the cartilage during placement of the initial guide pin and the cannulated reamer. If blow-out occurs or there are concerns regarding stability of the graft, absorbable pins, absorbable screws, or nonabsorbable headless compression screws can improve fixation of the graft until incorporation occurs.

Allograft fragmentation

Allograft fragmentation occurs in approximately 1.6% of OCAs.[68] Isolated fragmentation of the osteochondral allograft secondary to trauma is an extremely rare complication; however, fragmentation or damage of the graft during intraoperative seating of the graft is more common. The importance of gently seating the graft within the recipient site is evident because the deleterious effect of excessive force during insertion is well documented.[55,57,58] The surgeon should taper the edges of the graft before insertion, dilate the recipient site, and avoid using a mallet during seating of the graft. Frozen or fresh-frozen allografts should be avoided if a fresh allograft is available, because the former is more likely to fissure or delaminate due to chondrocyte death and extracellular matrix damage sustained during freezing.[69]

Graft overload

Graft overload resulting in failure secondary to malalignment is a commonly reported association. The benefits of unloading damaged cartilage are well-documented. Radin and coworkers[70] initially noted that a reduction in stress concentration around a cartilage defect induces cartilage healing, and Koshino and coworkers[71] noted a direct relationship between cartilage regeneration in the medial compartment with valgus alignment in patients 2 years following high tibial osteotomy. Clinical outcomes further support this association. Bugbee and Convery[65] found that lower-extremity malalignment is associated with failure of OCAs and Gross and colleagues[72] showed that varus or valgus malalignment of the knee is a negative clinical prognostic factor.[73]

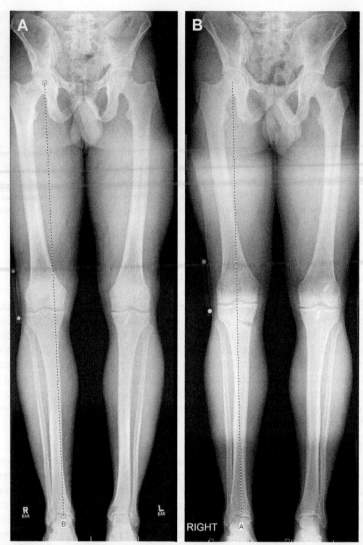

Fig. 15. Long-alignment radiographs. (*A*) Demonstrates preoperative varus alignment. (*B*) Demonstrates postoperative neutral alignment following high tibial osteotomy.

On account of these findings, a full evaluation of the patient's lower extremity alignment should be conducted before cartilage restoration procedures with consideration of corrective osteotomy in cases of lower extremity malalignment.

Graft prominence is an additional cause of graft overload. The normal geometry of the native articular surface must be matched using the donor graft. It is better to recess the graft slightly than to leave it prominent and thus create a stress concentration along the border of the graft. Tips to prevent articular surface mismatch or graft prominence include harvesting the allograft plug from an identical location of the native defect on the donor allograft condyle and making a mark in the 12-o'clock position to aid orientation on insertion and seating. In addition, initial guide pin insertion, articular surface cannulated reaming, and allograft harvest-core reaming must all be

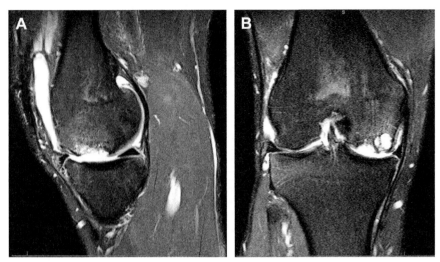

Fig. 16. MRI findings demonstrating 3.6-cm² cartilage lesion. (*A*) Sagittal. (*B*) Coronal.

perpendicular to the articular surfaces. Once the graft is harvested and removed from the reamer, the four quadrants of the graft must be marked and trimmed down to match the depths of the recipient site. Lastly, following final seating of the graft, viewing the recipient site from a perpendicular vantage point (see **Fig. 17**) helps assess the congruency of the implanted graft with the native cartilage.

Failure of graft incorporation
Failure of graft incorporation, such as subchondral collapse or nonunion of the graft, is a concern following OCA. An 86% healing or union rate has been reported at 1 year following surgery.[68] Several techniques are used to stimulate incorporation and healing of the graft into the native bone, including drilling multiple holes within the floor of the recipient site or using biologics (bone marrow aspirate) to encourage bony ingrowth. Bone grafting any present subchondral cysts before insertion of the new graft helps to prevent collapse of the graft. In addition, the patient should be restricted from high-impact activities (long distance running) for up to 1 year after allograft transplant to help reduce the risk of graft collapse during the phase of early creeping substitution.[74]

In summary, OCA is an excellent operation for restoring high-grade chondral and osteochondral defects within the constraints of appropriate surgical indications. Complications with this procedure are rare and the surgeon has a direct impact on the success of these surgical procedures by conducting a complete preoperative work-up and using the discussed surgical techniques (**Table 4**).

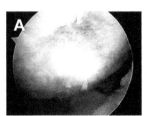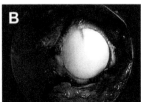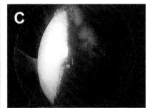

Fig. 17. Arthroscopic image of medial femoral condyle OCD. (*A*) Before OCA. (*B, C*) Coronal (*frontal*) profile and sagittal (*side*) profile images after OCA implantation.

Table 4
Technical pearls of OCA technique to reduce potentially encountered complications

Common Complications	Methods of Prevention
Graft early loosening	Use press-fit technique Develop adequate visualization Maintain perpendicular orientation to articular surface, during preparation and graft harvest Use supplemental fixation as needed
Allograft fragmentation	Taper edges of graft Dilate recipient site Avoid use of mallet or excessive force Use fresh allograft if available
Graft overload	Obtain long-alignment radiographs and address malalignment of the lower extremity before cartilage restoration procedure Harvest graft from allograft condyle in a location corresponding to defect in native knee Maintain orientation of graft and trim edges as needed to match depths of native recipient site
Subchondral collapse and nonunion	Drill "healing holes" into the recipient bone bed Consider use of biologics to stimulate incorporation, healing, and bony ingrowth Bone graft subchondral cysts before insertion of OCA Restrict patient from high-impact activities for up to 1 y following procedure

SUMMARY

Numerous techniques have been developed to repair and restore focal cartilage and osteochondral defects of the knee. No single best surgical strategy exists to treat these cartilage defects because patient characteristics, the location and nature of the defect, previous surgical history, and concurrent injury all play a role in surgical decision making and outcomes. It is important to know the common complications associated with these surgical techniques, because these too can play a role in patient education and decision making. This review has emphasized the most frequently encountered complications in the most commonly used procedures for management of focal cartilage defects of the knee. Some of these complications are shared among techniques, such as the potential for resorption with OAT and OCA, and graft hypertrophy with ACI, PJAC, and OAT. Other complications are unique to the surgical procedure. Clinically, most complications present as recurrent or persisting pain with mechanical symptoms. MRI with a low threshold for diagnostic arthroscopy is frequently used in the work-up of persisting symptoms after a cartilage repair or restorative procedure. Management of complications following these surgeries is varied, with outcomes of revision surgery worse than in the primary setting. Patient education and involvement in the decision-making process in these situations is important. Knowledge of how to recognize, prevent, and treat these complications, should they arise, is essential for any orthopedic surgeon managing focal cartilage lesions of the knee, which this review has sought to cover.

REFERENCES

1. Aroen A, Loken S, Heir S. Articular cartilage lesions in 993 consecutive knee arthroscopies. Am J Sports Med 2004;32:211–5.

2. Curl WW, Krome J, Gordon E, et al. Cartilage injuries: a review of 31,516 knee arthroscopies. Arthroscopy 1997;13:456–60.
3. Widuchowski W, Widuchowski J, Trzaska T. Articular cartilage defects: study of 25,124 knee arthroscopies. Knee 2007;14:177–82.
4. Heir S, Nerhus T, Rotterud J, et al. Focal cartilage defects in the knee impair quality of life as much as severe osteoarthritis: a comparison of knee injury and osteoarthritis outcome score in 4 patient categories scheduled for knee surgery. Am J Sports Med 2010;38:231–7.
5. Biant LC, McNicholas M, Sprowson A, et al. The surgical management of symptomatic articular cartilage defects of the knee: consensus statements from United Kingdom knee surgeons. Knee 2015;22(5):446–9.
6. Guettler JH, Demetropooulos C, Yang K, et al. Osteochondral defects in the human knee: influence of defect size on cartilage rim stress and load redistribution to surrounding cartilage. Am J Sports Med 2004;32:1451–8.
7. Shelbourne KD, Jari S, Gray T. Outcome of untreated traumatic articular cartilage defects of the knee: a natural history study. J Bone Joint Surg Am 2003;85:8–16.
8. Camp CL, Stuart MJ, Krych AJ. Current concepts of articular cartilage restoration techniques in the knee. Sports Health 2014;6:265–73.
9. Mankin HJ. The response of articular cartilage to mechanical injury. J Bone Joint Surg Am 1982;64:460–6.
10. Cole BJ, Lee SJ. Complex knee reconstruction: articular cartilage treatment options. Arthroscopy 2003;19(Suppl 1):1–10.
11. Gudas R, Gudaite A, Mickevicius T. Comparison of osteochondral autologous transplantation, microfracture, or debridement techniques in articular cartilage lesions associated with anterior cruciate ligament injury: a prospective study with a 3-year follow-up. Arthroscopy 2013;29:89–97.
12. Craig W, David JW, Ming HZ. A current review on the biology and treatment of the articular cartilage defects (part I & part II). J Musculoskelet Res 2003;7:157–81.
13. Richter DL, Schenck R, Wascher D, et al. Knee articular cartilage repair and restoration techniques: a review of the literature. Sports Health 2016;8(2):153–60.
14. Sgaglione NA. Decision-making and approach to articular cartilage surgery. Sports Med Arthrosc Rev 2003;11:192–201.
15. Farr J, Cole J, Sherman S, et al. Particulated articular cartilage: CAIS and DeNovo NT. J Knee Surg 2012;25:23–9.
16. Steadman JR, Rodkey WG, Singleton SB, et al. Microfracture technique for full thickness chondral defects: technique and clinical results. Oper Tech Orthop 1997;7:300–4.
17. Steadman JR, Rodkey WG, Rodrigo JJ. Microfracture: surgical technique and rehabilitation to treat chondral defects. Clin Orthop Relat Res 2001;(391 Suppl):S362–9.
18. Mithoefer K, McAdams T, Williams RJ, et al. Clinical efficacy of the microfracture technique for articular cartilage repair in the knee. Am J Sports Med 2009;37: 2053–63.
19. Bedi A, Feeley BT, Williams RJ. Management of articular cartilage defects of the knee. J Bone Joint Surg Am 2010;92:994–1009.
20. Steadman JR, Briggs KK, Rodrigo JJ, et al. Outcomes of microfracture for traumatic chondral defects of the knee: average 11-year follow-up. Arthroscopy 2003;19:477–84.
21. Gudas R, Kalesinskas RJ, Kimtys V, et al. A prospective randomized clinical study of mosaic osteochondral autologous transplantation vs microfracture for

the treatment of osteochondral defects in the knee in young athletes. Arthroscopy 2005;21:1066–75.

22. Knutsen G, Engebretsen L, Ludvigsen TC, et al. Autologous chondrocyte implantation compared with microfracture in the knee: a randomized trial. J Bone Joint Surg Am 2004;86:455–64.

23. Knutsen G, Drogset JO, Engebretsen L, et al. A randomized trial comparing autologous chondrocyte implantation with microfracture at five years. J Bone Joint Surg Am 2007;89:2015–22.

24. Rodrigo JJ, Steadman JR, Silliman JJ, et al. Improvement of full-thickness chondral defect healing in the human knee after debridement and microfracture using continuous passive motion. Am J Knee Surg 1994;7:109–16.

25. Mithoefer K, Venugopal V, Manaqibwala M. Incidence, degree, and clinical effect of subchondral bone overgrowth after microfracture in the knee. Am J Sports Med 2016;44:2057–63.

26. Mithoefer K, Williams RJ, Warren RF, et al. The microfracture technique for the treatment of articular cartilage lesions in the knee. A prospective cohort study. J Bone Joint Surg Am 2005;87:1911–20.

27. Frisbie DD, Oxford JT, Southwood L, et al. Early events in cartilage repair after subchondral bone microfracture. Clin Orthop Relat Res 2003;407:215–7.

28. Gobbi A, Nunag P, Malinowski K. Treatment of chondral lesions of the knee with microfracture in a group of athletes. Knee Surg Sports Traumatol Arthrosc 2005; 13:213–21.

29. Zaslav K, Cole B, Brewster R, et al. A prospective study of autologous chondrocyte implantation in patients with failed prior treatment for articular cartilage defect of the knee: results of the Study of the Treatment of Articular Repair (STAR) clinical trial. Am J Sports Med 2009;37:42–55.

30. Minas T, Von Keudell A, Bryant T, et al. A minimum 10-year outcome study of autologous chondrocyte implantation. Clin Orthop Relat Res 2014;472:41–51.

31. Wood JJ, Malek MA, Frassica FJ, et al. Autologous cultured chondrocytes: adverse events reports to the United States Food and Drug Administration. J Bone Joint Surg Am 2006;88:503–7.

32. Pietschmann MF, Niethammer TR, Horgn A, et al. The incidence and clinical relevance of graft hypertrophy after matrix-based autologous chondrocyte implantation. Am J Sports Med 2012;40:68–74.

33. Niemeyer P, Pestka JM, Kreuz PC, et al. Characteristic complications after autologous chondrocyte implantation for cartilage defects of the knee. Am J Sports Med 2008;36:2091–9.

34. Henderson I, Tuy B, Oakes B. Reoperation after autologous chondrocyte implantation: indications and findings. J Bone Joint Surg Br 2004;82:205–11.

35. Kreuz PC, Steinwachs M, Erggelet C, et al. Classification of graft hypertrophy after autologous chondrocyte implantation of full-thickness chondral defects in the knee. Osteoarthritis Cartilage 2007;15:1339–47.

36. Bahuaud J, Maitrot RC, Bouvet R, et al. Implantation of autologous chondrocytes for cartilagenous lesions in young patients. A study of 24 cases. Chirurgie 1998; 123:568–71.

37. Riboh JC, Cole BJ, Farr J. Particulated articular cartilage for symptomatic chondral defects of the knee. Curr Rev Musculoskelet Med 2015;8:429–35.

38. Bonner KF, Daner W, Yao JQ. 2-year postoperative evaluation of a patient with symptomatic full-thickness patellar cartilage defect repaired with particulated juvenile cartilage tissue. J Knee Surg 2010;23:109–14.

39. Tompkins M, Hamann JC, Diduch DR, et al. Preliminary results of a novel single-stage cartilage restoration technique: particulated juvenile articular cartilage allograft for chondral defects of the patella. Arthroscopy 2013;29:1661–70.

40. Solheim E, Hegna J, Øyen J, et al. Results at 10 to 14 years after osteochondral autografting (mosaicplasty) in articular cartilage defects in the knee. Knee 2013; 20:287–90.

41. Hangody L, Füles P. Autologous osteochondral mosaicplasty for the treatment of full-thickness defects of weight-bearing joints: ten years of experimental and clinical experience. J Bone Joint Surg Am 2003;85:25–32.

42. Barber FA, Chow JC. Arthroscopic chondral osseous autograft transplantation (COR procedure) for femoral defects. Arthroscopy 2006;22:10–6.

43. Krych AJ, Harnly HW, Rodeo SA, et al. Activity levels are higher after osteochondral autograft transfer mosaicplasty than after microfracture for articular cartilage defects of the knee: a retrospective comparative study. J Bone Joint Surg Am 2012;94:971–8.

44. Andrade R, Vasta S, Pereira H, et al. Knee donor-site morbidity after mosaicplasty - a systematic review. J Exp Orthop 2016;3:31.

45. Hangody L, Vásárhelyi G, Hangody LR, et al. Autologous osteochondral grafting-technique and long-term results. Injury 2008;39:S32–9.

46. LaPrade RF, Botker JC. Donor-site morbidity after osteochondral autograft transfer procedures. Arthroscopy 2004;20:69–73.

47. D'Lima DD, Chen PC, Colwell CW Jr. Osteochondral grafting: effect of graft alignment, material properties, and articular geometry. Open Orthop J 2009;3:61–8.

48. Huang FS, Simonian PT, Norman AG, et al. Effects of small incongruities in a sheep model of osteochondral autografting. Am J Sports Med 2004;32:1842–8.

49. Bentley G, Biant LC, Vijayan S, et al. Minimum ten-year results of a prospective randomised study of autologous chondrocyte implantation versus mosaicplasty for symptomatic articular cartilage lesions of the knee. J Bone Joint Surg Br 2012;94:504–9.

50. Patil S, Tapasvi SR. Osteochondral autografts. Curr Rev Musculoskelet Med 2015;8:423–8.

51. Hangody L, Dobos J, Baló E, et al. Clinical experiences with autologous osteochondral mosaicplasty in an athletic population: a 17-year prospective multicenter study. Am J Sports Med 2010;38:1125–33.

52. Sherman SL, Thyssen E, Nuelle CW. Osteochondral autologous transplantation. Clin Sports Med 2017;36:489–500.

53. Kock NB, Hannink G, van Kampen A, et al. Evaluation of subsidence, chondrocyte survival and graft incorporation following autologous osteochondral transplantation. Knee Surg Sports Traumatol Arthrosc 2011;19:1962–70.

54. Kock NB, Tankeren E, van Susante JL. Bone scintigraphy after osteochondral autograft transplantation in the knee. Acta Orthop 2010;81:206–10.

55. Borazjani BH, Chen AC, Bae WC, et al. Effect of impact on chondrocyte viability during insertion of human osteochondral grafts. J Bone Joint Surg Am 2006;88: 1934–43.

56. Ewers BJ, Dvoracek-Driksna D, Orth MW, et al. The extent of matrix damage and chondrocyte death in mechanically traumatized articular cartilage explants depends on rate of loading. J Orthop Res 2001;19:779–84.

57. Patil S, Butcher W, D'Lima DD. Effect of osteochondral graft insertion forces on chondrocyte viability. Am J Sports Med 2008;36(9):1726–32.

58. Kang RW, Friel NA, Williams JM. Effect of impaction sequence on osteochondral graft damage: the role of repeated and varying loads. Am J Sports Med 2010;38: 105–13.
59. Whiteside RA, Jakob RP, Wyss UP, et al. Impact loading of articular cartilage during transplantation of osteochondral autograft. J Bone Joint Surg Br 2005;7: 1285–91.
60. Hangody L, Kish G, Kárpáti Z, et al. Arthroscopic autogenous osteochondral mosaicplasty for the treatment of femoral condylar articular defects. A preliminary report. Knee Surg Sports Traumatol Arthrosc 1997;5:262–7.
61. Bodó G, Hangody L, Szabó Z, et al. Arthroscopic autologous osteochondral mosaicplasty for the treatment of subchondral cystic lesion in the medial femoral condyle in a horse. Acta Vet Hung 2000;48:343–54.
62. Hangody L, Feczkó P, Bartha L, et al. Mosaicplasty for the treatment of articular defects of the knee and ankle. Clin Orthop Relat Res 2001;391:S328–36.
63. Feczkó P, Hangody L, Varga J, et al. Experimental results of donor site filling for autologous osteochondral mosaicplasty. Arthroscopy 2003;19:755–61.
64. Pallante AL, Chen AC, Ball ST. The in vivo performance of osteochondral allografts in the goat is diminished with extended storage and decreased cartilage cellularity. Am J Sports Med 2012;40:1814–23.
65. Bugbee WD, Convery FR. Osteochondral allograft transplantation. Clin Sports Med 1999;18:67–75.
66. Levy LD, Gortz S, Pulido P, et al. Do fresh osteochondral allografts successfully treat femoral condyle lesions? Clin Orthop Relat Res 2013;471:231–7.
67. Krych AJ, Robertson CM, Williams RJ. Cartilage study group: return to athletic activity after osteochondral allograft transplantation in the knee. Am J Sports Med 2012;40:1053–9.
68. Chahal J, Gross A, Gross C, et al. Outcomes of osteochondral allograft transplantation in the knee. Arthroscopy 2013;29(3):575–88.
69. Demange M, Gomoll AH. The use of osteochondral allografts in the management of cartilage defects. Curr Rev Musculoskelet Med 2012;5:229–35.
70. Radin EL, Martin R, Burr D, et al. Effects of mechanical loading on the tissues of the rabbit knee. J Orthop Res 1984;2:221–34.
71. Koshino T, Wada S, Ara Y. Regeneration of degenerated articular cartilage after high tibial osteotomy for medial compartmental osteoarthritis of the knee. Knee 2003;10:229–36.
72. Gross AE, Shasha N, Aubin P. Long-term follow-up of the use of fresh osteochondral allografts for posttraumatic knee defects. Clin Orthop Relat Res 2005;(435): 79–87.
73. Ghazavi MT, Pritzker K, Davis A, et al. Fresh osteochondral allografts for posttraumatic osteochondral defects of the knee. J Bone Joint Surg Br 1997;79: 1008–13.
74. Gomoll AH, Cole BJ. Articular cartilage lesion. In: Miller MD, Thompson SR, editors. DeLee & Drez's orthopaedic sports medicine principles and practice. Philadelphia: Elsevier; 2015. p. 1134–48.

Foot and Ankle Surgery
Common Problems and Solutions

Lorena Bejarano-Pineda, MD[a],*, Annunziato Amendola, MD[b]

KEYWORDS

- Arthroscopy • Complications • Sports • Ankle joint • Achilles tendon • Instability
- Infection

KEY POINTS

- Complication rates in foot and ankle arthroscopy are slightly higher compared with other joint arthroscopies. The anatomy of the foot and ankle is surrounded by subcutaneous structures that are at risk, and a narrow joint space contributes to the risk of complications. Most of them are minor and neurologic.
- Ankle sprains contribute to chronic lateral ankle instability. After surgical treatment, recurrent instability is the main concern and has been reported in acute and delayed repairs. To prevent recurrence. Associated disorders must be assessed and treated within the same procedure if required.
- Wound complications after Achilles tendon repair can be significant generating negative long-term consequences. There are patient and procedure-related risk factors. Optimal conditions in terms of patient health and soft tissue status need to be considered to assure decreased rate of wound-related complications.

INTRODUCTION

Daily participation in sports and exercise in adults within the American population has increased significantly during the last decade. In competitive sport participation, injuries to the foot and ankle are the most common cause of time lost from sports.[1] Many of these injuries require surgical management but also, because of the spectrum of severity, understanding the pathophysiology and individualizing treatment are paramount.

Common foot and ankle injuries requiring surgical treatment include ankle instability (ankle sprains), tendon ruptures (most commonly Achilles), syndesmotic injuries, Lisfranc injuries, and high-risk stress fractures. In many of these injuries, arthroscopic techniques are used. Although the rate of complications among this type of operative

[a] Division of Foot and Ankle Surgery, Department of Orthopedic Surgery, Duke University Medical Center, 4709 Creekstone Drive - Suite 200, Durham, NC 27703, USA; [b] Division of Sports Medicine, Duke University Medical Center, Duke Sports Science Institute, 3475 Erwin Road, Durham, NC 27705, USA
* Corresponding author.
E-mail address: lorena.bejarano@duke.edu

Clin Sports Med 37 (2018) 331–350
https://doi.org/10.1016/j.csm.2017.12.009

sportsmed.theclinics.com

procedure is very low, foot and ankle and sports medicine surgeons should be acutely aware of their prevention, presentation, and effective management.

This article addresses these most frequent complications, in conjunction with the most commonly performed procedures in foot and ankle–related sport injuries.

FOOT AND ANKLE ARTHROSCOPY

Ankle arthroscopy was published as a surgical method by Takagi in 1939,[2] but it was not until the 1970s when arthroscopy became an important diagnostic and treatment tool for orthopedic surgeons.[3] Complication rates in foot and ankle arthroscopy vary from 6.8% to 9.8%.[4,5] Most of them are minor or neurologic and are caused by the procedure. The most common complications in foot and ankle arthroscopy are described in **Box 1**.

Neurologic Injuries

Neurovascular structures can be injured during the procedure because of improper portal placement, prolonged or inappropriate distraction, and extensive tourniquet use. The most common injured nerves are the superficial peroneal nerve because of its varied anatomic anterolateral ankle joint location, and the sural nerve because of its posterolateral location (**Figs. 1** and **2**). These injuries are usually associated with portal placement and at times with inappropriate or prolonged distraction.[6,7] Most of the nerve injuries are temporary paresthesias that resolve over time, but permanent paresis or paresthesias have been reported in a small number of patients.[4]

In order to minimize the risk of injury, surgeons should use vertical skin incisions for portals at the ankle because all structures longitudinally cross the ankle joint. Using a hemostat to spread the subcutaneous tissue avoids injury even if adjacent to a tendon or neurovascular structure. A protective interchangeable cannula helps to decrease the risk of repetitive soft tissue injury, including to neurovascular structures.

Tendon and Ligament Injuries

The numerous tendons and ligaments crossing the ankle and foot can easily be injured during portal and pin distraction placement (see **Fig. 1**). The use of a trans-Achilles portal during posterior arthroscopy is abandoned because it is

---

Box 1
Complications of ankle arthroscopy

Tourniquet complications

Neurovascular injury

Articular cartilage damage

Wound complications

Compartment syndrome

Hemarthrosis

Synovial fistula

Tendon and ligament injury

Stress fracture

Deep vein thrombosis

Complex regional pain syndrome

Instrument breakage

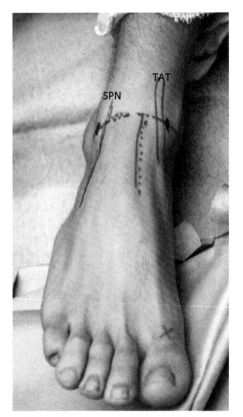

Fig. 1. Anterior arthroscopic portals placement. SPN, superficial peroneal nerve; TAT, tibialis anterior tendon.

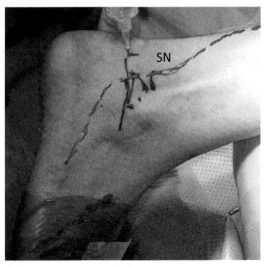

Fig. 2. Sural nerve (SN) in posterior portal placement.

unnecessary and because of its potential risk for rupture. Ligament injuries may occur because of extensive debridement, inappropriate distraction, or portal placement. Distraction for more than 2 hours with a force greater than 23 kg (50 lb) during ankle arthroscopy can place not only the nerves but the ligaments at risk.[7] Periodic relaxation and general anesthesia can minimize the distraction forces, thus diminishing the risk of injury.

Articular Injury

Damaging the articular cartilage is a frequently unreported complication of arthroscopy. Joints with narrow confines, such as those in the foot and ankle, are most susceptible to injury. Injury commonly occurs during the introduction of the arthroscope and the instruments. The use of a gentle technique avoiding sharp trocars and large-gauge needles can help in setting the appropriate location of the portals without articular cartilage damage. Carlson and Ferkel[6] recommend placing the anterior cannula in the anterior compartment first to evaluate the available space in the central and posterior compartments. The use of a distraction device can reduce the incidence of cartilage damage during arthroscopy in small joints such as the foot and ankle. The use of a smaller-diameter scope (ie, 2.7 mm) is helpful in avoiding injury.

The injury spectrum is wide, going from superficial scrapes and nicks to full-thickness injury to subchondral bone. However, the long-term sequelae of these injuries have not been well studied. Some investigators advocate avoiding intra-articular bupivacaine injections for postoperative pain control because of its potential effects of chondrotoxicity.[8]

Synovial Fistula

Sinus tract formation may occur in the ankle because the soft tissue envelope at the ankle is minimal and excessive early activity after surgery promotes fluid formation (**Fig. 3**). Observation and immobilization for a week or two generally suffice. Fistulas may occur with severely traumatized portals or in cases of postoperative infection. In cases of persistent drainage, the fluid should be cultured, the joint needs to be

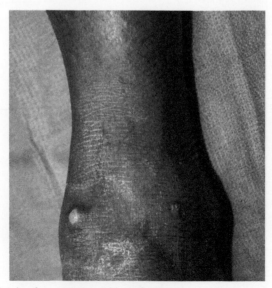

Fig. 3. Synovial fistula after anterior ankle arthroscopy.

immobilized, and oral antibiotics administered. If the initial treatment fails and the fistula persists, the patient undergoes surgical debridement, reclosure with suction drains, and immobilization should be instituted until it is completely healed.

Postoperative Effusion

Effusions are a result of bleeding or synovitis. Appropriate irrigation and removal of all intra-articular debris has decreased the incidence of postoperative effusion. In cases of recurrent effusion postoperatively, the fluid may need to be aspirated for analysis and culture. Hemarthrosis after arthroscopy is caused by the specific procedure or inadequate hemostasis during surgery. The use of aspirin or nonsteroidal anti-inflammatory medication may increase the risk of bleeding and should be discontinued before the procedure. Aspiration is indicated if the patient has severe pain or limited range of motion secondary to swelling.

Wound Complications

A variety of wound complications after ankle and foot arthroscopy can occur. Skin slough, necrosis, seroma, hematoma, and infection are potential complications. Anterior ankle arthroscopy is at higher risk because of the thinness of its skin with minimal subcutaneous tissue. The infection rate for ankle arthroscopy is 1.4%,[9] which is significantly higher compared with other joints.[10] Minimal subcutaneous tissue, thin skin around the ankle, and the use of absorbable sutures or surgical tape strips to close the wound are some of the predisposing factors that may be associated with the increased rate of infection.

Postoperative ankle arthroscopy infection is classified as superficial and deep infection. Most of these infections are considered superficial and they resolve with local wound care, removal of disturbing sutures, and oral antibiotics. In cases of deep infections, such as intra-articular infections, blood cultures, synovial fluid analysis, and culture should be obtained to confirm the diagnosis. Antibiotics should be initiated promptly after cultures are taken and the patient needs a second intervention for debridement and irrigation. To reduce the risk of infection, some investigators advocate the administration of prophylactic antibiotics, washing of the foot and ankle with antiseptic scrub brush that morning, and keeping the tourniquet and operative times as short as possible.[4,7]

There is some controversy regarding the advantage of postoperative immobilization as a protective factor against wound complications. Investigators such as Carlson and Ferkel[6] recommend immobilization in a splint for 5 to 7 days as part of the postoperative protocol. However, Zengerink and Van Dijk[11] advise that immediate mobilization in active dorsiflexion a few times per hour after the surgery is beneficial for the rehabilitation process. The authors prefer to immobilize the operated extremity for ambulation for a week or two after the procedure.

LATERAL ANKLE STABILIZATION

Ankle sprains are the most common injury in college athletes[12] and in recreational sports. Although most of these injuries are caused by acute trauma, 20% to 40% of the cases transition into chronic ankle instability.[13,14] Multiple surgical procedures have been described for restoring ankle stability.[15] Techniques can be categorized as anatomic or nonanatomic reconstructions. A modified Broström-Gould procedure was initially described in 1966 for direct ligament repair only. Gould then modified this technique, by also incorporating the inferior extensor retinaculum.[16–18] Now the modified Broström usually refers to taking down the anterior talofibular ligament and/or calcaneofibular ligament off the fibula directly and tensioning the ligaments back to bone with anchors, followed by the Gould addition. At present, this is the gold standard for surgical treatment.

Several studies have reported good and excellent outcomes after surgical treatment of lateral ankle instability. Surgical complications can be classified according to the time of presentation during the postoperative period. Early complications are related to wound healing and nerve injuries, and late complications to recurrent instability.

Early Complications

The published frequency of wound infection is 5%,[19] with most of complications being superficial infections. They usually respond to local treatment, as previously described. In cases of deep infection, such as septic arthritis or osteomyelitis, removal of foreign material and surgical debridement are mandatory. Culture-specific antibiotic treatment increases the chance of eradicating the infectious process promptly.[20]

Rates of nerve injury associated with ankle ligament reconstruction have been reported to be as high as 52%. However, this accounts for a range of subtle hyposensibility to severe disabling pain from nerve entrapment or neuroma. The overall incidence is reduced to a range of between 9% and 19% in terms of serious complications, including sensory deficits and severe pain.[19,21] Of note, the nerves at greatest risk to be injured during ankle ligament reconstruction are the superficial peroneal nerve and the sural nerve.[22] Understanding the topographic anatomy and avoiding the nerves altogether is the best way to prevent injury. Dissecting the nerves, if necessary, is also important, but, around the foot, any scarring around the nerves is likely to create some dysesthesias with shoe wear. Additional perioperative complications, such as reflex sympathetic dystrophy, neurogenic pain syndromes, deep venous thrombosis, and pulmonary embolus, have also been described.[23,24]

Late Complications

Recurrent instability is the main concern after ankle stabilization. Recurrent instability has been reported in acute and delayed primary repairs. The failure is classified into 4 groups according to the cause: (1) inadequate reconstruction; (2) functional instability regardless of a solid anatomic reconstruction; (3) reinjury to the ankle; and (4) overlooked medial instability or predisposing factors.[20] Identifying the nature of these failures allows appropriate treatment and better outcomes.

The aim of ankle reconstruction is to restore the ankle's stability; nevertheless, despite the procedure, recurrent ankle sprains may still occur with return to sport. Ankle bracing is recommended to prevent recurrence. Severe sprains after acute or delayed ligament repair are treated nonoperatively with protective immobilization and physical therapy, as with the initial treatment approach. Patients who do not respond to optimal rehabilitation (including bracing) may have mechanical laxity. In those cases, a revision repair or reconstruction ligament technique may be necessary.[25–28]

Patients with predisposing factors for chronic stability are at high risk of recurrence after surgery if these factors are not addressed. Conditions such as generalized joint hypermobility, cavovarus foot, peroneal tendon instability or tears, and anterior or posterior impingement should be treated simultaneously to decrease the risk of failure.[26] Generalized joint hypermobility, as defined by a Beighton score greater than 4, has been associated with recurrent instability and poor outcomes.[22] Therefore, some investigators advocate persistent nonoperative rehabilitation, and then as a surgical treatment to consider ligament reconstruction instead of repair as the first procedure, or to perform the Broström-Gould repair with an augmentation technique.[29,30]

In cavovarus deformity, either forefoot or hindfoot driven, the weight-bearing axis of the ankle is medialized, imposing higher demands on the lateral stabilizers. Sammarco[20] described ankle instability as the main complaint in 25% of patients with cavovarus foot deformity. If comorbidity is present, correction of the underlying deformity through calcaneal and/or metatarsal osteotomies needs to be simultaneously performed along with lateral ligament repair. Often peroneal tendon disease exists with cavovarus foot underlying the instability.[31]

A similar approach should be taken in cases of coexisting peroneal tendon disease or ankle impingement. Both disorders need to be addressed during the same procedure to diminish the incidence of recurrent instability or persistent pain.

Revision surgery has been described as revision anatomic reconstruction using grafts or revision repair with synthetic augmentation. Cho and colleagues[25] reported good results in 30 patients who underwent revision augmented with suture tape for persistent instability of the ankle after Broström procedure. At the final follow-up, the patients did not show a significant difference in talar tilt and anterior talar translation under stress radiographs compared with the contralateral ankle. They concluded that the revision procedure augmented with suture tape is a technique that provides stability and satisfactory clinical outcomes in patients with recurrent stability.[25]

Reconstructive procedures using autografts and allografts in assorted fixation techniques have been described.[32,33] Implanting the grafts in the anatomic footprint of the ligaments is crucial to reestablish the normal biomechanics of the ankle and subtalar joints. Matheny and colleagues[34] showed similar functional outcomes in patients with anatomic allograft reconstruction compared with those with ligament repair at 2 years postoperatively. However, 20% of the patients with anatomic allograft reconstruction required arthroscopy debridement because of arthrofibrosis.[34] Overtightening is a complication during reconstructive procedures, and surgeons need to be aware of this.

SYNDESMOTIC INJURY AND STABILIZATION

Injury to the distal tibiofibular syndesmosis occurs in up to 20% of ankle fractures and 10% of all ankle sprains.[35,36] Stable and unstable syndesmosis injuries are common in collision sports and occur primarily during direct contact, like tackling and blocking[37,38]; further, they have a higher incidence on artificial turf compared with natural grass.[39,40] Successful functional outcomes in patients with this injury rely on the ability to obtain an anatomic and stable reduction of the syndesmosis and the ankle mortise. Poor results following treatment can commonly be attributed to malreduction, even with surgery or chronic instability in neglected injuries or recurrent diastasis (**Fig. 4**).

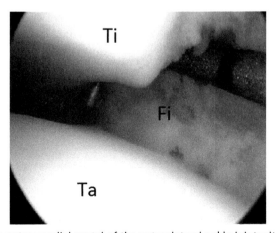

Fig. 4. View from anteromedial portal of the anterolateral ankle joint with probe showing absent anterior tibiofibular ligament. Instability of the tibiofibular joint following a high ankle sprain. Fi, fibula; Ta, talus; Ti, tibia.

Malreduction

Malreduction occurs at a high rate even after surgical treatment. Studies have described malreduction rates in 15% to 50% of postsurgical patients. Malposition has been attributed to an incorrect clamp location, eccentric screw placement, and associated posterior malleolus fracture.[41] Accurate assessment of syndesmotic reduction and stability intraoperatively is essential. Biomechanical studies have provided evidence of more sagittal instability than lateral instability in syndesmotic injuries.[42] The malposition is commonly encountered with the fibula having been anteriorly displaced and internally rotated.[43,44]

To achieve an anatomic reduction, the first step is to restore the length, alignment, and rotation of the fibula when there is an associated fracture.[45,46] Some investigators recommend performing an open reduction instead of a closed reduction of the syndesmosis.[19] The open technique allows direct visualization of the reduction and more control of the reduction's accuracy. In cases in which a clamp application is the chosen reduction technique, the medial clamp tine should be placed in the anterior third of the tibia when looking at a talar dome lateral image. Cosgrove and colleagues[47] provided evidence on how this position may contribute to lowering the rate of off-axis clamping and thereby ultimately decrease malreduction rates. Accurate assessment of reduction and achieving stability intraoperatively are necessary to ensure successful outcomes.

There are multiple fixation methods described, with the suture button techniques showing less risk of malreduction. Several studies have failed to show meaningful differences in clinical and functional outcomes regarding the material, number of screws, and fixed cortices in syndesmosis injuries.[48–51] An advantage of quadricortical fixation is the ability to access the screw from the medial side for removal if hardware breakage occurs. Nevertheless, further research is needed to determine optimal reduction, stability, and outcomes for the long term.

Screw fixation of the syndesmosis results in loss of physiologic motion at the distal tibiofibular joint. This restriction in motion places increased stress across the screws, leading to high breakage rates.[52,53] Most surgeons remove syndesmotic screws between 8 and 12 weeks after fixation; however, whether it is necessary to remove the screws remains controversial. In support of screw removal, some studies suggest that doing so allows the distal tibiofibular joint to return to normal motion, thereby improving functional outcomes.[53] Screw removal is an additional surgical procedure, with a wound infection rate as high as 9.2% and a recurrent diastasis of 6.6%.[54]

The suture button method is a dynamic fixation method now commonly used for syndesmotic injuries. Inge and colleagues,[55] in a systematic review comparing the traditional syndesmosis screw fixation with a dynamic fixation system, concluded that the dynamic fixation system had significantly better functional outcomes and lower complication and implant removal rates (10.5% vs 38.5%). However, complications, such as infection, skin irritation, and granuloma formation, have been reported using the suture button fixation method.[56] These complications may occur at a lower rate with newer implant modifications.

Chronic Instability

Chronic instability is defined as a persistent widening of the tibiofibular joint 3 months after initial injury.[57] This condition may occur in cases of neglected injuries, recurrent diastasis after hardware removal or breakage, and inadequate fixation. Distal tibiofibular instability causes an altered tibiotalar contact area, which leads to the development of ankle osteoarthritis.[43,58,59] Most patients present with lateral talar translation and increased medial clear space,[60] but occult instability may occur following syndesmotic sprains when there is no widening; radiographic relationships are normal; and diagnosis is based on clinical examination, MRI findings, and possibly arthroscopic evaluation.

Computed tomography (CT) scan is frequently used in a chronic setting. It allows evaluation of bone injury, healing status, and the presence of arthritis.[61] In addition, bilateral ankle CT scan is strongly recommended to analyze and compare the tibiofibular relationship and to detect latent diastasis.[62]

Once the diagnosis has been made, treatment options include screw fixation, arthroscopic debridement, reconstruction techniques, and arthrodesis.[63] Reconstruction techniques include tightening with advancement or ligament transposition, autograft substitution, and arthrodesis.[60] A meta-analysis on the management of chronic syndesmotic diastasis pooled data presented success rates of 87.9% for screw fixation, 79.4% for arthrodesis, and 78.7% for arthroscopic debridement.[64] According to these results, all such procedures have satisfactory outcomes, on the condition that an anatomic reduction and stability is obtained.

Ankle arthroscopy allows evaluation of tibiofibular joint stability, and debridement of interposed fibrous tissue if necessary, to help in reduction of the joint. In the scenario of clinical symptoms of anterolateral ankle impingement with normal radiological findings, isolated arthroscopic debridement without fixation can be considered as the treatment of choice.[65] However, some investigators advocate maximizing syndesmotic stability by using a suture button device during the same procedure.[60]

In the presence of frank diastasis, the underlying deformity needs to be corrected. If the fibula is malreduced or shortened, a fibular osteotomy is necessary to restore length. Open debridement of the syndesmosis is recommended to allow reduction of the fibula to the tibia. The authors' preference is to hold the reduced fibula with the usual syndesmotic fixation (ie, screws or 2 suture buttons), and then allow the syndesmosis to heal in this position with 6 weeks of immobilization and non–weight bearing. Suture tape may be used to reconstruct the anterior inferior tibiofibular ligament (AITFL) for additional stability.

Many soft tissue procedures have been described in the literature to stabilize the syndesmosis. If the AITFL is intact and lax, bone block advancement or repair and augmented fixation are viable options.[66] When the AITFL is ruptured and absent, reconstructive procedures using autografts, such as peroneous longus and hamstring autografts, have been described as having good functional outcomes.[67,68] Some investigators augment the reconstruction with suture button or screw fixation.[60]

As a last option, arthrodesis may be indicated in cases with chronic syndesmotic instability, and for patients with instability and associated syndesmotic arthritis. Pes planus may be the cause of chronic syndesmotic stress and latent widening, particularly in obese patients, in whom the usual syndesmotic fixation techniques may fail. Pena and Coetzee[69] recommend arthrodesis for patients with injuries older than 6 months, severe incongruity, and recurrence after removal of fixation. Arthrodesis of the distal tibiofibular joint has proven stability in the long term but might increase the risk of ankle arthrosis as well. This procedure should be reserved for low-demand patients and overcompression should also be avoided, because this creates a nonanatomic mortise.

LISFRANC INJURIES

The Lisfranc joint includes the tarsometatarsal joint among the metatarsals, the cuneiforms, and cuboid. The Lisfranc complex has osseous stability by the Roman arch configuration with the recessed second metatarsal base acting as a mortise. The tarsometatarsal, interosseous, and the transverse metatarsal ligaments confer ligamentous stability across the tarsometatarsal joint complex. The Lisfranc ligament is a thick and oblique ligament that extends from the base of the second metatarsal to the plantar aspect of the medial cuneiform. Its integrity is crucial for stability in the medial column because there is no transverse ligament between the first and second metatarsals.[70]

Other complications include infection, compartment syndrome, deep vein thrombosis, and neurovascular injury. Deol and colleagues[71] described deep peroneal nerve injury in 3 patients after surgical treatment. In the long term, joint instability caused by failed hardware, malreduction, or neglected injury may trigger pes planus deformity, midfoot posttraumatic arthritis, and persistent pain. Nevertheless, there is a weak correlation between the radiographic degenerative changes and symptoms. Only 7.8% of patients with arthritic changes are symptomatic enough to require an arthrodesis.[72]

Missed Diagnosis

Lisfranc joint fractures and dislocations are the most common type of severe injuries in the midfoot. Although these are not common orthopedic injuries, they do present a significant challenge in diagnosis and return to activity.[73] Approximately 20% of these injuries are missed or overlooked, especially in polytraumatized patients and in pure ligament injury in athletes (**Figs. 5** and **6**).[74] Therefore clinical suspicion is paramount in evaluating these injuries in detail to determine stability and need for treatment. Any widening on weight-bearing views of the Lisfranc joint requires a more detailed evaluation. This evaluation may be in the form of MRI to determine the extent of ligament injury[75] or performing stress views under fluoroscopy to determine stability. In the case of an unstable injury, surgical stabilization is indicated.

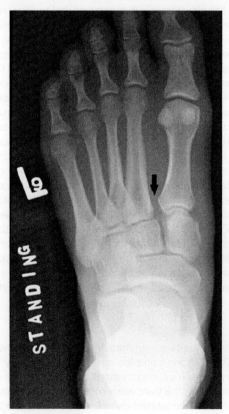

Fig. 5. Patient with a pure Lisfranc ligament injury (*black arrow*).

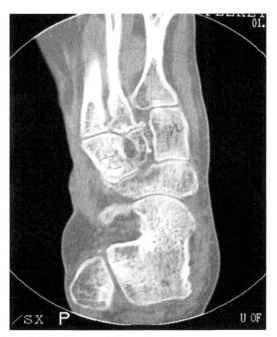

Fig. 6. Missed Lisfranc injury diagnosed 3 months after trauma.

Late Complications

In the long term, joint instability caused by failed hardware, malreduction, or neglected injury may trigger pes planus deformity, midfoot posttraumatic arthritis, and persistent pain. The prevalence of posttraumatic surgery increases up to 60% in cases of malreduction. The severity of the injury and its treatment contribute to the outcomes in both short-term and long-term cases. Malreduction and posttraumatic arthrosis are common and therefore anatomic reduction and stabilization are essential. Delayed weight bearing is important to prevent collapse, therefore non–weight-bearing immobilization for 6 weeks is recommended followed by careful mobilization. Type B injuries according to the Myerson classification are associated with a worse outcome compared with type A and C injuries.[76,77] The surgical treatment of unstable injuries includes open or percutaneous reduction and fixation. Primary arthrodesis has been advocated in severe unstable cases with multiple joints involved. At present, there is controversial evidence regarding the results with internal fixation and primary arthrodesis in patients with pure ligamentous injury and severely comminuted fracture-dislocations.[78]

Lisfranc complex injuries represent a broad spectrum. An early diagnosis is crucial to obtain an appropriate treatment and better outcomes. The goal of the surgical treatment is to achieve a stable and an anatomic reduction; however, in cases of adequate treatment the clinical outcomes do not correlate with the radiographic findings. Patients need to be aware of the severity of the injury and the spectrum of possible results.

ACHILLES TENDON REPAIR

The incidence of Achilles tendon rupture in the general population is 5 to 10 per 100,000, with some variation among regions.[79,80] Achilles tendinopathy affects competitive and recreational athletes, with more than 80% of ruptures occurring during recreational sports.[81] In addition, competitive athletes with a high incidence of tendon rupture include sprinters, decathletes, soccer players, and basketball players.[82]

The overall annual rate of surgical repair has declined dramatically during the last 15 years. This decline coincided with several publications showing equivalent declining rates of rerupture between surgical and nonsurgical treatment without the risk of wound-related complications.[80,83,84] However, this reduction did not persist in patients less than 20 years old. Patients within this age group showed early improvement in strength after surgical repair compared with nonsurgical treatment, making surgical repairs the preferred treatment of young patients and competitive athletes.[85–87]

Surgical treatment of Achilles tendon rupture can be performed by the classic open approach or by the percutaneous technique introduced by Ma and Griffith.[88] In the open approach, a medial incision is preferred with a careful dissection of the surrounding soft tissue, because the preservation of the paratenon is crucial to prevent healing complications. The most common complications following operative treatment of an acute rupture include infection and delayed wound-healing complications. Other complications following Achilles surgical treatment involve rerupture, healing in a lengthened position, sural nerve lesion, and peritendinous calcification.[89] Addressing chronic complications such as lengthened position or peritendinous calcification is beyond the scope of this article.

Infection and Wound-Healing Complications

The infection rate in open repairs varies from 4% to 20%. Bhandari and colleagues[90] described a relative risk of infection 5.2 times higher with an operative treatment compared with a conservative treatment. Among the risk factors related to the patient, diabetes, obesity, and smoking are strong and independent risk factors for infection and wound complications.[91,92] Patients with uncontrolled diabetes had a 7.25-fold increase of complications. Humphers and colleagues,[93] in 2014, attempted to determine the risk of postoperative infection after foot and ankle surgery, relative to the increase in hemoglobin A1c (HbA1c) level. They described a significant increase in infection rate in patients with HbA1c between 7.3% and 9.8%. The blood supply to the Achilles tendon is reduced in its distal part[94] and the soft tissue layer between the skin and the paratenon is minimal, compromising wound healing.

To minimize the chances of wound complications such as dehiscence, superficial infection, and seroma, the incision should be made sharply through the paratenon, thereby avoiding subcutaneous flaps, which can cause skin necrosis. Large nonabsorbable sutures and knots in the area of the repair site may promote a local reaction and poor healing response and should be avoided. The authors recommend suturing the paratenon once the repair is performed; this protects the tendon substance and decreases the incidence of foreign body reaction to the suture materials (**Fig. 7**). Superficial wound infection usually responds to a course of oral antibiotics and local wound care. Wound dehiscence or breakdown in small areas are susceptible of closure by secondary intention.

In the literature, the current rate of deep infection after an Achilles tendon repair is estimated to be 2% to 4%.[90,95] When there is evidence of a postoperative deep infection, an early and aggressive treatment intervention is paramount and the patient should be admitted for a course of intravenous antibiotics and surgical debridement. Often there is a local foreign body reaction around sutures, and suture removal may suffice as a treatment. If possible, tissue cultures should be processed to guarantee adequate antibiotic application and coverage. Positive cultures for *Staphylococcus aureus* are commonly isolated in patients with postoperative infection after ankle

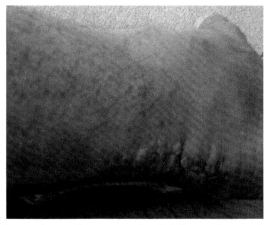

Fig. 7. Foreign body reaction to the sutures after Achilles tendon repair.

surgery.[96,97] All necrotic tissue and foreign material needs to be excised and repeated surgical debridement may be necessary until the infection is under control.

Rerupture

The historical rerupture rate for patients with Achilles tendon rupture surgically treated varies from 3% to 5%.[90,98] Aspects affecting a rerupture are discussed here.

Preoperative conditions

The presence of systemic disease such as peripheral arterial disease or diabetes needs to be addressed before surgery to decrease postoperative risks. Mohsenifar and colleagues[99] performed an experimental study in diabetic rats with tenotomized Achilles tendons. They showed significantly less elasticity and stress tensile load in the tendons of diabetic rats compared with controls. A similar experimental study reported a statistically significant lower peak force for failure and smaller amount of fibroblast and lymphocyte infiltration in diabetic rats compared with healthy rats.[100] These findings direct surgeons to be more cautions during the postoperative phase in diabetic patients and surgeons should strongly consider nonoperative treatment considering the success of current progressive nonoperative treatment regimens and results.[97]

Intraoperative aspects

During the repair the preservation of the blood supply is crucial to prevent rerupture. The central aspect of the tendon, which is described as a watershed zone, is vascularized from its ventral aspect.[101] Dissection in this area should be minimized. The suture technique needs to ensure the strongest repair possible. The initial technique used and described by Krackow,[102] and lately modified by Labib and colleagues[103] as the gift box technique, proved to increase the mean force to failure. Their modification, alternatively, moves the knots out of the defect site and simultaneously doubles the number of strands crossing the ruptured area.

Postoperative care

Most investigators advocate early onset of rehabilitation. Experimental studies have shown that early weight bearing induces essential changes in the healing process,[104] prevents muscle atrophy, and improves vascularization and immunologic response.[105]

Several surgical techniques have been prescribed to treat repeated ruptures of the Achilles tendon. These techniques include V-Y tendon lengthening and turndown flaps of the gastrocnemius,[97] and repair and augmentation by transfer of the peroneus brevis,[106] flexor digitorum longus,[107] flexor hallucis longus, gracilis, plantaris, and fascia lata.[108] The use of synthetic grafts has also been described as an alternative technique.[109] Independent of the use of these techniques, an optimal reconstruction requires achieving normal resting tension with healthy tissue. Surgeons need to be aware of all available options and to carefully plan in advance for any potential complications during the surgical procedure.

Sural Nerve Injury

Injury to the sural nerve is a common complication during surgical Achilles tendon repair. The sural nerve is a sensory branch of the tibial nerve that runs parallel to the distal third of the Achilles tendon in its lateral border.[101] Iatrogenic division, compression of the nerve during wound retraction, or suture ligation at the time of closure can cause long-term morbidity as chronic pain syndrome. Rates of sural nerve injury vary from 0% to 20% in open procedures.[91] Nistor[110] reported a lateral approach in 7 of 9 patients with postoperative sural neuritis. In order to minimize the risk of nerve injury, a medial or central incision over the tendon should be performed. Likewise, a straight dissection through the paratenon avoiding subcutaneous flaps decreases the risk of injury.

Regarding percutaneous procedures, rates of sural neuritis range from 3% to 40%.[111,112] During this technique the nerve is not visualized and it is inevitably at risk. To reduce the potential of sural nerve injuries, other investigators use a miniopen technique to either identify the nerve to protect it or avoid it by staying on the posteromedial side.[113] In case the nerve is divided or ligated and this is recognized intraoperatively, it should be buried deep within the peroneal muscles to prevent the formation of a neuroma and reduce the risk of postoperative pain.

Other complications related to Achilles tendon repair are scar adhesion, decreased ankle motion, overlengthening, deep venous thrombosis, and pulmonary embolus.[38] The risk of adhesions can be diminished by burying the intratendinous sutures and complete closure of the paratenon.[101] Elongation of the Achilles tendon is asymptomatic in most patients, except in high-demand athletes. To decrease the risk of intraoperative overlengthening, some investigators recommend preparing and draping both legs for the procedure. With the contralateral extremity in the field, the surgeon may be assured of the correct length and tension by comparing the degree of plantar flexion of both feet.[114]

REFERENCES

1. Lewis J Jr, Easley ME. Foot and ankle sports orthopaedics. New York: Springer; 2016.
2. Baker CL, Graham JM. Current concepts in ankle arthroscopy. Orthopedics 1993;16(9):1027–35.
3. Martin DF, Baker CL, Curl WW, et al. Operative ankle arthroscopy. Long-term followup. Am J Sports Med 1989;17(1):16–23 [discussion: 23].
4. Ferkel RD, Heath DD, Guhl JF. Neurological complications of ankle arthroscopy. Arthroscopy 1996;12(2):200–8.
5. Young BH, Flanigan RM, DiGiovanni BF. Complications of ankle arthroscopy utilizing a contemporary noninvasive distraction technique. J Bone Joint Surg Am 2011;93(10):963–8.
6. Carlson MJ, Ferkel RD. Complications in ankle and foot arthroscopy. Sports Med Arthrosc 2013;21(2):135–9.

7. Ferkel RD, Small HN, Gittins JE. Complications in foot and ankle arthroscopy. Clin Orthop Relat Res 2001;(391):89–104.

8. Gomoll AH, Kang RW, Williams JM, et al. Chondrolysis after continuous intra-articular bupivacaine infusion: an experimental model investigating chondrotoxicity in the rabbit shoulder. Arthroscopy 2006;22(8):813–9.

9. Barber FA, Click J, Britt BT. Complications of ankle arthroscopy. Foot Ankle 1990;10(5):263–6.

10. Complications of arthroscopy and arthroscopic surgery: results of a national survey. Committee on Complications of Arthroscopy Association of North America. Arthroscopy 1985;1(4):214–20.

11. Zengerink M, van Dijk CN. Complications in ankle arthroscopy. Knee Surg Sports Traumatol Arthrosc 2012;20(8):1420–31.

12. Hootman JM, Dick R, Agel J. Epidemiology of collegiate injuries for 15 sports: summary and recommendations for injury prevention initiatives. J Athl Train 2007;42(2):311–9.

13. Valderrabano V, Wiewiorski M, Frigg A, et al. Chronic ankle instability. Unfallchirurg 2007;110(8):691–9 [quiz: 700]. [in German].

14. Valderrabano V, Hintermann B, Horisberger M, et al. Ligamentous posttraumatic ankle osteoarthritis. Am J Sports Med 2006;34(4):612–20.

15. Peters JW, Trevino SG, Renstrom PA. Chronic lateral ankle instability. Foot Ankle 1991;12(3):182–91.

16. Broström L. Sprained ankles. VI. Surgical treatment of "chronic" ligament ruptures. Acta Chir Scand 1966;132(5):551–65.

17. Gould N, Seligson D, Gassman J. Early and late repair of lateral ligament of the ankle. Foot Ankle 1980;1(2):84–9.

18. Aydogan U, Glisson RR, Nunley JA. Extensor retinaculum augmentation reinforces anterior talofibular ligament repair. Clin Orthop Relat Res 2006;442: 210–5.

19. Mabit C, Tourné Y, Besse JL, et al. Chronic lateral ankle instability surgical repairs: the long term prospective. Orthop Traumatol Surg Res 2010;96(4):417–23.

20. Sammarco VJ. Complications of lateral ankle ligament reconstruction. Clin Orthop Relat Res 2001;(391):123–32.

21. Yeo ED, Lee KT, Sung IH, et al. Comparison of all-inside arthroscopic and open techniques for the modified Broström procedure for ankle instability. Foot Ankle Int 2016;37(10):1037–45.

22. Shakked RJ, Karnovsky S, Drakos MC. Operative treatment of lateral ligament instability. Curr Rev Musculoskelet Med 2017;10(1):113–21.

23. Larsen E, Angermann P. Association of ankle instability and foot deformity. Acta Orthop Scand 1990;61(2):136–9.

24. Sammarco GJ, Carrasquillo HA. Surgical revision after failed lateral ankle reconstruction. Foot Ankle Int 1995;16(12):748–53.

25. Cho BK, Kim YM, Choi SM, et al. Revision anatomical reconstruction of the lateral ligaments of the ankle augmented with suture tape for patients with a failed Broström procedure. Bone Joint J 2017;99-B(9):1183–9.

26. Tourné Y, Mabit C. Lateral ligament reconstruction procedures for the ankle. Orthop Traumatol Surg Res 2017;103(1S):S171–81.

27. Povacz P, Unger SF, Miller WK, et al. A randomized, prospective study of operative and non-operative treatment of injuries of the fibular collateral ligaments of the ankle. J Bone Joint Surg Am 1998;80(3):345–51.

28. Agoropoulos Z, Papachristou G, Efstathopoulos N, et al. Late results of surgical repair in recent ruptures of the lateral ligament of the ankle. Injury 1997;28(8): 531–4.
29. Karlsson J, Eriksson BI, Bergsten T, et al. Comparison of two anatomic reconstructions for chronic lateral instability of the ankle joint. Am J Sports Med 1997;25(1):48–53.
30. Huang B, Kim YT, Kim JU, et al. Modified Broström procedure for chronic ankle instability with generalized joint hypermobility. Am J Sports Med 2016;44(4):1011–6.
31. Bosman HA, Robinson AH. Treatment of ankle instability with an associated cavus deformity. Foot Ankle Clin 2013;18(4):643–57.
32. Caprio A, Oliva F, Treia F, et al. Reconstruction of the lateral ankle ligaments with allograft in patients with chronic ankle instability. Foot Ankle Clin 2006;11(3): 597–605.
33. Pagenstert GI, Hintermann B, Knupp M. Operative management of chronic ankle instability: plantaris graft. Foot Ankle Clin 2006;11(3):567–83.
34. Matheny LM, Johnson NS, Liechti DJ, et al. Activity level and function after lateral ankle ligament repair versus reconstruction. Am J Sports Med 2016; 44(5):1301–8.
35. Kellett JJ. The clinical features of ankle syndesmosis injuries: a general review. Clin J Sport Med 2011;21(6):524–9.
36. McCollum GA, van den Bekerom MP, Kerkhoffs GM, et al. Syndesmosis and deltoid ligament injuries in the athlete. Knee Surg Sports Traumatol Arthrosc 2013; 21(6):1328–37.
37. Gerber JP, Williams GN, Scoville CR, et al. Persistent disability associated with ankle sprains: a prospective examination of an athletic population. Foot Ankle Int 1998;19(10):653–60.
38. Clanton TO, Paul P. Syndesmosis injuries in athletes. Foot and ankle clinics 2002;7(3):529–49.
39. Hunt KJ, George E, Harris AH, et al. Epidemiology of syndesmosis injuries in intercollegiate football: incidence and risk factors from National Collegiate Athletic Association injury surveillance system data from 2004-2005 to 2008-2009. Clin J Sport Med 2013;23(4):278–82.
40. Osbahr DC, Drakos MC, O'Loughlin PF, et al. Syndesmosis and lateral ankle sprains in the National Football League. Orthopedics 2013;36(11):e1378–84.
41. Miller AN, Barei DP, Iaquinto JM, et al. Iatrogenic syndesmosis malreduction via clamp and screw placement. J Orthop Trauma 2013;27(2):100–6.
42. Candal-Couto JJ, Burrow D, Bromage S, et al. Instability of the tibio-fibular syndesmosis: have we been pulling in the wrong direction? Injury 2004;35(8): 814–8.
43. Sagi HC, Shah AR, Sanders RW. The functional consequence of syndesmotic joint malreduction at a minimum 2-year follow-up. J Orthop Trauma 2012; 26(7):439–43.
44. Miller AN, Carroll EA, Parker RJ, et al. Direct visualization for syndesmotic stabilization of ankle fractures. Foot Ankle Int 2009;30(5):419–26.
45. Choy E, Butrynski JE, Harmon DC, et al. Phase II study of olaparib in patients with refractory Ewing sarcoma following failure of standard chemotherapy. BMC Cancer 2014;14:813.
46. Marmor M, Kandemir U, Matityahu A, et al. A method for detection of lateral malleolar malrotation using conventional fluoroscopy. J Orthop Trauma 2013;27(12):e281–4.
47. Cosgrove CT, Putnam SM, Cherney SM, et al. Medial clamp tine positioning affects ankle syndesmosis malreduction. J Orthop Trauma 2017;31(8):440–6.

48. Symeonidis PD, Iselin LD, Chehade M, et al. Common pitfalls in syndesmotic rupture management: a clinical audit. Foot Ankle Int 2013;34(3): 345–50.
49. Lambers KT, van den Bekerom MP, Doornberg JN, et al. Long-term outcome of pronation-external rotation ankle fractures treated with syndesmotic screws only. J Bone Joint Surg Am 2013;95(17):e1221–7.
50. Hoiness P, Stromsoe K. Tricortical versus quadricortical syndesmosis fixation in ankle fractures: a prospective, randomized study comparing two methods of syndesmosis fixation. J Orthop Trauma 2004;18(6):331–7.
51. Beumer A, Campo MM, Niesing R, et al. Screw fixation of the syndesmosis: a cadaver model comparing stainless steel and titanium screws and three and four cortical fixation. Injury 2005;36(1):60–4.
52. Moore JA Jr, Shank JR, Morgan SJ, et al. Syndesmosis fixation: a comparison of three and four cortices of screw fixation without hardware removal. Foot Ankle Int 2006;27(8):567–72.
53. Hamid N, Loeffler BJ, Braddy W, et al. Outcome after fixation of ankle fractures with an injury to the syndesmosis: the effect of the syndesmosis screw. J Bone Joint Surg Br 2009;91(8):1069–73.
54. Schepers T, Van Lieshout EM, de Vries MR, et al. Complications of syndesmotic screw removal. Foot Ankle Int 2011;32(11):1040–4.
55. Inge SY, Pull Ter Gunne AF, Aarts CA, et al. A systematic review on dynamic versus static distal tibiofibular fixation. Injury 2016;47(12):2627–34.
56. Willmott HJ, Singh B, David LA. Outcome and complications of treatment of ankle diastasis with tightrope fixation. Injury 2009;40(11):1204–6.
57. Espinosa N, Smerek JP, Myerson MS. Acute and chronic syndesmosis injuries: pathomechanisms, diagnosis and management. Foot Ankle Clin 2006;11(3): 639–57.
58. de Souza LJ, Gustilo RB, Meyer TJ. Results of operative treatment of displaced external rotation-abduction fractures of the ankle. J Bone Joint Surg Am 1985; 67(7):1066–74.
59. Stiehl JB, Schwartz HS. Long-term results of pronation-external rotation ankle fracture-dislocations treated with anatomical open reduction, internal fixation. J Orthop Trauma 1990;4(3):339–45.
60. Fort NM, Aiyer AA, Kaplan JR, et al. Management of acute injuries of the tibiofibular syndesmosis. Eur J Orthop Surg Traumatol 2017;27(4):449–59.
61. Moravek JE, Kadakia AR. Surgical strategies: doubled allograft reconstruction for chronic syndesmotic injuries. Foot Ankle Int 2010;31(9):834–44.
62. Malhotra G, Cameron J, Toolan BC. Diagnosing chronic diastasis of the syndesmosis: a novel measurement using computed tomography. Foot Ankle Int 2014; 35(5):483–8.
63. Magan A, Golano P, Maffulli N, et al. Evaluation and management of injuries of the tibiofibular syndesmosis. Br Med Bull 2014;111(1):101–15.
64. Parlamas G, Hannon CP, Murawski CD, et al. Treatment of chronic syndesmotic injury: a systematic review and meta-analysis. Knee Surg Sports Traumatol Arthrosc 2013;21(8):1931–9.
65. Wagener ML, Beumer A, Swierstra BA. Chronic instability of the anterior tibiofibular syndesmosis of the ankle. Arthroscopic findings and results of anatomical reconstruction. BMC Musculoskelet Disord 2011;12:212.
66. Han SH, Lee JW, Kim S, et al. Chronic tibiofibular syndesmosis injury: the diagnostic efficiency of magnetic resonance imaging and comparative analysis of operative treatment. Foot Ankle Int 2007;28(3):336–42.

67. Grass R, Rammelt S, Biewener A, et al. Peroneus longus ligamentoplasty for chronic instability of the distal tibiofibular syndesmosis. Foot Ankle Int 2003; 24(5):392–7.

68. Morris MW, Rice P, Schneider TE. Distal tibiofibular syndesmosis reconstruction using a free hamstring autograft. Foot Ankle Int 2009;30(6):506–11.

69. Pena FA, Coetzee JC. Ankle syndesmosis injuries. Foot Ankle Clin 2006;11(1): 35–50, viii.

70. Lewis JS Jr, Anderson RB. Lisfranc injuries in the athlete. Foot Ankle Int 2016; 37(12):1374–80.

71. Deol RS, Roche A, Calder JD. Return to training and playing after acute Lisfranc injuries in elite professional soccer and rugby players. Am J Sports Med 2016; 44(1):166–70.

72. Stavlas P, Roberts CS, Xypnitos FN, et al. The role of reduction and internal fixation of Lisfranc fracture-dislocations: a systematic review of the literature. Int Orthop 2010;34(8):1083–91.

73. Desmond EA, Chou LB. Current concepts review: Lisfranc injuries. Foot Ankle Int 2006;27(8):653–60.

74. Perron AD, Brady WJ, Keats TE. Orthopedic pitfalls in the ED: Lisfranc fracture-dislocation. Am J Emerg Med 2001;19(1):71–5.

75. Raikin SM, Elias I, Dheer S, et al. Prediction of midfoot instability in the subtle Lisfranc injury. Comparison of magnetic resonance imaging with intraoperative findings. J Bone Joint Surg Am 2009;91(4):892–9.

76. Myerson MS, Fisher RT, Burgess AR, et al. Fracture dislocations of the tarsometatarsal joints: end results correlated with pathology and treatment. Foot Ankle 1986;6(5):225–42.

77. Hardcastle PH, Reschauer R, Kutscha-Lissberg E, et al. Injuries to the tarsometatarsal joint. Incidence, classification and treatment. J Bone Joint Surg Br 1982; 64(3):349–56.

78. Welck MJ, Zinchenko R, Rudge B. Lisfranc injuries. Injury 2015;46(4):536–41.

79. Suchak AA, Bostick G, Reid D, et al. The incidence of Achilles tendon ruptures in Edmonton, Canada. Foot Ankle Int 2005;26(11):932–6.

80. Huttunen TT, Kannus P, Rolf C, et al. Acute Achilles tendon ruptures: incidence of injury and surgery in Sweden between 2001 and 2012. Am J Sports Med 2014;42(10):2419–23.

81. Leppilahti J, Orava S. Total Achilles tendon rupture. A review. Sports Med 1998; 25(2):79–100.

82. Kujala UM, Sarna S, Kaprio J. Cumulative incidence of Achilles tendon rupture and tendinopathy in male former elite athletes. Clin J Sport Med 2005;15(3):133–5.

83. Ganestam A, Kallemose T, Troelsen A, et al. Increasing incidence of acute Achilles tendon rupture and a noticeable decline in surgical treatment from 1994 to 2013. A nationwide registry study of 33,160 patients. Knee Surg Sports Traumatol Arthrosc 2016;24(12):3730–7.

84. Mattila VM, Huttunen TT, Haapasalo H, et al. Declining incidence of surgery for Achilles tendon rupture follows publication of major RCTs: evidence-influenced change evident using the Finnish registry study. Br J Sports Med 2015;49(16):1084–6.

85. Olsson N, Silbernagel KG, Eriksson BI, et al. Stable surgical repair with accelerated rehabilitation versus nonsurgical treatment for acute Achilles tendon ruptures: a randomized controlled study. Am J Sports Med 2013;41(12):2867–76.

86. Heikkinen J, Lantto I, Flinkkila T, et al. Augmented compared with nonaugmented surgical repair after total Achilles rupture: results of a prospective

randomized trial with thirteen or more years of follow-up. J Bone Joint Surg Am 2016;98(2):85–92.

87. Lantto I, Heikkinen J, Flinkkila T, et al. Early functional treatment versus cast immobilization in tension after Achilles rupture repair: results of a prospective randomized trial with 10 or more years of follow-up. Am J Sports Med 2015;43(9):2302–9.

88. Ma GW, Griffith TG. Percutaneous repair of acute closed ruptured Achilles tendon: a new technique. Clin Orthop Relat Res 1977;(128):247–55.

89. Krahe MA, Berlet GC. Achilles tendon ruptures, re rupture with revision surgery, tendinosis, and insertional disease. Foot Ankle Clin 2009;14(2):247–75.

90. Bhandari M, Guyatt GH, Siddiqui F, et al. Treatment of acute Achilles tendon ruptures: a systematic overview and metaanalysis. Clin Orthop Relat Res 2002;(400):190–200.

91. Barp EA, Erickson JG. Complications of tendon surgery in the foot and ankle. Clin Podiatr Med Surg 2016;33(1):163–75.

92. Burrus MT, Werner BC, Park JS, et al. Achilles tendon repair in obese patients is associated with increased complication rates. Foot Ankle Spec 2016;9(3):208–14.

93. Humphers J, Shibuya N, Fluhman BL, et al. The impact of glycosylated hemoglobin and diabetes mellitus on postoperative wound healing complications and infection following foot and ankle surgery. J Am Podiatr Med Assoc 2014; 104(4):320–9.

94. Carr AJ, Norris SH. The blood supply of the calcaneal tendon. J Bone Joint Surg Br 1989;71(1):100–1.

95. Khan RJ, Fick D, Keogh A, et al. Treatment of acute Achilles tendon ruptures. A meta-analysis of randomized, controlled trials. J Bone Joint Surg Am 2005; 87(10):2202–10.

96. Bowler PG, Duerden BI, Armstrong DG. Wound microbiology and associated approaches to wound management. Clin Microbiol Rev 2001;14(2):244–69.

97. Pajala A, Kangas J, Ohtonen P, et al. Rerupture and deep infection following treatment of total Achilles tendon rupture. J Bone Joint Surg Am 2002; 84-A(11):2016–21.

98. Wilkins R, Bisson LJ. Operative versus nonoperative management of acute Achilles tendon ruptures: a quantitative systematic review of randomized controlled trials. Am J Sports Med 2012;40(9):2154–60.

99. Mohsenifar Z, Feridoni MJ, Bayat M, et al. Histological and biomechanical analysis of the effects of streptozotocin-induced type one diabetes mellitus on healing of tenotomised Achilles tendons in rats. Foot Ankle Surg 2014;20(3):186–91.

100. Egemen O, Ozkaya O, Ozturk MB, et al. The biomechanical and histological effects of diabetes on tendon healing: experimental study in rats. J Hand Microsurg 2012;4(2):60–4.

101. Dalton GP, Wapner KL, Hecht PJ. Complications of Achilles and posterior tibial tendon surgeries. Clin Orthop Relat Res 2001;(391):133–9.

102. Krackow KA, Thomas SC, Jones LC. A new stitch for ligament-tendon fixation. Brief note. The Journal of bone and joint surgery American 1986;68(5):764–6.

103. Labib SA, Rolf R, Dacus R, et al. The "Giftbox" repair of the Achilles tendon: a modification of the Krackow technique. Foot Ankle Int 2009;30(5):410–4.

104. Palmes D, Spiegel HU, Schneider TO, et al. Achilles tendon healing: long-term biomechanical effects of postoperative mobilization and immobilization in a new mouse model. J Orthop Res 2002;20(5):939–46.

105. Andersson T, Eliasson P, Aspenberg P. Tissue memory in healing tendons: short loading episodes stimulate healing. J Appl Physiol (1985) 2009;107(2):417–21.

106. Pérez Teuffer A. Traumatic rupture of the Achilles tendon. Reconstruction by transplant and graft using the lateral peroneus brevis. Orthop Clin North Am 1974;5(1):89–93.

107. Mann RA, Holmes GB, Seale KS, et al. Chronic rupture of the Achilles tendon: a new technique of repair. J Bone Joint Surg Am 1991;73(2):214–9.

108. Chan JY, Elliott AJ, Ellis SJ. Reconstruction of Achilles rerupture with peroneus longus tendon transfer. Foot Ankle Int 2013;34(6):898–903.

109. Parsons JR, Weiss AB, Schenk RS, et al. Long-term follow-up of Achilles tendon repair with an absorbable polymer carbon fiber composite. Foot Ankle 1989; 9(4):179–84.

110. Nistor L. Surgical and non-surgical treatment of Achilles tendon rupture. A prospective randomized study. J Bone Joint Surg Am 1981;63(3):394–9.

111. Lim J, Dalal R, Waseem M. Percutaneous vs. open repair of the ruptured Achilles tendon–a prospective randomized controlled study. Foot Ankle Int 2001; 22(7):559–68.

112. Cretnik A, Kosanović M, Smrkolj V. Percutaneous suturing of the ruptured Achilles tendon under local anesthesia. J Foot Ankle Surg 2004;43(2):72–81.

113. Lansdaal JR, Goslings JC, Reichart M, et al. The results of 163 Achilles tendon ruptures treated by a minimally invasive surgical technique and functional after-treatment. Injury 2007;38(7):839–44.

114. Molloy A, Wood EV. Complications of the treatment of Achilles tendon ruptures. Foot Ankle Clin 2009;14(4):745–59.

Pediatric Sports Medicine Injuries
Common Problems and Solutions

Joel B. Huleatt, MD[a], Carl W. Nissen, MD[b],
Matthew D. Milewski, MD[c],*

KEYWORDS

- Physeal arrest • Overgrowth • Arthrofibrosis • Medial epicondyle • Nonunion
- Osteochondritis dissecans • Pediatrics • Sports medicine

KEY POINTS

- Anterior cruciate ligament (ACL) tears in the skeletally immature are best treated with early reconstruction, with skeletal age used to help guide technique choices that range from physeal sparing to transphyseal graft placement. Patients should be monitored for growth deformity until skeletal maturity.
- Arthrofibrosis after tibial spine fracture fixation can be reduced by initiating immediate range of motion postoperatively. If arthrofibrosis occurs, treat it early with consideration of lysis of adhesions before a gentle manipulation monitored with fluoroscopy.
- Nonunions of medial epicondyle elbow fractures are to be expected in at least half of patients treated nonoperatively and occur less frequently with surgical fixation, but seldom lead to clinical problems outside of certain athletes. If symptomatic, they can be treated successfully with open surgical techniques.
- Fixation of osteochondritis dissecans lesions with metal screws often requires a secondary surgery for screw removal, whereas the use of bioabsorbable screws can be complicated by breakage that may cause mechanical symptoms and cartilage damage.

INTRODUCTION

The treatment of sports injuries in skeletally immature patients has a unique set of complications, including growth deformity after anterior cruciate ligament (ACL) reconstruction, arthrofibrosis after tibial spine fracture fixation, nonunion of medial epicondyle elbow fractures, and hardware issues with fixation of osteochondritis

Disclosure Statement: M.D. Milewski receives compensation for editorial work for Elsevier, Inc along with research support from Allosource and Vericel. C.W. Nissen receives research support from Allosource and Vericel.
[a] Orthopedics and Sports Medicine, University of Connecticut School of Medicine, 263 Farmington Avenue, Farmington, CT 06030, USA; [b] Elite Sports Medicine, Connecticut Children's Medical Center, 399 Farmington Avenue, Farmington, CT 06032, USA; [c] Division of Sports Medicine, Boston Children's Hospital, 300 Longwood Avenue, Boston, MA 02115, USA
* Corresponding author.
E-mail address: mdmilewski@gmail.com

dissecans (OCD) lesions. These complications can be best avoided, recognized, and managed with an understanding of their incidence, risk factors, clinical relevance, and treatment results.

ANTERIOR CRUCIATE LIGAMENT RECONSTRUCTION IN THE SKELETALLY IMMATURE: GROWTH DEFORMITY

Growth deformity is an important complication to recognize and avoid when surgically addressing ACL deficiency in skeletally immature patients. The true incidence of this problem is difficult to discern, as many of the current surgical techniques have been recently developed or modified and surgeons are becoming more aggressive with surgical treatment of the ACL-insufficient knee in this young population. Additionally, the risk of developing a clinically relevant deformity decreases as patients progress toward skeletal maturity. In a survey by Kocher and colleagues[1] of American surgeon members of the Herodicus Society and ACL Study Group published in 2002, only 11% reported having seen growth deformities. Of these, 80% were on the femoral side and were mostly genu valgum but also included cases of leg shortening and lengthening, whereas 20% were tibial recurvatum due to closing of the tibial tubercle apophysis.[1] An overall rate of 1.8% was reported in a 2010 meta-analysis including 935 ACL reconstructions performed via an assortment of physeal sparing and transphyseal techniques, with a limb length discrepancy greater or equal to 1 cm and axis deviation greater than 3° defined as pathologic.[2] This finding is likely an underestimation of the true incidence because few of the included studies monitored for and reported on leg-length discrepancy or angular deformity. Of the growth disturbances reported, leg-lengthening deformities were twice as common as shortening and genu valgum was twice as common as genu recurvatum and 4 times more common than genu varum.[2] A more significant growth disturbance rate of 10.7% was reported in a French multicenter study of 102 patients treated with varying techniques, measured on long-leg radiographs following physeal closure at the knee. Of the 11 growth deformities, only one patient was symptomatic. This patient developed a femoral valgus that became apparent at 3 months and reached 13° of valgus with 9° of flexion deformity by 18 months. The cause of the growth deformity in this case was attributed to technical error. The 10 asymptomatic cases included 3 femoral valgus, 3 tibial valgus, 2 tibial varus, one leg shortening of 13 mm, and one leg lengthening of 11 mm.[3] In summary, skeletally immature patients undergoing ACL reconstruction are at risk for a variety of growth deformities about the knee that range from subtle and asymptomatic to more problematic abnormalities that require further treatment.

Much of the lower extremity longitudinal growth takes place at the knee, with the distal femoral physis responsible for 70% of femoral growth, averaging 1.2 cm per year, and the proximal tibial physis producing 60% of tibial growth, averaging 0.9 cm per year.[4] Premature arrest of the open physis resulting in either angular deformity or limb shortening is a well-known phenomenon after injuries or fractures involving the physis or placement of hardware across the physis. However, both animal and clinical studies attempting to elucidate the growth disturbances caused by physeal-respecting ACL reconstruction techniques have provided inconsistent results. In rabbit and canine models, growth disturbances have been reported with soft tissue grafts tensioned across the physis.[5–7] However, in another canine model, no growth disturbances were noted with grafts placed across the physis; but growth arrest occurred when similar tunnels were created and left empty.[8] Clinical factors reported to be associated with growth disturbances include the placement of fixation hardware and/or bone plugs across the physis or apophysis (such as using BTB, or bone-tendon-bone patellar tendon as opposed to hamstring autografts), fixation close to the physis as opposed to farther away, large (12 mm) tunnels, extra-articular tenodesis, and suturing or periosteal elevation near the apophysis.[2,9,10] It has been suggested that growth disturbances that occur after physeal-sparing techniques could be due to heat damage from tangential drilling close to an open physis.[2] Fractures or surgery near the physis can also stimulate overgrowth, possibly through a hyperemic response (**Fig. 1**). In the case of ACL reconstructions in the skeletally immature, this overgrowth phenomenon seems to be more common than complete physeal arrest resulting in limb shortening.[2,10,11] Other potential risk factors for growth deformity, such as skeletal age, sex, and associated secondary pathologies, have not been adequately assessed in the current literature.

Altering the treatment of ACL injuries in the skeletally immature has been proposed as a way to avoid or reduce growth disturbance. Although renewed interest in scaffold assisted repair of the ACL has promising early results,[12] suture repair of the ACL has historically failed to demonstrate the success of ACL reconstruction techniques. On the other hand, delaying ACL reconstruction until skeletal maturity increases the risk of further cartilage and meniscal injuries.[13-16] Therefore, physeal-sparing or at least physeal-respecting reconstruction techniques have been developed in an attempt to avoid growth disturbances, which the authors highly recommend. Generally accepted principles are that fixation or bone blocks should not cross the open physis and tunnels or drill holes that cross the physis should be centrally located, as small as possible, and as close to perpendicular to the grow plate as possible.[2,17] Milewski and colleagues[18] suggest an algorithmic approach based on skeletal age with the use of the Michele-Kocher combined extra-articular intra-articular iliotibial band procedure that avoids tunnel drilling at all in patients around 8 years of age; physeal-sparing techniques, such as the Anderson and Ganley-Lawrence all-epiphyseal techniques around 8 to 12 years of age; a hybrid all-epiphyseal femoral transphyseal tibial technique in around 12 years of age; and lastly transphyseal techniques that avoid bone blocks or hardware crossing the physis in 14 years of age or older. Kocher and colleagues[9,19] have reported no angular deformity or leg-length discrepancy and excellent functional outcomes with their physeal-sparing technique in Tanner stage 1 or 2 patients (mean skeletal age of 10.1 years) at a mean of 5.3 years after surgery and with a transphyseal technique in Tanner stage 3 patients (mean skeletal age 14.4) at a mean of 3.6 years after surgery. In apparent contradiction to the widely accepted belief that physeal-sparing techniques should be used in patients with significant growth remaining, the meta-analysis by Frosch and colleagues[2] reported that transphyseal techniques had a statistically significant lower risk of leg-length difference or axis deviation (1.9%) compared with physeal-sparing techniques (5.8%). This discrepancy is perhaps due to the transphyseal technique being used more commonly in older adolescents who have a lower risk of significant growth deformity, and will hopefully be clarified in future studies.

It should also be noted that the potential for growth disturbance is just one of many factors that complicate the treatment of children or adolescents with ACL tears. These patients have an increased risk of ACL graft failure and contralateral ACL tear compared with skeletally mature patients. In a study documenting outcomes and complications at an average of 3.6 years after 27 all epiphyseal ACL reconstructions, Wall and colleagues[10] reported that although no patients had growth arrest or abnormal Lachman examinations, with 81% returning to full activities and sports, one-third reported pain, 15% of grafts failed, and overall there was a 48% rate of complications with 37% requiring secondary procedures. Knee reinjury was found to be more common in patients with concomitant injuries at the time of index ACL reconstruction. Therefore, it is important to anticipate and consider all potential injuries

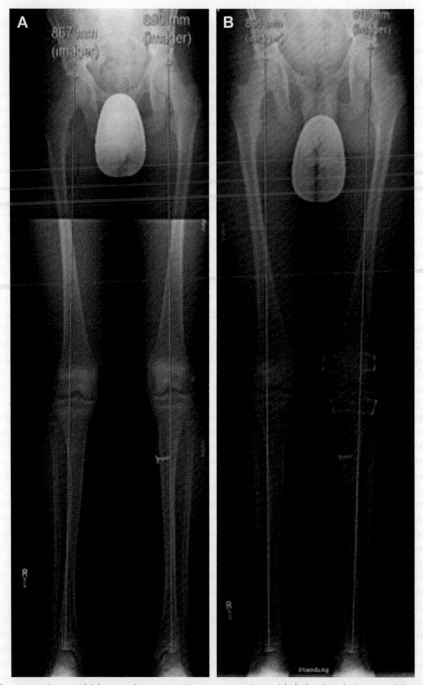

Fig. 1. A 10-year-old boy underwent ACL reconstruction with hybrid technique and lateral meniscal repair. (*A*) Four years later at 14 years of age, still skeletally immature, an overgrowth deformity had caused a 23-mm leg-length discrepancy. (*B*) The patient was treated with epiphysiodesis of both the distal femur and proximal tibia, which resulted in an improved leg-length discrepancy of 20 mm at 7 months postoperatively before moving out of state and transferring care to another pediatric orthopedic surgeon for further care.

and complications to help guide treatment choices and educate patients and families about likely outcomes.

The first step in treating growth disturbances after ACL reconstruction is monitoring for their occurrence. Patients should be followed regularly until skeletal maturity with clinical examinations and full-length lower-extremity radiographs. If growth arrest has occurred with growth potential remaining, any fixation device that crosses the physis should be removed if possible. Hemi-epiphysiodesis may be considered for angular deformities with open growth plates.[10] If there is a significant angular deformity present at skeletal maturity, an osteotomy may be beneficial.[20] In cases of overgrowth, monitoring is often the first step, as it may spontaneously resolve.[10] If overgrowth persists, epiphysiodesis may be performed before skeletal maturity (see **Fig. 1**), or a shoe lift on the contralateral side may be adequate for leg-length discrepancies less than 2 cm.[11]

TIBIAL SPINE FRACTURE FIXATION: ARTHROFIBROSIS

Tibial spine fractures represent an avulsion of the ACL from its insertion on the tibia, most common in 8 to 14 year olds and accounting for up to 5% of knee injuries associated with a knee effusion in the pediatric population.[21] Completely displaced fractures are typically treated with arthroscopically assisted or open reduction and fixation to reduce the rate of nonunion and increased laxity. The incidence of arthrofibrosis after surgical reduction and internal fixation of displaced tibial spine fractures varies considerably in the literature. However, it is recognized as one of the most common complications after tibial spine fracture fixation and is difficult to successfully treat. In the largest published case series consisting of 205 patients treated arthroscopically with sutures or transepiphyseal screws by Vander Have and colleagues,[22] 10% developed arthrofibrosis that was defined as lacking 10° of extension and/or less than 90° of flexion at 3 months after surgery. The authors noted that, in particular, lack of extension was poorly tolerated, with noticeable limps associated with a loss of even 5°. Most of the stiff patients were lacking both flexion and extension and required surgical intervention to satisfactorily improve their range of motion. In a recent meta-analysis by Gans and colleagues,[21] arthrofibrosis that was defined as a 10° extension deficit and/or 25° flexion loss at 3 months after treatment that persisted despite physical therapy and was not caused by nonunion, malunion, a new injury, a ligamentous or meniscal injury, or a bony deformity occurred in 7.1% of type I and II fractures and 14.2% of type III and IV fractures.

The risk of developing arthrofibrosis after treatment of tibial spine fractures is influenced by the displacement of the fracture, associated injuries, surgical technique, and rehabilitation.[21–23] With increasing fracture displacement and classification, the risk of developing both flexion and extension deficits increases.[21] And in similarity to ACL tears, the risk of postoperative stiffness increases with the magnitude of soft tissue and bony injury to the knee.[22] The literature is inconclusive as to whether arthroscopic versus open fixation and use of suture versus screw fixation leads to a greater risk of arthrofibrosis, but many investigators comment on the importance of reducing and fixing the fracture in a stable enough fashion to withstand early range of motion.[21,22] It is important to consider the possibility of an entrapped structure acting as a block to reduction and/or motion. In a study by Kocher and colleagues,[24] 26% of type 2 fractures and 65% of type 3 fractures were found to have an entrapped anterior horn of the medial meniscus (most common), intermeniscal ligament, or anterior horn of the lateral meniscus at the time of surgery and a 4% rate of meniscal tear. Although preoperative MRI imaging is not always needed, it is highly suggested if displaced fractures are treated through an open arthrotomy without arthroscopy, as it may be more difficult to identify such meniscal pathologies.

The goal of early mobilization is well supported in the literature. Patel and colleagues[25] reported that knee range of motion initiated within 4 weeks of surgical fixation resulted in a 12-fold reduction in the rate of arthrofibrosis. Several case series have reported lower rates of arthrofibrosis with arthroscopic treatment and knee motion started either immediately or within 2 weeks, as compared with the 10% rate of arthrofibrosis in the study by Vander Have and colleagues,[22] in which most patients were immobilized in a long leg cast or knee brace locked in full extension for the first 4 to 6 weeks after surgery.[22,23,26,27] With earlier motion protocols, it is especially important to follow tibial spine fracture healing closely with radiographs to assess for loss of reduction and fixation.

If arthrofibrosis develops after tibial spine fracture fixation and fails to respond appropriately to emphasized mobilization protocols and physical therapy, the treatment of choice is to perform arthroscopic lysis of adhesions and manipulation under anesthesia around 12 weeks after fracture fixation. In the study by Vander Have and colleagues,[22] 24 patients underwent arthroscopic lysis of adhesions, with adhesions noted in all knees, and manipulation under anesthesia, followed by immediate mobilization and physical therapy. In the 8 patients treated with manipulation under anesthesia without lysis of adhesions 18 to 24 weeks after tibial spine fixation, 3 sustained iatrogenic distal femoral physeal fractures, 2 of which developed growth arrest and angular deformity requiring further surgery and never regained full extension.[22] To lessen the risk of fracture with manipulation (**Fig. 2**), the authors recommend returning to the operating room early if arthrofibrosis develops, performing an arthroscopic lysis of adhesion before a gentle manipulation, and using fluoroscopy during the manipulation to potentially diagnosis any iatrogenic fracture as early as possible.

NONUNION OF MEDIAL EPICONDYLE FRACTURE

Medial epicondyle fractures of the elbow make up approximately 12% of elbow injuries in the pediatric population and may occur in the setting of elbow dislocation.[28] When treated nonoperatively, the incidence of nonunion was 69% in fracture

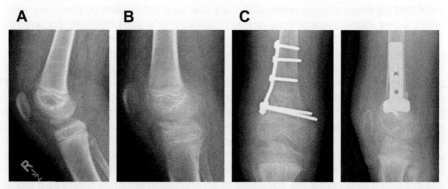

Fig. 2. (*A*) Right knee lateral radiograph of a 9-year-old boy who sustained a tibial spine fracture that remained displaced after attempted closed reduction. (*B*) Lateral radiograph after the patient underwent arthroscopic reduction and internal fixation with transosseous sutures. (*C*) At 2 months after fixation, the patient had developed arthrofibrosis with knee range of motion limited to 15° to 70°. The patient was taken to the operating room for a manipulation under anesthesia, where flexion of 90° was obtained. However, on attempting to gain better extension, an iatrogenic fracture of the distal femur occurred, which was treated with open reduction and internal fixation.

dislocations and 49% in isolated fractures according to a recent systematic review including 81 pediatric patients by Knapik and colleagues.[28] Although decreased elbow motion was reported in 43% and 15% of these patients, respectively, overall the investigaotrs reported minimal clinical or functional disabilities in the patients at the final follow-up, whether or not they had a bony union. In a systematic review by Kamath and colleagues,[29] the nonunion rate in 122 nonoperatively treated patients was 51%, compared with 8% in 281 operatively treated patients.[29] Although not statistically significant, there was a trend toward increased pain and ulnar symptoms in the operatively treated patients, with other outcomes difficult to compare. When comparing the rates of union and other outcomes in medial epicondyle fracture studies, it should be noted that there is a lack of randomized trials, and so the present literature is subject to considerable selection bias.

The displacement criteria used to determine conservative versus operative management has not been standardized. Although many surgeons base treatment recommendations on initial fracture displacement, with a common threshold of greater than 5 mm used to recommend operative treatment in throwing athletes and athletes involved in upper-extremity weight-bearing sports, such as gymnastics and wrestling, the measurement of displacement on radiographs is inaccurate; therefore, its effect on nonunion and outcomes is not clear.[28–30] Other factors, such as the mechanism or extent of injury to the elbow, time to surgery, fixation method, rehabilitation protocol, and stress placed on the elbow following surgery, may have some influence on the risk of nonunion; but this has yet to be verified.

Most nonunions of medial epicondyle fractures are asymptomatic and will require no further treatment, as the fibrous union is sufficient for most activities. Occasionally, however, nonunions will be painful and/or contribute to the feeling of instability, especially with provocative activities, such as throwing, gymnastics, and weightlifting.[31] Regardless of the initial fracture management, symptomatic nonunions can be treated effectively with open reduction and internal fixation. Smith and colleagues[31] reported improved pain and good outcomes at a minimum follow-up of 1 year for 8 nonunions that were revised on average 1 year after the initial injury and fixation. The revision technique included screw fixation with varying use of suture augmentation, demineralized bone matrix or bone graft, ulnar nerve transposition if nerve instability or impingement was present, and capsular release if joint contracture was an issue.[31] Although fracture fragment excision at the time of the initial injury and suture fixation of the avulsed flexor tendons and medial collateral ligament to the adjacent periosteum has produced poor results and is inadvisable,[32] Gilchrist and colleagues[33] reported successful results with excision of nonunion fragments and medial collateral ligament repair at an average of 10 years after the initial injury. The authors recommend treating symptomatic nonunions with open reduction and internal fixation with as large a screw as feasible, with additional use of a washer, augmenting sutures, and an iliac crest bone graft as needed (**Fig. 3**).

OSTEOCHONDRITIS DISSECANS FIXATION: HARDWARE COMPLICATIONS

Internal fixation of OCD lesions of the knee is indicated for unstable lesions and is often supplemented with transarticular or retro-articular drilling and possible bone grafting.[34] When internal fixation is used to treat unstable or at-risk OCD lesions, it is important to recognize that the common fixation techniques have distinct complication profiles. Using headless, variable-pitch metal compression screws is one common option. The proposed advantages are rigid, compressive fixation that should optimize bony union while minimizing the area of cartilage damage at the insertion site.[34,35] It is often recommended to remove these screws after healing has occurred to reduce the risk of eventual

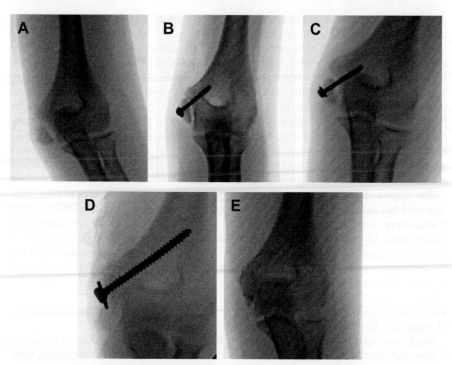

Fig. 3. (*A*) Anteroposterior radiograph of a 12-year-old girl who presented 6 months after a left elbow medial epicondyle fracture, which had failed to unite with nonoperative treatment by an outside physician. The patient had continued pain and difficulty returning to sports. (*B*) The symptomatic nonunion was treated with open reduction and internal fixation using a screw and washer. (*C*) Four months later, the fragment had redisplaced and the patient had discomfort over the medial epicondyle and ulnar nerve. (*D*) The patient underwent revision open reduction and internal fixation with iliac crest bone grafting and anterior subcutaneous nerve transposition. (*E*) At 15 months, the patient had healed the nonunion but complained of prominent hardware, which was removed.

backing out of the screws or gradual cartilage wear that may lead to prominent screws and rapid cartilage damage. In a study of 15 knees that included both skeletally immature and mature patients, Makino and colleagues[35] reported a 93% rate of healing with secondary surgery performed in all patients on average 101 days later. With increasing age and skeletal maturity, the success rate of operative treatment declines. Barrett and colleagues[36] reported an 18% OCD nonunion rate in skeletally mature individuals with unstable lesions treated with headless metal compression screws. In their series of 22 patients, 4 knees required loose fragment excision and hardware removal; 2 patients required screw advancement for the screws backing out past the subchondral bone; and 15 patients had planned screw removal performed at 6 months, with only one patient not undergoing a secondary surgery. Although it is possible that many patients would do well without hardware removal, the authors recommend that metal screws are removed after healing of the lesion because of the rapid cartilage damage that can occur if a screw becomes prominent.

Using bioabsorbable screw fixation is another common option that obviates a planned secondary surgery for screw removal. However, multiple studies have reported on higher rates of screw breakage as well as cases of synovitis possibly due to a foreign body immune reaction.[34,37–39] Camathias and colleagues[38] report a

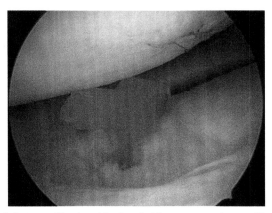

Fig. 4. Arthroscopic image of broken bioabsorbable screw causing cartilage damage within the knee joint 14 months after fixation of an OCD lesion. The patient had radiographic healing at 6 months but after a year developed pain, swelling, and mechanical symptoms. (*From* Camathias C, Gögüs U, Hirschmann MT, et al. Implant failure after biodegradable screw fixation in osteochondritis dissecans of the knee in skeletally immature patients. Arthroscopy 2015;31(3):413; with permission.)

23% rate of absorbable poly-ʟ-lactic acid screw breakage in a series of 30 knees treated with 61 screws. The investigators proposed that there was a quicker decomposition of the part of the screw within bone than of the part within the cartilage, which was evident on MRI scans performed at 6-month intervals, and could lead to dislodged screw heads (**Fig. 4**).[38] Webb and colleagues[37] reported a higher rate of failure with bioabsorbable implants compared with metal screw fixation in a study of 20 juvenile knees. On the other hand, investigators such as Tuompo and colleagues[39] reported reliable fixation and good long-term results without routine implant removal and no noted implant breakage with the use of self-reinforced polylactide (PLLA) rods. As bioabsorbable materials continue to evolve, the issue of implant breakage and inflammatory reaction may be improved; but at present, both surgeons and patients should be aware of these potential risks when electing this option.

SUMMARY

ACL tears in the skeletally immature should be treated with early reconstruction because of the increased risk of further meniscal and cartilage damage with delayed or nonoperative treatment. However, this carries a risk of inducing growth deformities, including overgrowth, growth arrest, and angular deformity. An algorithm based on skeletal age can help guide technique choices that range from physeal avoiding to physeal sparing to transphyseal tunnel and graft placement. Patients should be monitored for growth deformity until skeletal maturity. Tibial spine fracture fixation is often complicated by the development of arthrofibrosis; therefore, it is recommended to start range of motion immediately. If arthrofibrosis occurs, the authors recommend treating it early with consideration of performing a lysis of adhesions before a gentle manipulation with fluoroscopy because of the risk of an iatrogenic fracture. Nonunions of medial epicondyle elbow fractures are to be expected in at least half of patients treated nonoperatively and occur at a lower rate with surgical fixation, but seldom lead to clinical problems outside of certain athletes. In both nonoperative and operative cases, if a symptomatic nonunion occurs, it can be treated successfully with an open surgical technique using a large screw, washer, suture augmentation, and bone grafting as needed. Fixation of OCD lesions with metal screws often requires a secondary surgery for screw removal, whereas the use of bioabsorbable screws introduces the possibility of broken screws that may cause mechanical symptoms and cartilage damage.

REFERENCES

1. Kocher MS, Saxon HS, Hovis WD, et al. Management and complications of anterior cruciate ligament injuries in skeletally immature patients: survey of the Herodicus Society and the ACL Study Group. J Pediatr Orthop 2002;22(4):452–7.
2. Frosch KH, Stengel D, Brodhun T, et al. Outcomes and risks of operative treatment of rupture of the anterior cruciate ligament in children and adolescents. Arthroscopy 2010;26(11):1539–50.
3. Bonnard C, Chotel F. Knee ligament and meniscal injury in children and adolescents. Rev Chir Orthop Reparatrice Appar Mot 2007;93(6 SUPPL. 1):95–139. Available at: https://www.scopus.com/inward/record.uri?eid=2-s2.0-37149011459&partner ID=40&md5=3c3ab54acf3a323e958ab4d238e5c03b.
4. Larsen MW, Garrett WE, Delee JC, et al. Surgical management of anterior cruciate ligament injuries in patients with open physes. J Am Acad Orthop Surg 2006; 14(13):736–44.
5. Guzzanti V, Falciglia F, Gigante A, et al. The effect of intra-articular ACL reconstruction on the growth plates of rabbits. J Bone Joint Surg Br 1994;76(6):960–3. Available at: http://www.ncbi.nlm.nih.gov/pubmed/7983128. Accessed December 11, 2012.
6. Edwards TB, Greene CC, Baratta RV, et al. The effect of placing a tensioned graft across open growth plates. A gross and histologic analysis. J Bone Joint Surg Am 2001;83-A(5):725–34. Available at: http://www.ncbi.nlm.nih.gov/pubmed/11379743. Accessed December 11, 2012.
7. Houle JB, Letts M, Yang J. Effects of a tensioned tendon graft in a bone tunnel across the rabbit physis. Clin Orthop Relat Res 2001;(391):275–81. Available at: http://www.ncbi.nlm.nih.gov/pubmed/11603681.
8. Stadelmaier DM, Arnoczky SP, Dodds J, et al. The effect of drilling and soft tissue grafting across open growth plates. A histologic study. Am J Sports Med 1995; 23(4):431–5. Available at: http://www.ncbi.nlm.nih.gov/pubmed/7573652.
9. Kocher MS, Smith JT, Zoric BJ, et al. Transphyseal anterior cruciate ligament reconstruction in skeletally immature pubescent adolescents. J Bone Joint Surg Am 2007;89(12):2632–9.
10. Wall EJ, Ghattas PJ, Eismann EA, et al. Outcomes and complications after all-epiphyseal anterior cruciate ligament reconstruction in skeletally immature patients. Orthop J Sports Med 2017;5(3). 2325967117693604.
11. Zimmerman LJ, Jauregui JJ, Riis JF, et al. Symmetric limb overgrowth following anterior cruciate ligament reconstruction in a skeletally immature patient. J Pediatr Orthop B 2015;24(6):530–4.
12. Murray MM, Flutie BM, Kalish LA, et al. The bridge-enhanced anterior cruciate ligament repair (BEAR) procedure: an early feasibility cohort study. Orthop J Sports Med 2016;4(11):2325967116672176.
13. Lawrence JT, Argawal N, Ganley TJ. Degeneration of the knee joint in skeletally immature patients with a diagnosis of an anterior cruciate ligament tear: is there harm in delay of treatment? Am J Sports Med 2011;39(12):2582–7.
14. Millett PJ, Willis AA, Warren RF. Associated injuries in pediatric and adolescent anterior cruciate ligament tears: does a delay in treatment increase the risk of meniscal tear? Arthroscopy 2002;18(9):955–9.

15. Henry J, Chotel F, Chouteau J, et al. Rupture of the anterior cruciate ligament in children: early reconstruction with open physes or delayed reconstruction to skeletal maturity? Knee Surg Sports Traumatol Arthrosc 2009;17(7):748–55.

16. Engebretsen L, Svenningsen S, Benum P. Poor results of anterior cruciate ligament repair in adolescence. Acta Orthop Scand 1988;59(6):684–6.

17. Lawrence JTR, Bowers AL, Belding J, et al. All-epiphyseal anterior cruciate ligament reconstruction in skeletally immature patients. Clin Orthop Relat Res 2010; 468(7):1971–7.

18. Milewski MD, Beck NA, Lawrence JT, et al. Anterior cruciate ligament reconstruction in the young athlete: a treatment algorithm for the skeletally immature. Clin Sports Med 2011;30(4):801–10.

19. Kocher MS, Garg S, Micheli LJ. Physeal sparing reconstruction of the anterior cruciate ligament in skeletally immature prepubescent children and adolescents. J Bone Joint Surg Am 2005;87(11):2371–9.

20. Robert HE, Casin C. Valgus and flexion deformity after reconstruction of the anterior cruciate ligament in a skeletally immature patient. Knee Surg Sports Traumatol Arthrosc 2010;18(10):1369–73.

21. Gans I, Baldwin KD, Ganley TJ. Treatment and management outcomes of tibial eminence fractures in pediatric patients: a systematic review. Am J Sports Med 2013;42:1743–50.

22. Vander Have KL, Ganley TJ, Kocher MS, et al. Arthrofibrosis after surgical fixation of tibial eminence fractures in children and adolescents. Am J Sports Med 2010; 38(2):298–301.

23. Hunter RE, Willis JA. Arthroscopic fixation of avulsion fractures of the tibial eminence: technique and outcome. Arthroscopy 2004;20(2):113–21.

24. Kocher MS, Micheli LJ, Gerbino P, et al. Tibial eminence fractures in children: prevalence of meniscal entrapment. Am J Sports Med 2003;31(3):404–7.

25. Patel NM, Park MJ, Sampson NR, et al. Tibial eminence fractures in children. J Pediatr Orthop 2012;32(2):139–44.

26. Mah JY, Adili A, Otsuka NY, et al. Follow-up study of arthroscopic reduction and fixation of type III tibial-eminence fractures. J Pediatr Orthop 1998;18(4):475–7.

27. Senekovič V, Veselko M. Anterograde arthroscopic fixation of avulsion fractures of the tibial eminence with a cannulated screw: five-year results. Arthroscopy 2003; 19(1):54–61.

28. Knapik DM, Fausett CL, Gilmore A, et al. Outcomes of nonoperative pediatric medial humeral epicondyle fractures with and without associated elbow dislocation. J Pediatr Orthop 2016;37(4):1.

29. Kamath AF, Baldwin K, Horneff J, et al. Operative versus non-operative management of pediatric medial epicondyle fractures: a systematic review. J Child Orthop 2009;3(5):345–57.

30. Lee H-H, Shen H-C, Chang J-H, et al. Operative treatment of displaced medial epicondyle fractures in children and adolescents. J Shoulder Elbow Surg 2005; 14(2):178–85.

31. Smith JT, McFeely ED, Bae DS, et al. Operative fixation of medial humeral epicondyle fracture nonunion in children. J Pediatr Orthop 2010;30(7):644–8.

32. Farsetti P, Potenza V, Caterini R, et al. Long-term results of treatment of fractures of the medial humeral epicondyle in children. J Bone Joint Surg Am 2001;83(9): 1299–305.

33. Gilchrist AD, McKee MD. Valgus instability of the elbow due to medial epicondyle nonunion: treatment by fragment excision and ligament repair-a report of 5 cases. J Shoulder Elbow Surg 2002;11(5):493–7.

34. Grimm NL, Ewing CK, Ganley TJ. The knee: internal fixation techniques for osteo-chondritis dissecans. Clin Sports Med 2014;33(2):313–9.
35. Makino A, Muscolo DL, Puigdevall M, et al. Arthroscopic fixation of osteochondri-tis dissecans of the knee: clinical, magnetic resonance imaging, and arthro-scopic follow-up. Am J Sports Med 2005;33(10):1499–504.
36. Barrett I, King AH, Riester S, et al. Internal fixation of unstable osteochondritis dis-secans in the skeletally mature knee with metal screws. Cartilage 2016. https://doi.org/10.1177/1947603515622662.
37. Webb JE, Lewallen LW, Christophersen C, et al. Clinical outcome of internal fixa-tion of unstable juvenile osteochondritis dissecans lesions of the knee. Orthope-dics 2013;36(11):e1444–9.
38. Camathias C, Gögüs U, Hirschmann MT, et al. Implant failure after biodegradable screw fixation in osteochondritis dissecans of the knee in skeletally immature patients. Arthroscopy 2015;31(3):410–5.
39. Tuompo P, Landtman M, Sandelin J, et al. Operative treatment of osteochondritis dissecans of the knee: a retrospective comparison of fixation with autologous bone pegs vs. bioabsorbable rods. Knee 2000;7(1):31–8.

Rehabilitation
Common Problems and Solutions

Kevin E. Wilk, PT, DPT, FAPTA[a,b], Christopher A. Arrigo, MS, PT, ATC[c,d,*]

KEYWORDS

• Prevention • Physical therapy • Surgery • Musculoskeletal • Sports medicine

KEY POINTS

- There are numerous complications that can occur following a musculoskeletal injury or surgery in the sporting population.
- Many of these complications include stiffness, pain, and/or movement dysfunction.
- Prevention of the most frequent complications is the key in any successful rehabilitation program, but occasionally problems do occur.
- A thorough well-designed postoperative or postinjury rehabilitation program may prevent most of these problems.
- However, if complications do arise, a team approach among all of the parties involved in the process (physician, physical therapist, athletic trainer, strength and conditioning specialist, coach, and athlete) working to develop an evidenced-based treatment program designed specifically for the underlying complication can successfully treat these issues.

Rehabilitation plays a significant role in the successful results and positive outcomes following any orthopedic and sports medicine injury or surgical procedure. Complications following even what are generally regarded as the most successfully managed conditions are common and far more prevalent than desired. For example, following anterior cruciate ligament (ACL) surgery it has been reported that 7% to 15% of patients will exhibit a loss of normal motion.[1,2] The authors of this article think the incidence of motion loss in these instances is much higher when range of motion (ROM) is carefully and accurately measured. The same complication is evident following rotator cuff (RTC) repair surgery. Koo and colleagues[3] have reported that 5% to 16% of patients will exhibit a loss of motion

[a] Champion Sports Medicine, A Select Medical Facility, 805 Street Vincents Drive, STE G-100, Birmingham, AL 35205, USA; [b] Rehabilitation Research, American Sports Medicine Institute, 833 Street Vincents Drive, STE 205, Birmingham, AL 35205, USA; [c] Advanced Rehabilitation, 4539 South Dale Mabry, Suite 100, Tampa, FL 33611, USA; [d] MedStar Sports Medicine, MedStar Orthopaedics and Sports Medicine at Lafayette Centre, 1120 20th Street, NW, Building 1 South, Washington, DC 20036, USA
* Corresponding author. 4539 South Dale Mabry, Suite 100, Tampa, FL 33611.
E-mail address: carrigo@advancedrehab.us

Clin Sports Med 37 (2018) 363–374
https://doi.org/10.1016/j.csm.2017.12.010
0278-5919/18/© 2017 Elsevier Inc. All rights reserved.

sportsmed.theclinics.com

or shoulder stiffness following RTC repair. Likewise, other surgeries may also exhibit similar incidences of motion loss. Motion loss is not the only common postoperative complication. Reinjury following ACL reconstruction occurs in up to 25% of patients.[4–6] Surgical failure after RTC repair is evident in 29% to 94% of patients.[7,8] Shoulder instability following shoulder stabilization surgery has been shown to be present in approximately 15% of all patients. The purpose of this article is to discuss rehabilitation strategies specifically designed to avoid and successfully treat postoperative and postinjury complications that frequently occur in sports medicine.

There are several rehabilitation principles and strategies effective in minimizing complications. These principles should be routinely used to successfully reduce and prevent the incidence of postoperative or postinjury complications. The essential key to treating complications is not allowing them to occur at all. The first strategy is to use early motion and mobility in the rehabilitation process. Early motion has been shown to reduce postoperative stiffness and motion loss at the knee joint.[9] The second principle is beginning rehabilitation immediately following injury or surgery. This practice ensures patients are doing the proper exercises and receiving accurate education regarding their condition and the activities that they both must perform and avoid. Next, it is important for the rehabilitation team to establish proper milestones and goals, ensuring patients are not falling behind, becoming stiff, or in some cases moving too fast. A team approach to treatment and rehabilitation is the critical key, with the orthopedic surgeon, physical therapist, athletic trainer, and strength and conditioning specialist all being included in treatment planning. Communication among these team members is vital and invaluable to ensure everyone remains on the same page throughout the process. Lastly, developing a proper treatment plan (protocol) is vital to a successful outcome. This plan serves as the treatment guideline for patients so that all members of the team are aware of what is or should be happening and when it is expected to occur. The authors now discuss several areas of the body, their specific types of complications, and treatment.

KNEE JOINT

The knee joint is frequently injured. Common injuries include patellofemoral pain, medial collateral ligament injuries, ACL injuries, and meniscus lesions. The ACL is one of the most frequently reconstructed ligaments in the orthopedic and sports medicine population. Wilk[10] reported that approximately 148,000 ACL reconstructions are performed annually. The most common complication following ACL reconstruction is a loss of motion or stiffness.[1,9] There are several strategies to prevent postoperative knee stiffness and motion loss following ACL reconstruction, including (1) delaying surgery until the knee has returned to homeostasis, (2) immediate motion following ACL surgery, (3) proper rehabilitation, and (4) patient compliance.

As mentioned, loss of knee motion and stiffness occurs in approximately 7% to 15% of all ACL reconstructions.[1] For the most part, this postoperative complication is preventable. Delaying surgery until the knee joint calms down and returns to a normal state assists in minimizing the development of arthrofibrosis and motion loss.[1] Shelbourne and colleagues,[1] in a classic article, reported that by delaying surgery until after the knee joint calms down following ACL injury the development of arthrofibrosis was reduced from 17% in the immediate surgery group to 0% in the delayed surgery group. In the authors' opinion, returning the knee to a normal homeostatic state means

(1) reducing swelling to minimal levels, (2) restoring full passive knee extension, (3) reestablishing quadriceps activation, (4) obtaining sufficient knee flexion (usually 130° or more), and (5) reestablishing a functional level of neuromuscular control of the lower extremity. In addition, the authors think the knee joint should be protected from the risk of additional damage and further injury. To facilitate this, the authors recommend placing patients in a drop-locked knee brace in full extension for ambulation and weight-bearing functional activities until adequate quadriceps tone and neuromuscular control of the knee joint are present and ambulation is nonantalgic. This practice prevents giving-way episodes and reduces further damage to the menisci. Failla and colleagues[11] reported that delaying surgery longer to participate in a complete prehabilitation program improved functional knee scores by 12% to 15% when compared with a group that participated in a shorter prehabilitation program.

Additional strategies to reduce knee stiffness include the initiation of immediate knee joint motion following ACL reconstruction. Several investigators, and leaders in knee surgery, advocate immediate knee joint motion following ACL reconstruction.[12–15] Immediate motion should be included in proper rehabilitation of the postoperative knee joint, regardless of the procedure. Immediately following ACL surgery, the physical therapist may initiate passive movement through an arc of motion tolerated by patients, based on their swelling and pain. The authors recommend full passive knee extension immediately following ACL surgery to prevent the development of scar tissue in the front of the knee joint. Knee flexion should be gradually increased during the initial 8 to 12 weeks following surgery progressing sequentially to the restoration of full knee flexion. The milestones the authors recommend facilitating the restoration of knee flexion include 90° by the end of week 1; 105° by the end of week 2; 125°/130° by the end of week 4; 135° to 140° by week 6 to 8; and heel to gluteal muscle knee flexion by the end of week 12. Restoring knee flexion reduces the incidence of anterior knee pain following knee surgery. Patient compliance in the regular performance of an independent persistent motion program is critical to preventing knee stiffness following ACL surgery.

Immediately following ACL surgery and during the first 7 postoperative days, the goals of a successful complication prevention program include the following:

1. Reduction of swelling and pain via the use of ice, compression, laser therapy, elevation, and gentle motion
2. Restoration of full knee extension using an extension overpressure program in combination with patellar and tibiofemoral mobilization
3. Restoration of knee flexion through a gradual program of passive knee flexion exercises
4. Restoration of quadriceps activation using electrical muscle stimulation (EMS) to the quadriceps muscle group during exercise
5. Improved neuromuscular control of the lower kinetic chain via balance drills
6. Restoration of a moderate level of functional activity by the use of gait training, ambulation, and balance drills

If a complication occurs, the treatment of an individual who has developed knee stiffness must follow a rigid treatment regimen performed several times per day at home, in conjunction with clinical physical therapy. This program includes the following:

1. Heating with overpressure into extension for 10 to 15 minutes
2. Patellar mobilizations (superior/inferior and medial/lateral directions)
3. EMS applied to quads during quadriceps setting and straight leg raise flexion

4. Hamstring and gastrocnemius stretching
5. Light knee flexion ROM exercises (passive ROM [PROM], bicycle, and so forth)
6. Retrograde walking over cups or cones
7. Overpressure into extension (10–15 minutes in duration)
8. Repeated overpressure program at home for at least a total of 60 minutes per day

The overpressure program is designed to provide a low-load, long-duration (LLLD)–type stretch to the soft tissues around the knee, in particular the posterior joint capsule. McClure and colleagues[16] have reported that LLLD programs were the best to elongate soft tissue around joints. This finding has been advocated by several other investigators.[17,18] The authors recommend performing the LLLD stretches into extension in the supine position with the use of a cuff weight (Fig. 1) or an external device (Figs. 2 and 3) to facilitate the desired LLLD result.

Another complication following ACL reconstruction surgery is ACL graft failure. This complication occurs in 0% to 25% of patients. Patients who are most commonly susceptible to graft failure and reinjury are the 16- to 19-year-old girls or boys involved in level 1 sports that have returned to play early (before 9 months following surgery). Grindem and colleagues[19] have reported that delaying the return to play until 9 months or later can significantly reduce the reinjury rate in the ACL reconstructed knee. Athletes who pass a battery of return-to-play testing examinations with specific criteria before returning to activity exhibit reinjury rate reductions of 84%.[19] In addition, patients who have returned to sport early (before 6 months following reconstruction) exhibit a higher rate of contralateral ACL injury.[20] Paterno and colleagues[21,22] have stated that patients with an ACL reconstructed knee are more susceptible for a second ACL injury to the contralateral knee than they are for a second injury to the ipsilateral knee. The strategies the authors recommend to incorporate to successfully decrease the risk of a second ACL injury in young athletic individuals include an emphasis on neuromuscular and perturbation training in both lower extremities, the establishment of strict criteria that must be fulfilled before any return to sports, the inclusion of rehabilitation exercises for both extremities, and delaying the return to play until patients are functionally ready with a concerted effort to de-emphasize an early return to play.

Another complication frequently seen at the knee joint is patellar tendinopathy. This complication may develop as a primary disorder or secondarily to knee surgery, such as ACL reconstruction with a patellar tendon graft. In the case of chronic patellar

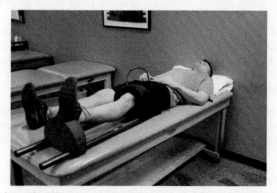

Fig. 1. Low-load, long-duration overpressure using a weight to restore knee extension.

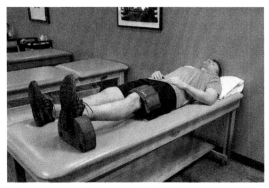

Fig. 2. Low-load, long-duration overpressure device to restore knee extension.

tendinopathies, the authors have found the most successful approach is to emphasize eccentric muscle training, flexibility exercises, modalities and techniques to increase blood flow to the involved area, along with the correction of any biomechanical factors present. The program the authors have found most successful begins with moist heat applied to knee joint followed by soft tissue techniques to both the patellar tendon and retinaculum and static stretching of the quadriceps, hip, and calf musculature followed by an active warm-up on the bicycle. After the active warm-up, an eccentric training program is incorporated. The exercises the authors emphasize are a leg press, wall slides, step downs, and knee extensions performed with an emphasize on contractions. Langberg and colleagues[23] have shown that heavy slow resistance is successful in treating chronic tendinopathies. In addition, hip strengthening is performed, especially for the hip external rotators, abductors, and extensors. Balance training is also incorporated, followed by more stretching with the focus on the quadriceps and gastrocnemius/soleus muscles. Witvrouw and colleagues[24] have reported that quadriceps tightness is also a substantial risk factor for developing patellar tendinitis and should be aggressively addressed with appropriate stretching interventions. The treatment program is completed with class 4 laser therapy and home exercise instructions. If patellofemoral or tendon pain is too intense during the performance of eccentric exercises, the authors use pain stimulation to neuromodulate the patients' pain complaints. Pain stimulation is EMS applied to inert tissue on both sides of the patellar tendon (on the fat pad). The goal of EMS is to create a noxious stimulation to the

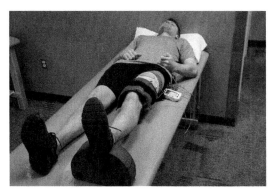

Fig. 3. Low-load, long-duration overpressure device to restore knee extension.

structure, and patients will then release endorphins to neuromodulate their pain. The EMS parameters are important, as this determines the sensation felt by patients. The authors use EMS with the following parameters: a frequency of 2500 Hz, 50 pulses per second, a duty cycle of 10 seconds on/10 seconds off, and an intensity to tolerance but noxious and slightly painful.

The last complication at the knee joint the authors discuss is patellofemoral pain and dysfunction. The authors' approach for this lesion begins with a careful assessment and determination of what type of disorder patients are exhibiting. Wilk and colleagues[25] have classified patellofemoral disorders into 8 categories. Based on the type of disorder present, the appropriate condition-specific treatment program would be initiated. The patellofemoral disorder most frequently encountered by the authors is that of a lower extremity biomechanical disorder. This condition is usually due to excessive femoral anteversion and an increase tibial torsion leading to a high Q angle. The excessive, uncontrolled dynamic Q angle (seen during walking, step downs, or running), not a non–weight-bearing measurement, is the primary concern because it indicates poor dynamic hip control in functional positions. The authors' focus is to control the increased dynamic Q angle via activation and retraining the hip abductors, external rotators, and extensors. In addition, hip flexibility exercises, stretching the gastrocnemius/soleus muscle complex, and proprioception drills are also emphasized. Powers and colleagues[26,27] have reported that a program focused on hip strengthening and retraining reduced patellofemoral pain in patients. The authors have found this type of program to be clinically useful and effective.

SHOULDER JOINT COMPLEX

The complications most commonly seen at the shoulder joint complex can occur secondary to surgery, following an injury, or even be completely insidious in onset. Postoperative complications, such as glenohumeral joint stiffness, can occur following RTC repair surgery. This complication occurs in approximately 5% to 16% of patients.[3,28,29] Patients who demonstrate specific risk factors are more likely to exhibit stiffness; these include calcific tendinitis, preexisting adhesive capsulitis, partial articular supraspinatus tendon avulsion (PASTA)-type lesion repairs, concomitant superior labrum anterior to posterior (SLAP) repairs, and single tendon repairs.[3] To prevent motion complications from occurring in these high-risk patients, Koo and colleagues[3] recommended patients perform a table slide exercise to allow glenohumeral joint motion with minimal muscle recruitment. The addition of this exercise has been shown to reduce postoperative motion loss in patients who are at a high risk for developing stiffness. Others have suggested allowing RTC-repaired patients to become stiff during the postoperative rehabilitation phase to allow healing and reduce retear rates. Parsons and colleagues[30] retrospectively reported outcomes on 43 patients who underwent RTC repair surgery. These patients were instructed to wear their postoperative sling full time (never take it off) for 6 weeks and encouraged to allow their shoulder to get stiff. At 6 weeks following surgery, approximately 23% of the patients (n = 10) did get stiff; when these patients were evaluated at 1 year and compared with the group of patients who did not get stiff, the stiff patients exhibited a better outcome (higher American Shoulder and Elbow Surgeons' functional scores, similar ROM). Thus, the dilemma continues whether to allow patients who have undergone RTC repair to get stiff or not, but either way appropriate interventions to regain motion and function are essential for a successful outcome.

In some cases, patients get stiff after RTC repair and do not regain their motion spontaneously. These patients typically require physical therapy to assist in regaining the motion that has been lost. It has been the authors opinion for quite some time that the rate of rehabilitation and stresses applied to the repair should be based on several factors, including (1) size of tear, (2) tissue quality, (3) location of tear, (4) type of repair, (5) chronicity of tear, (6) concomitant lesions/surgeries, (7) patient variables, and (8) patients' response to surgery (host tissue response). Thus, if the surgeon and physical therapist decide that physical therapy is indicated to restore motion following RTC repair, the authors recommend basing the degree of aggressiveness of stretching and mobilization on several factors: (1) time of surgery, (2) size of the tear, (3) tissue quality, (4) the patients' PROM, and (5) joint end feel. The authors often begin ROM exercises with light PROM movements and gentle joint mobilizations. In many instances of shoulder joint stiffness, the focus is on restoring inferior capsular mobility; this is especially true in middle-aged shoulder patients. The authors do not believe in using aggressive stretching and PROM until adequate tissue healing has occurred; this should be recommended and directed by the patients' surgeon.

It is often difficult to restore motion in patients with adhesive capsulitis, especially when patients have exhibited this condition for longer than 4 to 5 months. The authors recommend basing the treatment on the stage of adhesive capsulitis (**Box 1**). Based on the stage of adhesive capsulitis, the authors would perform specific and different treatment techniques to address this condition and its associated motion complications. In stage I adhesive capsulitis, the treatment approach would be based on reducing inflammation and easy frequent ROM exercises; but the specific focus is light motion and no aggressive stretching. The authors recommend easy motion exercises performed for 5 to 10 minutes maximum, 8 to 10 times per day. Conversely, patients with stage 4 adhesive capsulitis are treated with heat, grade III and IV joint mobilization techniques, and LLLD stretching (**Figs. 4** and **5**). The purpose of the LLLD stretching is to create plastic deformation of the mature collagen scar tissue.[16]

Patients who have undergone other types of surgeries, such as glenohumeral joint stabilization, SLAP repairs, or open reduction internal fixation of humeral fractures, may become stiff as well. If at an appropriate time frame the physician has determined patients are stiff and behind in their recovery, he or she may recommend physical therapy to restore motion. Based on the amount (degree) of stiffness and the time frame from surgery, an appropriate condition-specific treatment program would be developed. If patients are determined to be extremely stiff and the duration from surgery is longer than 12 to 14 weeks, the physician may recommend aggressive physical therapy. In these instances, the authors recommend the use of LLLD stretching, followed by joint mobilizations with sustained holds and laser therapy to produce tissue deformation and assist in collagen remodeling.

Box 1
Stages of adhesive capsulitis

Stage I: Preadhesive stage

Synovial inflammation, pain with minimal loss of motion, spasm end feel

Stage II: Acute adhesive stage

Synovial inflammation present, early adhesions forming, spasm end feel

Stage III: Maturation stage

Loss of axillary fold, minimal synovitis, firm end feel

Stage IV: Chronic stage

Mature adhesions, pronounced stiffness, hard end feel

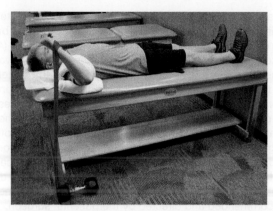

Fig. 4. Low-load, long-duration stretching for a loss of shoulder external rotation.

ELBOW JOINT

Complications following elbow joint injuries or surgeries may likewise occur; as with the other joints discussed, the most commonly seen complication is a loss of motion. Motion loss complications are often seen in postoperative ulnar collateral ligament (UCL) reconstruction or repair, following fracture/dislocation of the elbow complex or after periods of prolonged immobilization. Following UCL reconstruction or repair, the authors' experience has been 2% to 3% of patients will develop some degree of stiffness during the rehabilitation process, most predominantly a loss of elbow extension.[31,32] The authors have found the optimal treatment to restore elbow extension in these patients to be

1. Heat to the elbow joint complex
2. PROM and joint mobilizations (posterior glides to the radiohumeral and ulna-humeral joints)
3. LLDD stretching (**Fig. 6**)
4. Muscle energy techniques (contract/relax, hold/relax techniques)
5. PROM and joint mobilization
6. Laser therapy

Occasionally, patients may experience elbow stiffness into flexion. The authors have found that an easy way to address this complication is to use a wall slide

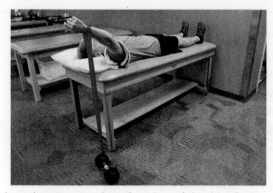

Fig. 5. Low-load, long-duration stretching for a loss of shoulder flexion.

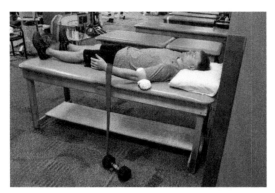

Fig. 6. Low-load, long-duration stretch to restore elbow extension.

technique performed both in the clinic and at home using patient-controlled body weight to gradually improve elbow flexion (**Fig. 7**). Patients stand against the wall with a flexed elbow and then gradually slide their arm down the wall to produce more elbow flexion. Patients can also add in the performance of contract-relax exercises along with the wall slide to further enhance elbow flexion.

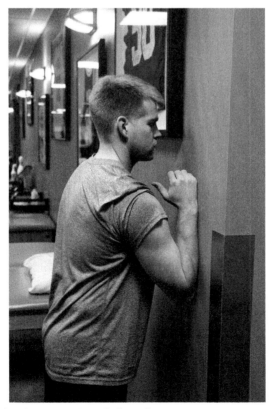

Fig. 7. Wall slide for the restoration of elbow flexion.

FOOT AND ANKLE JOINTS

As already described in the knee, shoulder, and elbow joints, the number one compli-cation in the foot and ankle complex is also a loss of motion and stiffness. Most frequently, there is the loss of both active and passive talocrural joint dorsiflexion. This loss of ankle dorsiflexion can occur following virtually any ankle or foot injury from simple, uncomplicated sprains to complex fractures. The loss of ankle dorsiflex-ion is often exacerbated by any period of extended immobilization and/or reduced weight bearing. Additionally, a functional loss of passive great toe or combined first ray extension may also complicate the return to functional athletic activities and is typically seen in first metatarsophalangeal (MTP) joint sprains or turf toe. Treatment of loss of ankle dorsiflexion and first ray extension follows the same guidelines previ-ously outlined for the knee, with early motion, mobility, and controlled weight bearing favored over non–weight bearing and delayed motion.

The treatment program for ankle and foot stiffness also follows a firm set of treat-ment guidelines performed several times a day and in conjunction with clinical inter-ventions like the program outlined earlier for the knee. This program includes

1. Heat with overpressure into dorsiflexion and/or first ray extension for 10 to 15 minutes
2. Mobilizations focused on posterior talocrural glides, coupled with combined motion mobilization of the subtalar and midtarsal joints, as well as posterior glides of the first MTP joint and posterolateral mobilization of the first metatarsal-cuneiform joint
3. EMS applied to the posterior tibialis, peroneals, and/or gastrocnemius/soleus musculature during isometric setting exercises of ankle movements and resisted band exercises focused on eccentric activation of the involved musculature
4. Gastrocnemius, soleus, plantar fascia, and flexor hallicus longus stretching
5. Light ankle and foot ROM exercises (PROM, bicycle, active knee to wall, passive combined toe extension and ankle dorsiflexion exercises, and so forth)
6. Retrograde walking over cups, cones, or on a treadmill
7. Reverse standing on a slant board (10–15 minutes)
8. Overpressure into extension (10–15 minutes in duration)
9. Repeat overpressure program at home for at least a total of 60 minutes per day

Tendinopathy complications are also prevalent about the foot and ankle complex and, like their counterparts in the knee and shoulder, can be primary or secondary dis-orders. The most frequent tendinopathies complicating a return to athletic participa-tion are those involving the Achilles complex, the posterior tibialis tendon, the peroneal tendons, and the flexor hallicus longus. The same treatment program that the authors have found successful in managing patellar tendinopathies is incorporated for the treatment of Achilles tendinopathies in the foot and ankle beginning with the application of moist heat to the involved foot, ankle, and lower leg, followed by soft tissue techniques to the involved tendon and surrounding soft tissues, static stretch-ing of the Achilles complex, plantar fascia and flexor hallicus along with the thigh and hip musculature followed by an active warm-up on the bicycle. Following the active warm-up, an eccentric training program is initiated emphasizing eccentric movements of the associated structures involved. These exercises are performed with an empha-size on a slow, heavy resistance eccentric contraction. In addition, hip strengthening is performed, especially for the hip external rotators, abductors, and extensors. Balance training is then performed, followed by more stretching exercises and the use of a deep tissue laser and home exercise instructions. As with the knee, if pain is too intense during the eccentric exercises, pain stimulation is used to neuromodulate pa-tients' pain complaints for successful performance of eccentric exercise activities.

SUMMARY

Complications following common orthopedic and sports injuries or surgeries occur more frequently than anyone desires. Even when small instances of complication rates are prevalent, the patients involved are 100% affected and require a slightly different approach to their rehabilitation care than the interventions typically used with uncomplicated patient conditions. Although the best course of care is a proactive program that minimizes the development of complications in the first place, the clinician must be cognizant of the complications possible, diligent in assessing for their presence, and ready to adapt a different treatment approach as soon as any complication becomes evident.

REFERENCES

1. Shelbourne KD, Wilckens JH, Mollabashy A, et al. Arthrofibrosis in acute anterior cruciate ligament reconstruction. The effect of timing of reconstruction and rehabilitation. Am J Sports Med 1991;19:332–6.
2. Harner CD, Irrgang JJ, Paul J, et al. Loss of motion after anterior cruciate ligament reconstruction. Am J Sports Med 1992;20:499–506.
3. Koo SS, Parsley BK, Burkhart SS, et al. Reduction of postoperative stiffness after arthroscopic rotator cuff repair: results of a customized physical therapy regimen based on risk factors for stiffness. Arthroscopy 2011;27(2):155–60.
4. Wright RW, Dunn WR, Amendola A. Risk of tearing the intact anterior cruciate ligament in the contralateral knee and rupturing the anterior cruciate ligament graft during the first 2 years after anterior cruciate ligament reconstruction: a prospective MOON cohort study. Am J Sports Med 2007;35(7):1131–4.
5. Sward P, Kostogiannis I, Roos H. Risk factors for a contralateral anterior cruciate ligament injury. Knee Surg Sports Traumatol Arthrosc 2010;18(3):277–91.
6. Shelbourne KD, Gray T, Haro M. Incidence of subsequent injury to either knee within 5 years after anterior cruciate ligament reconstruction with patellar tendon autograft. Am J Sports Med 2009;37(2):246–51.
7. Boileau P, Brassart N, Watkinson DJ, et al. Arthroscopic repairs of full thickness supraspinatus tears: does the tendon really heal? J Bone Joint Surg Am 2005; 87(6):1229–40.
8. Galatz LM, Ball CM, Teefey SA, et al. The outcome and repair integrity of completely arthroscopically repaired large and massive rotator cuff tears. J Bone Joint Surg 2004;86-A(2):219–24.
9. Noyes FR, Mangine RE, Barber S. Early knee motion after open and arthroscopic anterior cruciate ligament reconstruction. Am J Sports Med 1987;15:149–60.
10. Wilk KE. Anterior cruciate ligament injury prevention and rehabilitation: let's get it right. J Orthop Sports Phys Ther 2015;45(10):729–30.
11. Failla MJ, Logerstedt DS, Grindem H, et al. Does extended preoperative rehabilitation influence outcomes 2 years after ACL reconstruction?: a comparative effectiveness study between the MOON and Delaware-Oslo ACL cohorts. Am J Sports Med 2016;44(10):2608–14.
12. Clancy WG Jr, Nelson DA, Reider B, et al. Anterior cruciate ligament reconstruction using one-third of the patellar ligament, augmented by extra-articular tendon transfers. J Bone Joint Surg Am 1982;64:352–9.
13. Shelbourne KD, Gray T. Anterior cruciate ligament reconstruction with autogenous patellar tendon graft followed by accelerated rehabilitation. A two-to-nine-year follow-up. Am J Sports Med 1997;25:786–95.

14. Mangine RE, Noyes FR. Rehabilitation of the allograft reconstruction. J Orthop Sports Phys Ther 1992;15:294–302.

15. Wilk KE, Andrews JR. Current concepts in the treatment of anterior cruciate ligament disruption. J Orthop Sports Phys Ther 1992;15:279–93.

16. McClure PW, Blackburn LG, Dusold C. The use of splints in the treatment of joint stiffness: biologic rationale and an algorithm for making clinical decisions. Phys Ther 1994;74:1101–7.

17. Kottke FJ, Pauley DL, Ptak RA. The rationale of prolonged stretching for connective tissue. Arch Phys Med Rehabil 1966;47:345–52.

18. Warren CG, Lehmann JF, Koblanski JN. Elongation of rat tail tendon: effect of load and temperature. Arch Phys Med Rehab 1971;52:465–74.

19. Grindem H, Snyder-Mackler L, Moksnes H, et al. Simple decision rules can reduce reinjury risk by 84% after ACL reconstruction: the Delaware-Oslo ACL cohort. Br J Sports Med 2016;50(13):804–8.

20. Schilaty ND, Nagelli C, Bates NA, et al. Incidence of second anterior cruciate ligament tears and identification of associated risk factors from 2001 to 2010 using a geographic database. Orthop J Sports Med 2017;5(8):1–8.

21. Paterno MV, Rauh MJ, Schmitt LC, et al. Incidence of second ACL injuries 2 years after primary ACL reconstruction and return to sport. Am J Sports Med 2014; 42(7):1567–73.

22. Paterno MV, Rauh MJ, Schmitt LC, et al. Incidence of contralateral and ipsilateral anterior cruciate ligament (ACL) injury after primary ACL reconstruction and return to sport. Clin J Sports Med 2012;22(2):116–21.

23. Langberg H, Ellingsgaard H, Madsen T, et al. Eccentric rehabilitation exercise increases peritendinous type I collagen synthesis in humans with Achilles tendinosis. Scand J Med Sci Sports 2007;17(1):61–6.

24. Witvrouw E, Lysens R, Bellemans J, et al. Intrinsic risk factors for the development of anterior knee pain in an athletic population. A two-year prospective study. Am J Sports Med 2000;28(4):480–9.

25. Wilk KE, Davies GJ, Mangine RE, et al. Patellofemoral disorders: a classification system and clinical guidelines for nonoperative rehabilitation. J Orthop Sports Phys Ther 1998;28(5):307–22.

26. Powers CM. The influence of altered lower-extremity kinematics on patellofemoral joint dysfunction: a theoretical perspective. J Ortho Sports Phys Ther 2003; 33(11):639–46.

27. Powers CM, Bolgla LA, Callaghan MJ, et al. Patellofemoral pain: proximal, distal, and local factors, 2nd International Research Retreat. J Ortho Sports Phys Ther 2012;42(6):A1–54.

28. Chung SW, Huong CB, Kim SH, et al. Shoulder stiffness after rotator cuff repair: risk factors and influence on outcome. Arthroscopy 2013;29(2):290–300.

29. Franceschi F, Papalia R, Palumbo A, et al. Management of postoperative shoulder stiffness. Sports Med Arthrosc 2011;19(4):420–7.

30. Parsons BO, Gruson KI, Chen DD, et al. Does slower rehabilitation after arthroscopic rotator cuff repair lead to long-term stiffness? J Shoulder Elbow Surg 2010;19(7):1034–9.

31. Cain EL Jr, Andrews JR, Dugas JR, et al. Outcome of ulnar collateral ligament reconstruction of the elbow in 1281 athletes: results in 743 athletes with minimum 2-year follow-up. Am J Sports Med 2010;38(12):2426–34.

32. Wilk KE, Macrina LC, Cain EL, et al. Rehabilitation of the athlete's elbow. J Sports Health 2012;4(5):404–14.

Moving?

Make sure your subscription moves with you!

To notify us of your new address, find your **Clinics Account Number** (located on your mailing label above your name), and contact customer service at:

Email: journalscustomerservice-usa@elsevier.com

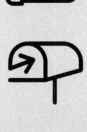

800-654-2452 (subscribers in the U.S. & Canada)
314-447-8871 (subscribers outside of the U.S. & Canada)

Fax number: 314-447-8029

Elsevier Health Sciences Division
Subscription Customer Service
3251 Riverport Lane
Maryland Heights, MO 63043

*To ensure uninterrupted delivery of your subscription, please notify us at least 4 weeks in advance of move.

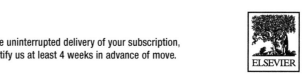

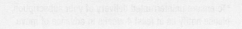

Printed and bound by CPI Group (UK) Ltd, Croydon, CR0 4YY

08/05/2025

01864711-0002